health
administration
press

The Press was established in 1972 with the support of the W. K. Kellogg Foundation as a joint endeavor of the Association of University Programs in Health Administration (Washington, D.C.) and The University of Michigan Program and Bureau of Hospital Administration.

INFORMATION SYSTEMS for HOSPITAL ADMINISTRATI

The U

Asso

U

R

Universi

University

Nor

Charles J. Austin

INFORMATION SYSTEMS for HOSPITAL ADMINISTRATION

Second Edition

with contributions by William J. Harvey

Health Administration Press Ann Arbor, Michigan 1983

Library of Congress Cataloging in Publication Data
Austin, Charles J.
Information systems for hospital administration.

Includes bibliographies and index.
1. Hospitals—Administration—Data processing.
I. Title. [DNLM: 1. Hospital administration. 2. Information systems. WX 150 A935i]
RA971.6.A93 1983 362.1'1'068 83-8495
ISBN 0-914904-91-4

Health Administration Press
School of Public Health
The University of Michigan
Ann Arbor, Michigan 48109
(313) 764-1380

This second edition is dedicated to my children:
Lynn, Charles, Christopher, Andrew, and Carroll Jane.

Contents

List of Figures

Preface

This book is intended to aid hospital and health administrators in understanding the intricacies of information systems and how such systems can become effective management tools in their organizations. Sufficient technical detail on computer systems and design techniques is included to enable the administrator to become conversant with modern technology and its use in the hospital. However, the basic perspective of this book is an administrative one, and the emphasis is on the intelligent use of information for management planning and control.

The book is suitable as a textbook for a one semester graduate or advanced undergraduate course in the design and management of hospital information systems. It can serve also as a reference for hospital administrators and others involved in the design of hospital systems. Extensive citations are included for those desiring additional technical information on the major topics covered.

I am indebted to my colleague, William J. Harvey, for contributing Chapters 4, 5 and 6 of this second edition. I also appreciate the assistance of my former faculty colleagues and students in the Department of Health Care Administration at Trinity University who helped me test many of the concepts included in the book. Particular thanks go to Mike Cagle, Rosalie Presti, Cecilia Stubbs, Carolyn Trezevant, and Kay Harvey for assistance in manuscript preparation using the East Texas State University word processing system. The responsibility for any errors or oversights lies solely with the author.

Charles J. Austin

I

Introduction and Background Concepts

1

Introduction

This book is about management and how the management of hospitals can be improved by *intelligent* use of information. Some management theorists discount the value of information in the management process, stating that management is still more of an art than a science. They argue that experience, judgment, intuition, and a good sense of the political environment are the critical skills involved in administrative decisions. On the other end of the spectrum are the technocrats, who argue that management and information are completely inseparable, that all management decisions need to be completely rational and based entirely on analysis of information collected to support the decision to be made. The focus of this book lies between these two extreme views of the managerial world. The use of information by hospital managers has both costs and benefits associated with it. These need to be carefully assessed, and administrators need to develop their skills in using information intelligently.

The intelligent use of information in hospital management doesn't just happen. Rather, the hospital administrator must insure that it occurs in a systematic, formally planned way. This book, then, deals with two important matters: the management of the information-processing function in hospitals and the effective use of information in institutional management.

Careful distinction should be drawn between data and information. As used in this book, *data* refers to raw facts and figures which are collected as part of the normal functioning of the hospital. *Information*, on the other hand, is defined as data which have been processed and analyzed in a formal, intelligent way, so that the results are directly useful to those involved in the operation and management of the hospital. Some hospitals collect masses of data which are never effectively transformed into intelligence—useful, processed information. All too often, voluminous computer printouts gather dust on the desks or shelves of hospital personnel because insufficient thought went into the preparation of useful reports, both in form and content. Alternatively, computerized databanks, accessible through terminals or microprocessors, may exist but be little used because of lack of planning in the retrieval and analysis of the information for purposes of management planning and control. In order to insure that information rather than data will be available to support management planning and decision making, hospital administrators must insist that a careful process of planning, analysis, and design precede the implementation of information systems in their organizations.

An essential element for the successful development of hospital information systems is carefully planned teamwork by administrative and technical (systems) personnel in information systems development. Information systems designed by technical personnel in isolation may be "technically pure and elegant in design," but rarely will they pass the test of reality in meeting organizational needs. On the other hand, very few hospital administrators possess the technical knowledge and skills of systems analysis and design which are equally important, and the amateur analyst cannot hope to avoid the havoc that will result from a poorly designed system. What is needed, therefore, is a balanced effort at all stages of a systems development project, in which hospital operating and administrative personnel contribute ideas on systems requirements and the realities of operations, and technical personnel employ their skills in analysis and design.

It should also be noted that computers are in a sense only incidental to the entire process of information systems development. Many very useful information systems have been and can be developed without using computers for data-processing purposes. On the other hand, the size and complexity of many hospitals necessitate the use of computers for data communications and analysis, but it must always be remembered that computers are only tools to aid in the accomplishment of a broader set of goals. The analysis of information requirements should always take precedence over a rush to computerize.

ALTERNATIVE APPROACHES TO MANAGEMENT DECISIONS

Management theorists have disagreed on the extent to which information can and should be used to support administrative decisions in organizations. The "purely rational" approach suggests that no decision should be made without complete information and an exhaustive analysis of all costs and benefits involved. The rational model was in vogue in the 1960's, partly as the result of the application of systems analysis techniques in the U.S. Department of Defense, later mandated for all government agencies.[1] Strong arguments were advanced for thorough, data-based analysis to support management planning and control. Some of the resulting methodologies (cost-benefit analysis, planning-programming-budgeting systems) were advocated as the solution to all of management's problems and the panacea for organizational problem solving.

On the opposite end of the spectrum are those management theorists who argue that most, indeed the vast majority of, administrative decisions are arrived at through judgment, intuition, and inference on the part of an experienced administrator. Proponents of the "nonrational" model argue that most, if not all, decisions of major import are situation-specific, heavily influenced by political factors, and that the rational approach, while methodologically elegant, adds very little to the actual decision process.[2]

As is the case with most human activities, neither of these two extreme views seems to be adequate in answering the fundamental question: to what extent should information be used to support management planning and control? The purely rational model has been criticized as impractical in most real world situations and impossible to apply in a strict sense. For example, Kuhn describes a planning or policy decision involving only five kinds of benefits and five kinds of costs. If the systems analyst were to assign three dimensions to each cost and benefit (the dimensions of magnitude, duration, and probability of occurrence) and if each dimension were ranked according to a five-point scale (e.g., very probable, likely, uncertain, unlikely, very improbable), then the resultant decision matrix is of size 625 by 625, or 390,625 alternatives to be evaluated.[3] Such an approach is obviously unrealistic.

Does this mean, however, that *no* information is better than *some* information in support of major policy decisions? It can be argued that many, if not most, decisions could be improved through the judicious use of information by the decision maker. Even a decision which is heavily entrenched in political factors and special interests can likely be improved if the political actors involved are required to justify their respective positions in the face of certain fundamental facts about the costs and potential benefits of alternatives available. Suboptimal decisions are often required in the face of reality, but a board of trustees and hospital administrator are still wise to keep as well informed as possible about the costs to the organization of suboptimization in the face of special interests or special problems. The recommended middle ground approach, then, is to suggest that hospital administrators and their subordinate supervisors be trained in the *intelligent use of information*, to develop the ability to identify those problems in which additional information can be of real value in seeking solutions but also to be sensitive to those situations in which information would add very little to the deliberations and in which the costs of gathering the relevant information would exceed the benefits to be gained in improved analysis.

Etzioni presents cogent arguments for this middle ground approach in his mixed scanning theory of policy decision making.[4] The theory represents a compromise between the purely rational and purely situational models. He argues that management policymaking should be separated into *funda-*

mental decisions involving major organizational goals and resultant long-range policies which guide operations and *short-range operational decisions* which deal with procedures that can be readily changed without doing violence to institutional purposes. Fundamental decisions, Etzioni would argue, should be subjected to thorough analysis with complete information, while short-range procedural decisions can be more situational and arrived at incrementally through trial and error approaches.

The basic message of this book is not that more information is better information, but rather that administrative decision making in hospitals can be improved through more judicious and intelligent use of information. It is the responsibility of the chief executive officer of the hospital to insure that the hospital's information systems and processes are adequate for the task.

VALUE OF MANAGEMENT INFORMATION

Information, intelligently used, and information systems, carefully planned, can be great assets to the hospital administrator. In general, management information can be used in several important ways in the operational setting. Information should be an important aid to the hospital board and administrator in strategic planning and setting of goals for the institution. Clinical information and information on the quality of care rendered by the hospital is essential to an effective process of quality assessment and improvement. Perhaps the most pressing problem of hospitals today is the containment of costs, and current, relevant, and reliable financial information is a necessary ingredient in the management system of any hospital. Hospitals must also continually monitor and evaluate their performance, both for internal purposes and to satisfy external regulators and accreditors. Up-to-date management information is an essential part of this process of evaluation and performance monitoring.

The basic management process within a hospital can be described in cyclical terms:

Basic Management Cycle in Hospitals

- establish goals and objectives
- estimate demand for services
- allocate resources to meet demand
- control the quality of performance
- evaluate programs

Cycle repeated after each evaluation

Major policy decisions follow this cycle in roughly sequential fashion.

Policy decisions must first be made with regard to the establishment of institutional goals and objectives. Once goals have been established, those responsible for implementing the goals must estimate the demand for specific services to be rendered. Demand can only be met through efficient allocation of limited resources, which is the third element of the management decision cycle. Allocation of resources in response to demand for services results in the establishment of operational procedures for providing patient care. The quality of performance in the rendering of patient care must be constantly watched and improved. And finally, the effects of those services upon the community must be measured through evaluation of program impact—the "So what?" question. Impact analysis usually results in reevaluation and modification of organizational goals; hence, the cycle is completed and repeated once again.

Management information should play an important role in each element of this basic management cycle. Figure 1-1 presents examples of some of the kinds of information which, used intelligently, can help to improve decision making in each category. For example, problem indicators are an important element in setting goals and objectives. What are the major health problems of the population to be served by the hospital? How can these be measured? Direct indicators include health status measures, but certain indirect measures can be useful as well, particularly demographic characteristics of the population and past utilization patterns. Realistic goal setting also requires information on resources available to the hospital, such as manpower resources, income to be generated, and capital requirements. Goal setting also requires information about what others are doing in the community to meet the need for improved health care, and it cannot be done solely in an institutional context. Hence, community profile and resource data are important.

Demand estimation and forecasting require additional information, including historical data on population characteristics and previous utilization of services by type of service available. Demographic projections must also be made for the planning period. In addition, forecasters must take into account social and cultural determinants of demand and attempt to develop demographic indicators which will aid in predicting how these determinants may change during the period of the forecast. Hence, information is an essential part of the demand estimation process.[5]

Health administrators spend a considerable amount of time deciding how to allocate limited resources to meet seemingly unlimited demand. Information is useful to this activity as well. Data are needed on manpower presently available and on projected requirements for the planning period. Financial information and projections are an essential element, as are estimates of capital requirements. Short-term demand forecasting is important to the immediate process of resource allocation.[6]

FIGURE 1-1
Management Decisions and Related Information Requirements

1. Establishment of Institutional Goals and Objectives
   - problem indicators, direct and indirect (morbidity and mortality data, social indicators, economic data on the community, data on personal health habits of members of the community)
   - resources available
2. Demand Estimation
   - historical data on utilization of health services
   - demographic data
   - community projections
3. Resource Allocation
   - manpower data
   - financial information
   - capital requirements
   - short-term demand forecasts
4. Performance and Quality Control
   - output measures (program statistics)
   - quality control data
   - work sampling and measurement
   - medical audit
5. Evaluation of Program Impact
   - changes in problem indicators, direct and indirect
   - cost-benefit analysis
   - change in community capability to provide services

Hospital administrators must frequently evaluate their institutional performance, both in order to improve the delivery of services and to meet the inspections of external regulators. Program statistics are commonly used to aid in performance monitoring and evaluation. These include output measures such as inpatient days of care rendered, patient encounters in the outpatient department, and counts of procedures carried out in the service departments of the hospital. Quality control systems are in use in most hospitals, and these systems are data-dependent for their functioning. Work sampling and measurement along with medical audit procedures are often used to generate information for quality control purposes. In completion of the management cycle, hospitals need to gather data to support studies of program impact. The same kind of data used in the initial establishment of goals and objectives—problem indicators (before and after), costs incurred, etc.—assist management in the process of evaluation and usually lead to modifications in program goals for the future.

PERIODIC AND NONPERIODIC MANAGEMENT DECISIONS

Management decisions in hospitals fall into two categories: (1) one-time decisions or decisions which arise infrequently at irregular time intervals; and (2) periodic decisions which occur regularly. The proper approach to information system design is obviously influenced by the periodicity or nonperiodicity of the decision.

Two general approaches are possible in obtaining management information to support one-time or infrequent management decisions. The first approach is to conduct a special study to obtain the necessary information to aid the decision process. This usually involves assignment of a staff analyst to organize the study, obtain the data, process it, and prepare an analysis based upon the results. Such studies involve considerable time and effort, and careful consideration must be given to costs and benefits before embarking on the special study. A second alternative is available only if the hospital has in operation a generalized management information system. If such a system is in existence and if the relevant data have been collected and stored in master data files, then the process becomes a simple one of retrieval and analysis of pertinent facts from the general database. Techniques for the design and development of generalized management information systems will be discussed later in this book. Although the initial investment of time and funds in the development of generalized systems is substantial, these costs can be offset by eliminating the need for innumerable special studies each time a major planning or policy decision must be faced.

In the case of periodic decisions, the special study approach is ordinarily not cost-effective. That is, it probably does not make sense to repeat a special study and gather new data each time the decision must be made. Three other alternatives are available to the system designer.

If there is an information system in operation in the area in which the periodic decision is required, then the existing system can perhaps be expanded to produce the relevant management information on a regular basis. For example, a hospital administrator is required to conduct a periodic review of the status of accounts receivable from various third-party payers to be sure that the hospital is not approaching a cash flow problem caused by an inordinately high level of outstanding revenue. If the hospital has installed an operational data-processing system for processing patient charges and billing accounts, then the necessary management reports on aged accounts receivable should be a logical and readily available extension of that system.

A second approach would be to draw information for the periodic decision from a generalized management information system, if one exists in the hospital. In the example just cited, the availablity of additional information might help to improve the decision. Assume that the generalized management information system included both the data on aged accounts receivable previously mentioned *and* additional data on the current cash position of the hospital, perhaps with regard to fixed commitments and other accounts payable. Management action might then be improved through the use of this additional information from an expanded and coordinated management database covering all major areas of the hospital.

The third alternative in dealing with periodic decisions is to program the decision itself into an ongoing information system. This can be done through the development of a set of generalized decision rules which becomes part of the system itself. For example, in the accounts receivable situation described above, a decision rule might be developed in which the information system automatically generates a detailed statement of overdue accounts to be sent to a third-party payer whenever the aged accounts receivable total from that payer exceeds a certain maximum threshold figure. Automatic reordering systems for inventory control and purchasing are another example of the programmed decision approach. Obviously not all management decisions lend themselves to the development of generalized decision rules, but the designers of information systems could go much further in the creative use of information in this way.

HOSPITAL INFORMATION SYSTEM OBJECTIVES

Hospital administrators, board members, and medical staff members look to information systems to provide support in the following areas: (1) medical quality assurance, (2) cost control and productivity enhancement, (3) utilization analysis and demand estimation, (4) program planning and evaluation, (5) simplification of external reporting, (6) clinical research, and (7) education. The last two areas, research and education, are not universal and apply primarily to larger hospitals, often those associated with a university or those carrying major teaching responsibilities.[7]

Medical Quality Assurance. Clinical information abstracted from patient medical records provides the basic material utilized by health professionals in peer review systems to assess diagnostic and treatment practices within the hospital. One goal of a computerized hospital information system is to make such data readily accessible and retrievable from a central patient data file for purposes of quality assessment and initiation of necessary corrective action.

Cost Control and Productivity Enhancement. Hospitals are under increasing pressure to contain increases in the cost of services. Computerized information systems offer the potential for providing cost analyses and productivity reports for use by hospital management and board members in improving the efficiency of operation. Such systems require the ability to integrate clinical and financial information systems.

Utilization Analysis and Demand Estimation. A complete hospital information system should provide current and historical data on utilization of hospital services. Such data systems serve to assist in current analysis of the efficiency of utilization of resources and also provide a basis for predicting future demand for services.

Program Planning and Evaluation. Information obtained for the above purposes—quality assurance, cost control, utilization analysis, and demand estimation—serves as the basic input for management decisions related to evaluation of present programs and services. When combined with projections about future changes in the demographic characteristics of the service population, the hospital information system can provide an important resource for planning future programs and services.

Simplification of Internal and External Reporting. Information-processing costs consume a substantial portion of a hospital's budget. Every hospital service rendered requires concurrent recording of accurate medical and financial information. External reporting requirements are growing exponentially, with a multiplicity of reports needed to satisfy local, state, and federal governmental agencies; accrediting bodies; third-party financing agencies; and the like. An important goal for a hospital information system is to simplify the preparation of these various reports, often a difficult task.

Clinical Research. Larger hospitals, particularly those affiliated with an educational institution, utilize computerized systems for aggregating patient records in support of clinical research conducted by investigators on the medical staff or at affiliated institutions. Such records must be properly indexed according to a uniform classification system with data files maintained over long periods of time for longitudinal and comparative studies.

Education. Related to the above, computerized patient record systems can aid in the training of physicians and other health professionals by making current and historical clinical records readily available for educational purposes.

Categories of Information Systems in Hospitals

There are three general categories of information systems available to hospitals: clinical or medical information systems, information systems to support administrative operations, and management planning and control systems. Taken together, these three categories of information systems provide all elements of information required for the development of a total hospital information system. Efforts at designing such "total systems" are discussed in Chapter 13.

Clinical or medical information systems are designed primarily to support direct patient care activities in the hospital. Specific applications range from direct computerized monitoring of the vital functions of critically ill patients in intensive care, to records retrieval systems designed to aid the medical audit process in the hospital to insure that quality standards are being maintained.

Operational administrative systems are designed to assist in the necessary non-patient care activities of the hospital. Examples include financial information systems, personnel and payroll systems, purchasing and inventory control systems, bed census and control, and numerous others.

Management planning and control systems are designed to deal with strategic policy matters that transcend daily administrative or patient care activities. They are designed to assist in long-range planning, evaluation of hospital performance, and analysis of the impact of programs offered to the community. As Davis and Freeman describe the purposes of a management information system:

> Properly structured, the MIS (management information system) will provide indices which enable the manager to relate resources to results, i.e. to convert various alternative programs or program levels to resource requirements. Thus, the MIS not only supports both the control function and the planning function; it also serves as the link between the two.[8]

The efficiency of information processes in hospitals will be directly proportional to the degree of integration among these various information systems. If individual clinical and administrative systems are designed in isolation, they will be unable to communicate with one another. Since information transfer is necessary among all the major functional areas of the hospital, failure to follow an integrated approach will be very costly. Most (if not all) data needed to support management policy decisions should be available from operational clinical and administrative information systems in the hospital, if these systems are designed with management information requirements in mind. The very important subject of information system integration will be discussed in much more detail later. Systems integration constitutes one of the most important concepts introduced in this book.

HISTORICAL REVIEW

Four time intervals have been selected for this brief historical review of the evolution of hospital information systems: the period from 1950 to 1959, which constitutes the pre-computer era; the developmental period in computer technology from 1960 to 1969; the period from 1970 to 1979, in which attention shifted from preoccupation with computer equipment (or "hardware") to a greater concentration on development of systems which can utilize the new technology; and the post-1980 period characterized by microprocessor development and distributed processing of hospital information. The time periods chosen are not meant to be exact measures of specific events, but rather present a simple scheme for classifying trends over a period of recent history. The chronology of events is summarized in Figure 1-2.

Before 1960, electronic computers were not in general use in hospitals. Most hospital information systems operated on a manual basis and were, for the most part, totally self-contained within an organizational unit such as the admitting department, emergency room, nursing service, or the patient accounting department. Stated differently, there was no attempt to develop *integrated systems*, in which a given element of data is captured only once, centrally stored, and communicated to various service centers of the hospital on demand. In fact, such an integrated approach was not practical, and in most cases not possible, before the development of electronic data-processing capabilities. Some mechanical aids for data processing were in use, including posting and bookkeeping machines, punched card equipment, and mechanical data recorders such as embossing systems utilizing metal identification plates. Although punched card machines, including sorters, collators, calculators, and tabulators, had been available for some time, their use in hospitals was quite limited, usually to assist with accounting functions and in a few cases for medical records controls.

The decade of the 1960's saw the rapid development of the electronic computer as an aid to information processing throughout the world. Hospitals increased their use of computer equipment during this period. Batch processing was the hallmark of initial computer systems, in hospitals and most other industries: that is, data generated over a given period (one day,

FIGURE 1-2
Information Systems in Hospitals: Historical Overview

	Time Period			
	1950–1959	*1960–1969*	*1970–1979*	*1980 and Later*
Data-Processing Equipment	Primarily manual systems for information handling	Initial use of computers, oriented to batch processing	Increased computer use, on-line processing orientation	Rapid development of microprocessor technology
	Some mechanical aids, such as bookkeeping machines and punched card equipment		Development of minicomputer technology	Improvement of data communications capabilities (fiber optics, laser transmission, etc.)
Systems Design Approaches	Individual departmental systems	Mostly batch processing; focus on administrative applications	Shifts to on-line applications	Shift back to distributed processing in hospital applications
	No integration of systems	Attempts to tie related systems together	Interest in fully integrated systems	
Focus of Hospital Administration	Insuring that individual departmental information needs were met	Interest in computer systems to support operating departments of the hospital	More attention to system planning and use of information for management control and medical quality assurance	Concern with proliferation of microcomputers and problems of system integration caused by decentralization of computing to hospital departments

FIGURE 1-3
Punched Card Machines

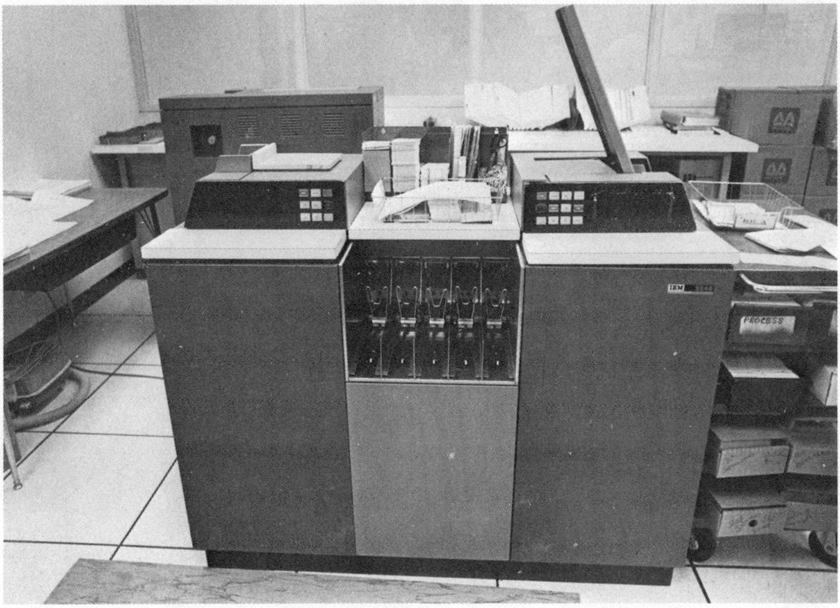

one week, one month) were collected at a central point, appropriate coding was added for computer processing, the data forms were keypunched, and the resultant machine readable records were processed in a group, or batch, with reports delivered to users of the information on a periodic basis. Hospital batch processing systems were usually developed on an application-by-application basis—payroll first, followed by accounts receivable, followed by inventory control, and so on—with no serious efforts to achieve systems integration throughout the hospital.

This time period also was marked by amazingly rapid increases in the sophistication of electronic computer hardware. The early vacuum tube computers, which were large and somewhat unreliable, gave way to the more efficient and less costly transistorized machines of the mid-1960's. Faster and better input and output units were developed for reading data into the computer and printing the results of processing. Significant and rapid improvements occurred in the development of mass storage devices for rapid access to data stored in electronic form, and all of these impressive technological improvements were accompanied by a continuous decrease in the unit costs of computing and data-processing power.

FIGURE 1-4
Electronic Computer

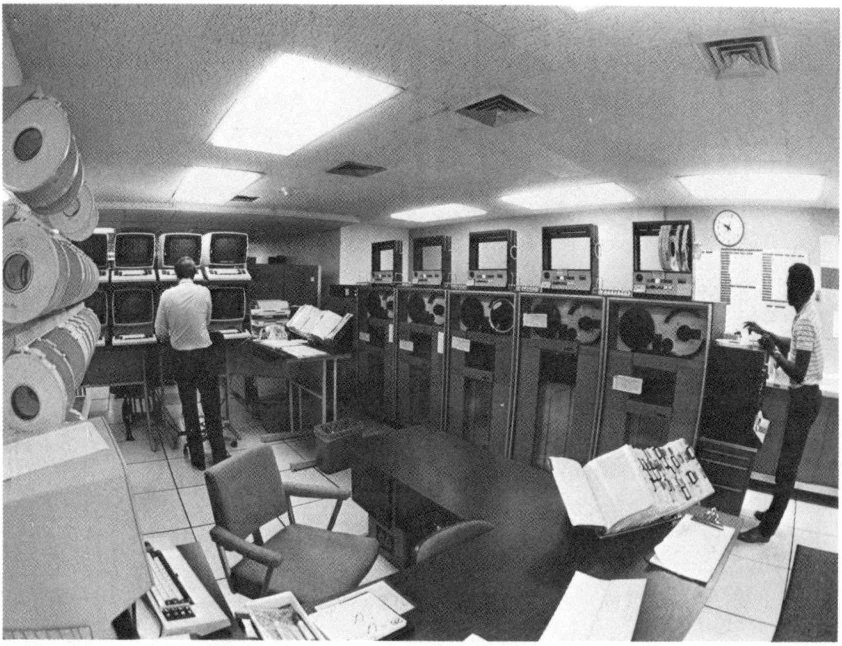

Some hospitals experimented with the development of total systems during the 1960's. The basic approach was to develop a fully integrated, single system which would meet all hospital information requirements, administrative and clinical. Although a limited number of such systems functioned for experimental purposes, the concept proved to be an idea whose time had not yet come, at least for practical applications in hospitals.

There were many bad experiences with computer systems in hospitals during this time. Some hospitals rushed to computerize without fully understanding the capabilities and limitations of such systems. Often they received considerable encouragement from vendors who were understandably anxious to penetrate the growing hospital computer market. Unfortunately, this rush to automate often was not accompanied by adequate systems planning in advance of equipment installation, and many "horror stories" of poor experiences with computers circulated in U.S. hospitals during the 1960's.

Fortunately, most hospitals have learned from these early mistakes (which were also common in other industries since computer technology was so new), and in the post-1970 era infatuation with hardware was superseded by more consideration of the information system itself, with hardware decisions flowing from carefully stated information system requirements.

The major advance in hardware technology during the 1970's was the increasing availability of on-line computer systems, which provide hospital personnel access to computerized data files through communications terminals. Although batch processing systems are still common in hospitals, more and more institutions are converting to systems which provide direct access to data files.* So, for example, a central computer file of patient information might be established to provide direct access to patient information for physicians, nurses, and others involved in treatment and patient care. As services are ordered for patients, the computer system prices them automatically, and the same central data file is used to generate billing information for the hospital's business office.

The second major advance in computer technology during this period was the development of inexpensive minicomputers. There was emerging interest in the possible use of multiple minicomputers to meet hospital information requirements by installing individual small computers in various functional areas of the hospital. The term *distributed processing* has been applied to the concept of multiple small computers used in separate locations to meet an organization's information-processing requirements. Although this approach appears to be attractive from a cost viewpoint, there are still questions about whether or not effective integration of information systems is possible when following a multiple-mini approach.

The decade of the 1970's also saw the increasing availability of "packaged" systems for hospitals, that is, generalized computer systems designed to fill the information-processing needs of any hospital. These are marketed by a number of companies specializing in the development of such systems; and they have been developed both on an individual application basis (accounts receivable, admissions and bed census, inventory control, medical records indexing) as well as on a total system basis. A number of companies are now marketing fully integrated hospital communications systems.**

In addition, growing attention concentrated on the development of

---

* Systems of this kind operate in a time-shared, real-time mode. That is, multiple users simultaneously share time on the computer, but each user receives an immediate, or *real-time*, response to his request for information from the computer's data files. The term *interactive computing* is also used to describe this kind of operation.

** Some packaged systems involve the installation of computer equipment (hardware) as well as the provision of specific computer programs (software) for the various hospital applications included in the package. Others are based on the assumption that the hospital has computer equipment installed, and the packaged system includes only software.

FIGURE 1-5
Picture of Microcomputer

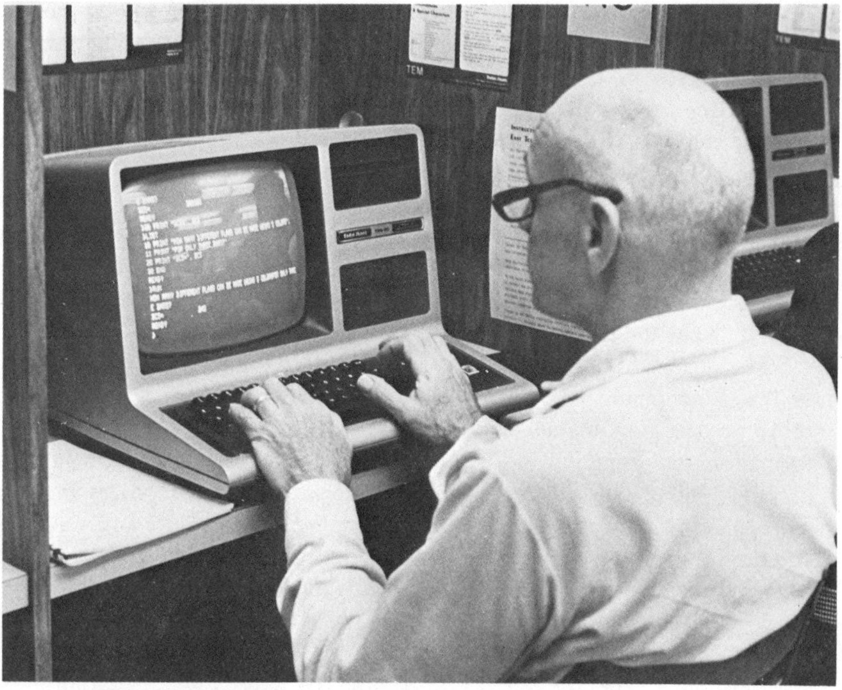

shared computer systems for hospitals. A central system is installed at one location, and data communications devices are placed in each participating hospital to transmit data to and from the central computer. Shared systems have been developed under a variety of auspices, ranging from central systems serving a chain of investor-owned hospitals to voluntary cooperation by a group of hospitals in a local community.

The final trend to be noted during the 1970's was a particularly encouraging one. Hospitals began to consider the development of information systems which are designed not only to support day-to-day operations, but also to provide information to support management planning and control and quality assurance within their organizations.

The post-1980 era has been marked by rapid advances in technology, particularly improvements in microcomputers, small and inexpensive but powerful systems which bring the costs of dedicated computer hardware within the budgetary reach of many hospital departments. This has led to a shift away from total system development back to data processing which is distributed throughout the hospital. As a result, many hospital administrators are now faced with the problem of computer proliferation and the more serious concern of how to integrate distributed systems from throughout the hospital, particularly those developed through departmental initiative without central planning and control.

As a counterbalance to this most recent trend, dramatic improvements in computer terminals and data communications make large databases more feasible than before, even for medium-sized hospitals.

CURRENT STATUS

The evolution of information systems in hospitals has followed the pattern of development of such systems in other industries, although perhaps a bit more slowly. Initial efforts have been directed toward the design of single-application systems to support administrative and clinical functions in the hospital. Most hospitals have given attention to administrative functions before moving into the area of clinical applications. Only modest progress has been made in the design and implementation of management planning and control systems.

A 1976 survey by the Hospital Financial Management Association (HFMA) documented the state of the art of information processing in hospitals.[9] Data drawn from a statistically representative sample of 2,300 U.S. hospitals indicated that about 50 percent of the hospitals had computers installed or on order and were well into the process of information systems design. The most common applications were in administrative areas, with 75 percent of the respondent hospitals involved in the design of patient accounting information systems, 75 percent working in the area of census reporting and facility utilization, 60 percent involved in payroll and personnel records systems, and 50 percent working on the development of cost accounting and general ledger accounting systems. Clinical applications were much less common. Although 40 percent of the responding hospitals had medical records information systems of some type, no other clinical computer application was installed in more than 10 percent of the responding hospitals.

A 1979 study of 250 community hospitals indicated that 216 were computer users. These hospitals spent $98.5 million on computer costs in 1979, 21 percent of total hospital operating expenses. Computer costs per bed ranged from $1,718 for large hospitals (500 beds and over) to $984 for hospitals with under 100 beds. Hospitals employing in-house computers spent $69 million (70 percent of the total); those participating in shared computer services spent $18.3 million (19 percent); and hospitals utilizing a combination of in-house equipment and shared services spent $11.2 million (11 percent).[10]

Following the pattern of other industries, hospitals are beginning to shift their attention from a sole focus on operational information systems and are beginning to work on the design of institutional management information systems. However, at the time of this writing, these efforts are still in a developmental stage.

In discussing the current state of management information systems in hospitals, Herzlinger argues that "what one sees in most health organizations are systems that aren't systematic; information which doesn't inform; and a managerial level which is functioning without the benefit of the sorts of data that a routinized, accurate, well-established management information system can provide."[11] She goes on to point out that management information needs in hospitals are greater than in most other industries, since the very functioning of the hospital is information-dependent and since hospitals are beset by reporting requirements from myriad external agencies. Hospital administrators must assume some of the responsibility for the present low state of development of management information systems, since they often have not taken the leadership necessary for the careful design, implementation, and operation of such systems.

SUMMARY

Hospitals by their very nature are information-dependent. The management of hospitals can be improved substantially by the intelligent use of information, but, for this to occur, hospital administrators must take direct responsibility for the careful planning and management of information systems in their institutions.

Although not all decisions in hospitals require it, most major policy decisions can be improved through the judicious use of information. Information can and should be available to assist administrators and policymakers in the basic management tasks faced by all hospitals: establishment of institutional goals and objectives, estimation of demand for services, allocation of limited resources, monitoring and control of performance, and evaluation of the impact of programs offered to the community served by the hospital.

Management decisions can be supported by information derived in different ways. Special studies can be carried out to obtain data to support decisions which occur infrequently. Periodic or frequently repetitive decisions can be aided by data drawn from specific operational data systems or from a generalized management information system, if one exists in the hospital.

Hospital information system objectives include: (1) medical quality assurance, (2) cost control and productivity enhancement, (3) utilization analysis and demand estimation, (4) program planning and evaluation, (5) simplification of external reporting, (6) clinical research, and (7) education.

Operational data systems should be designed with management information requirements always in mind; and since all functional areas of the hospital are interdependent, integration of information systems becomes an essential design criterion.

Hospitals are most advanced in the design of single-application, administrative information systems. Some progress has also occurred in the development of clinical information systems. However, fully integrated, or total, hospital information systems are still in developmental stages. The major challenge facing hospital administrators is to provide leadership in the design and development of effective management information systems within their organizations.

Many important concepts have been introduced in this chapter, but they are only discussed in a most general way. The chapters which follow are designed to provide specific guidance to administrators on the effective use of information in hospital management as well as techniques for managing the information-processing function in their institutions.

DISCUSSION QUESTIONS

1-1 Define *information*. What is the difference between data and information?

1-2 Describe some of the alternative approaches to decision making as discussed by management theorists. What is the role of information in these alternative approaches?

1-3 Describe the basic management cycle in hospitals. What categories of information can assist the hospital administrator in carrying out his responsibilities in relation to the activities embodied in the cycle?

1-4 How do the frequency and periodicity of a management decision influence the manner in which information can be obtained to support the decision? What alternative approaches are available to the system designer?

1-5 What are some of the major objectives which hospitals have in mind in the development of hospital information systems?

1-6 Describe the three categories of information systems in hospitals (clinical information systems, information systems to support administrative operations, and management planning and control systems). How important is integration of information in each of these three categories of systems?

1-7 Describe in a general way the state of the art of information systems development in U.S. hospitals.

1-8 Provide an example which demonstrates how the planned integration of several systems could result in improved information for a hospital.

NOTES

1. See, for example, Charles J. Hitch and Roland N. McKean, *The Economics of Defense in the Nuclear Age* (New York: Atheneum, 1967) for an elegant theoretical statement in support of the rational model.
2. See, for example, David Braybrooke and Charles E. Lindblom, *A Strategy of Decision* (New York: The Free Press, 1970) or Aaron Wildavsky, *The Politics of the Budgetary Process* (Boston: Little, Brown, 1964).
3. Alfred Kuhn, *The Study of Society: A Unified Approach* (Homewood, Illinois: Irwin-Dorsey Press, 1963), pp. 277-80.
4. Amitai Etzioni, "Mixed Scanning: A Third Approach to Decision-Making," *Public Administration Review*, December 1967, pp. 385-92.
5. For a discussion of various forecasting methods see Michael B. Harrington, "Forecasting Areawide Demand for Health Care Services: A Critical Review of Major Techniques and Their Application," *Inquiry*, September 1977, pp. 254-268.
6. See John R. Griffith, "Short-Term Forecasting Techniques," in *Quantitative Techniques for Hospital Planning and Control* (Lexington, Massachusetts: Lexington Books, 1972), pp. 50-55.
7. Charles J. Austin, "Hospital Information Systems and the Development of a National Health Information System," *Journal of Medical Systems*, Vol. 6, No. 1, 1982, pp. 4-5.
8. Samuel Davis and John R. Freeman, "Hospital Managers Need Management Information Systems," *Health Care Management Review*, Fall 1976, pp. 65-74.
9. Hospital Financial Management Association, *The State of Information Processing in the Health Care Industry* (Chicago: The Association, 1976).
10. Sheldon I. Dorenfest, "Information Systems: Hospitals' Computer Costs Will Rise Dramatically During Next Five Years," *Modern Healthcare*, May 1980, pp. 73-76.
11. Regina Herzlinger, "Management Noninformation Systems in Health Care Organizations," *Health Care Management Review*, Spring 1976, pp. 71-76.

ADDITIONAL READINGS

Alter, Steven L. "How Effective Managers Use Information Systems." *Harvard Business Review*, November-December 1976, pp. 97-104.

Ball, Marion J. and Boyle, Thomas M. "Hospital Information Systems: Past, Present, and Future." *Hospital Financial Management*, February 1980, pp. 12-24.

Davis, Samuel and Freeman, John R. "Hospital Managers Need Management Information Systems." *Health Care Management Review*, Fall 1976, pp. 65-74.

Hospital Financial Management Association. *The State of Information Processing in the Health Care Industry*. Chicago: The Association, 1976.

Koza, Russell C., ed. *Health Information Systems Evaluation*. Boulder, Colorado: Colorado Associated University Press, 1974.

Levey, Samuel and Loomba, N. Paul. *Health Care Administration: A Managerial Perspective*. Philadelphia: J.B. Lippincott, 1973. Note particularly Chapter 8, "Health Information Systems."

Lindberg, Donald A. B. *The Growth of Medical Information Systems in the United States*. Lexington, Massachusetts: Lexington Books, 1979.

Mecklenburg, Gary A. "Types and Uses of Hospital Information Systems Expand." *Hospitals*, April 1, 1981, pp. 112-119.

Murdick, Robert G. *Management Information Systems, Concepts and Design*. Englewood Cliffs, New Jersey: Prentice-Hall, 1980.

Riley, M. J. *Management Information Systems*. San Francisco: Holden-Day, Inc., 1981.

Schmitz, Homer H. *Hospital Information Systems*. Germantown, Maryland: Aspen Systems Corp., 1979.

Shuman, Larry J., Speas, R. Dixon, Jr., and Young, John P., eds. *Operations Research in Health Care*. Baltimore: Johns Hopkins University Press, 1975. See particularly Chapter ll, "Information Systems," by Ronald L. Gue and John R. Freeman.

Stimson, David H. and Stimson, Ruth H. *Operations Research in Hospitals: Diagnosis and Prognosis*. Chicago: Hospital Research and Educational Trust, 1972. Note particularly "Computer Applications and Total Hospital Information Systems," pp. 26-35.

2

General Systems Concepts

A variety of systems comprises the functioning of a modern hospital. These can be categorized into three groups: mechanical systems, human systems, and man-machine systems. *Mechanical systems* are an integral part of the physical plant, serving such purposes as heating and cooling, monitoring temperature, pressure, and humidity, and supplying chilled and heated water. Some hospitals employ pneumatic tube systems for transporting documents and small objects, and a variety of mechanical systems has been developed for transporting supplies and materials throughout the hospital.

Most of the essential functions of the hospital are carried out through *human systems*—organized relationships among patients, physicians, hospital employees, family members of patients, and others. Many of these systems are formally defined. For example, nursing care is provided in accordance with a scheduled set of predetermined procedures, and nursing service personnel are trained and supervised in the proper execution of this "system of care." Many things also happen in hospitals (as in other organizations) through informal relationships, which often become well-defined and known to those in the organization. Thus certain activities get accomplished by "knowing the right person" or sending informal signals to key individuals about actions that need to be taken.

With the development of modern technology, many systems in hospitals fall into the third category, *man-machine systems*. These are formally defined systems in which human effort is assisted by various kinds of automated equipment. For example, many hospitals now operate intensive care units for critically ill patients in which highly trained personnel provide diagnosis and treatment with the aid of a variety of machines designed to monitor continuously the vital signs of patients in the unit. Many hospitals also employ computers for assisting hospital personnel with both patient care and non-patient care activities.

Information systems in hospitals fall into the second and third cate-

FIGURE 2–1
The Hospital as a System

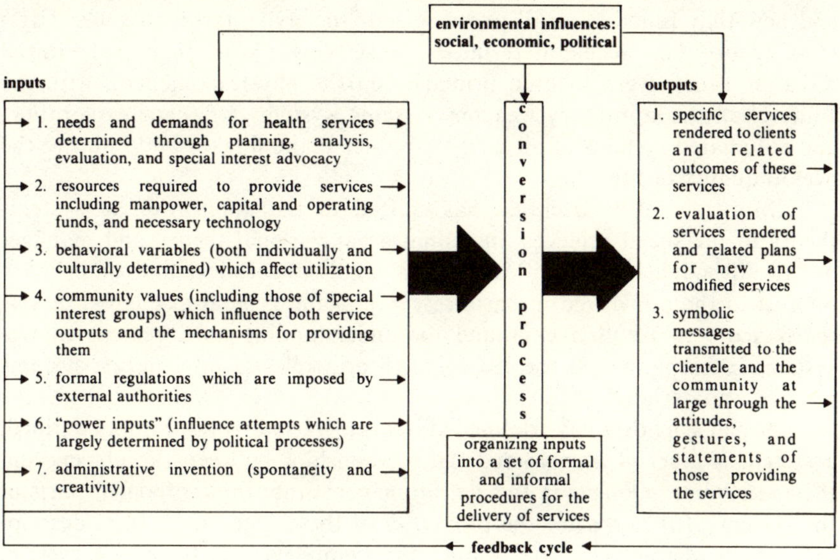

Reprinted from Charles J. Austin, "Current Status of Education for Health Administration" in *A Future Agenda: Education for Health Administration,* Volume III (Ann Arbor, Michigan: Health Administration Press, 1977).

gories of this simple taxonomy; that is, information systems will either be human systems or man-machine systems designed to support hospital operations. Information systems which operate without any type of machine processing of data are described as *manual* systems in the jargon of the computer and data-processing industry. Although much of this book deals with machine-aided information processing in hospitals, most of the principles which are set forth, particularly those dealing with systems analysis and design, have equal applicability to the development of manual systems for processing of information.

The hospital also can be described in a broader context. Figure 2-1 is a systems diagram for the entire hospital, showing the relationships among various inputs and environmental factors as these factors influence the provision of services to the community. In this context, mechanical, human, and man-machine systems would constitute elements, or subsystems, of the conversion process. The theoretical concepts on which this diagram is based are described in the section on general systems theory, which follows.

GENERAL SYSTEMS THEORY

Considerable research has been carried out by scientists on systems and how they function in all phases of our society. Interest in general systems theory has accelerated in the post-World War II period. Initial research efforts were focused primarily on the physical sciences, with the study of strategic military weapons systems, systems for space exploration, and automated systems of all kinds to reduce manual labor and improve the overall quality of life.

More recently, attention has shifted to the application of systems theory to the social sciences, including organizational theory and management.[1] Although much of this work is highly theoretical and of primary interest to those involved in basic research, some general discussion of systems theory is useful background for understanding management control systems in hospitals and for setting forth principles of information systems analysis and design.

Social scientists have defined systems in various ways. Simply defined, a system is a set of objects and the relationships between the objects and their attributes.[2] *Objects* in this definition constitute the component parts of the system. *Attributes* are the properties of these objects, abstract descriptors which characterize and define the component parts of the system. Essential to the concept of a system are defined relations, which tie the component parts together, thus enabling the parts to equal some greater unity rather than simply constituting an uncoordinated assemblage of objects or people. Relationships can be planned or unplanned, formal or informal, but they must exist if the collection of components is to constitute a system.

Certain basic concepts are central to a general understanding of systems and how they function.[3] First, a system must have *unity*, or *integrity*. That is, the system must be something which can be viewed as an entity in its own right, with unity of purpose in the accomplishment of some goal or function. Thus a team of skilled personnel at work in the operating suite of a hospital would constitute a system, whereas an assemblage of people sitting in the waiting room in the hospital's lobby could not be similarly described. Stated differently, a system must have an identity and must have describable boundaries which allow it to be defined without reference to external events or objects.

Systems at work in hospitals are for the most part very *complex*. The intricate web of complex relationships that constitutes most social systems often makes it difficult to describe simple cause and effect relationships among individual components of the system. The phenomenon of system complexity is often described by stating that a system is more than the sum of its parts.

FIGURE 2–2
Hospital System Hierarchy

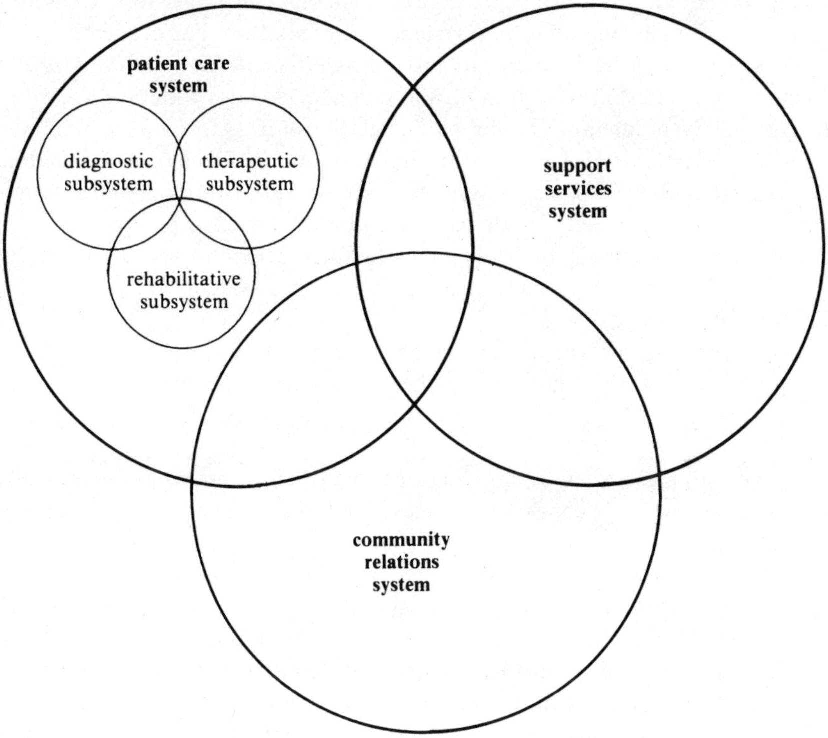

Complex systems are further defined by their *hierarchical structure*. That is, large systems in hospitals can be divided into several subsystems, and these subsystems in turn are subject to further subdivision in a nested format. For example, the patient care system of a hospital is composed of several subsystems: a diagnostic subsystem, a therapeutic subsystem, a rehabilitative subsystem, and so forth. Each of these subsystems in turn can be further described by a series of smaller systems. The entire network of systems and subsystems nests together in a structured way to describe the patient care system of the hospital (see Figure 2-2).

Although most hospital systems are dynamic and subject to frequent change, they nonetheless must possess some *stability* and *equilibrium*. That is, the system must continue to function in the face of changing requirements and changes in the external environment in which it operates. To accomplish this, procedures must be sufficiently generalized to accommodate a variety of situations which can be expected to develop. Complex systems must be self-adapting and possess control functions which are continuous and automatic. At that time when the system can no longer adapt to changing requirements or major changes in the external environment, it no longer functions as a system and breakdown has occurred.

Systems can be further categorized as either *deterministic* or *probabilistic*. In a deterministic system, the component parts function according to completely predictable or definable relationships. Most mechanical systems are deterministic. On the other hand, human systems or man-machine systems (including information systems) are probabilistic, since all relationships cannot be perfectly predicted. In hospitals, for example, most operating systems are subject to fairly extreme fluctuations in the quantity and nature of the demand for patient services. Hospital systems are probabilistic by their very nature.

Systems theory, then, provides a perspective, a way of viewing not just the parts, not just the whole, but rather the spectrum of relationships of the parts viewed in the context of the unitary purposes of the system as a whole.

The simplest of all systems will consist of three essential components: one or more inputs, a conversion process, and one or more outputs (see Figure 2-3).

Consider for a moment the inpatient admissions process of a hospital as a simple system. Inputs to the system consist of elective admission requests from physicians; emergency admission requirements; beds currently available; and admitting department resources, including personnel, procedures, and supporting materials. The conversion process includes a set of actions in which the admitting clerks collect information from incoming patients, match patient requirements to available beds, and make room assignments. Output of this simple system consists of patients admitted to the inpatient services of the hospital. Note that the output of this system becomes the input for several other functional systems of the hospital—nursing care, diagnostic services, and others.

Most systems also involve *feedback*, a process by which one or more items of output information "feeds back" and influences future inputs (Figure 2-4).

In the example just cited, feedback would occur in the form of adjusted information on the number of beds available as patients are admitted to the hospital. Each time such an admission occurred, input data on bed availability would be revised and updated.

Systems are either *open* or *closed*. A closed system is completely self-contained and is not influenced by external events. In an open system, the components of the system exchange materials, energies, or information with their environment (see Figure 2-5). That is, they are influenced by, and

FIGURE 2–3
Diagram of a Simple System

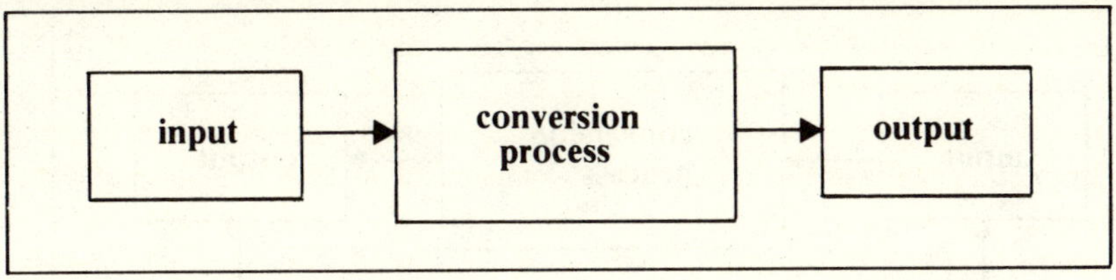

themselves influence, the environment in which they operate. All closed systems eventually die (cease to function as a system). Only open systems which adjust to the environment can survive as systems over time.

Hospital systems, with the exception of certain purely mechanical systems in the physical plant, fall into the category of open systems. Human or man-machine systems in hospitals are influenced by a variety of environmental factors (sometimes referred to as exogenous factors, or variables), and these are important to consider in understanding how a system functions. These environmental factors fall into four broad categories.

FIGURE 2–4
Simple System with Feedback

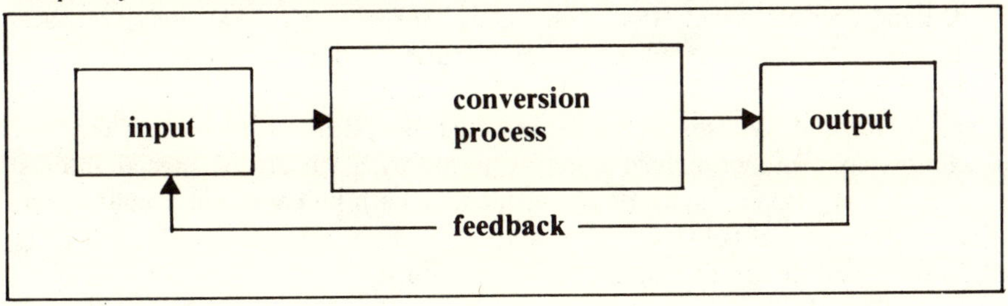

Hospital systems are influenced by *social factors*, characteristics of individuals and groups of people involved in the transactions that hospitals undertake. Social factors affect patient behavior and patterns of utilization of services. Informal patterns of behavior develop among hospital employees, and these have definite effects on the way hospital systems function. Role playing by physicians and other health professionals interacts with the formal functioning of systems. Social factors are important determinants of system functioning, and systems analysts need to be well versed in the art of human-factors engineering when designing systems for their hospitals.

FIGURE 2–5
Open System Diagram

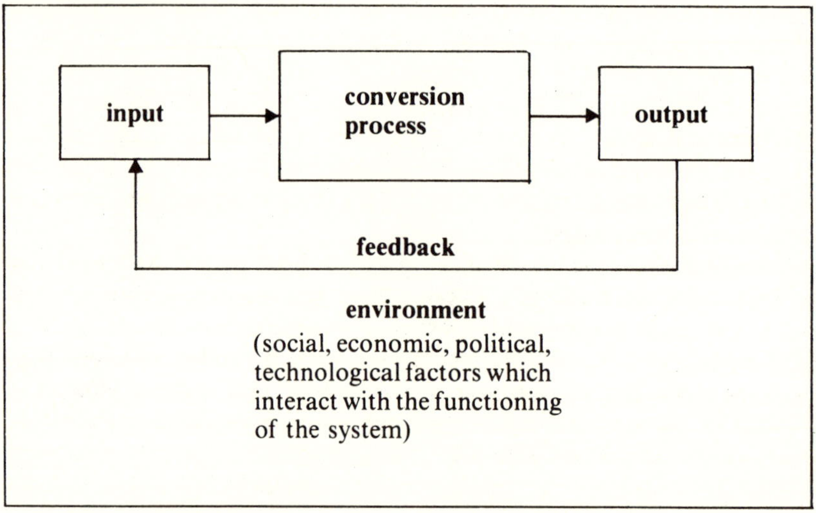

A second major category of environmental factors is *economic* in nature. Systems are directly dependent upon the availability of resources, and fluctuations in the local and national economy will influence both demand and resources. It is well known, for example, that elective procedures are often deferred by hospital patients during times of economic recession.

Hospital systems are also affected by *political factors*. There are competing demands placed upon hospitals by a variety of special interest groups, and hospital systems are influenced both by community politics and by organizational politics. These political realities must be considered in the analysis and design of systems for the institution.

The *physical environment* constitutes the final category of environmental factors affecting hospital systems. The amount of space available and the way in which system components relate physically to each other will influence the effectiveness of a system.

To summarize briefly, hospital systems are open systems influenced by a variety of social, economic, and political factors and by the physical environment within which they function. In the example of the hospital admission system referred to earlier in this chapter, it is easy to conceive of environmental factors which might affect the system. Social factors would include the characteristics of the patient population served by the hospital, as well as the kinds of people employed to work in the admitting department. The "culture of the enterprise" will affect the system and how it functions. Current economic conditions will influence demand patterns of patients and of physicians in their admitting practices. The system will also be influenced by political factors, particularly the need to meet the requirements of key members of the medical staff who admit large numbers of patients to the hospital. Finally, the physical layout of the admitting department will affect the system; the degree of crowding of the physical work space, the amount of privacy for confidential discussion with patients and their family members, and other physical conditions will be important determinants of system effectiveness.

The final concept to be introduced in this brief review of general systems theory is the concept of a cybernetic, or self-regulating, system.[4] Figure 2-6 is a generalized diagram of a cybernetic system. Feedback in a cybernetic system is controlled in order to adjust the future functioning of the system within a predetermined set of standards. The following elements are added to the general system components in order to provide this automatic control:

1. A *sensor* element continuously gathers data on system outputs.
2. Data from the sensor are fed into a *monitor* for continuous matching of the quantity or quality, or both, of performance against *standards*, predetermined expectations of system performance.
3. Error signals from the monitor are sent to a *control unit* whose purpose is to generate correctional signals which automatically modify inputs and conversion processes to bring the functioning of the system back into control.

The most often cited example of a cybernetic system is a thermostatic control system for the automatic heating and cooling of a building. Continuous sensing of the temperature in the building is monitored against a preset temperature, and automatic correction signals are sent back to the heating/cooling units of the system to keep the temperature within control limits.

Management Control Systems in Hospitals

Organized systems in hospitals should be designed as cybernetic systems with formal management controls built in as an integral part of the design. Figure 2-7 is a conceptual diagram of a generalized hospital cybernetic system.

The inputs to this generalized system include demand for services by patients and those who represent them and also the resources required to provide services—labor, materials, capital, and technology. The conversion

FIGURE 2–6
Cybernetic System

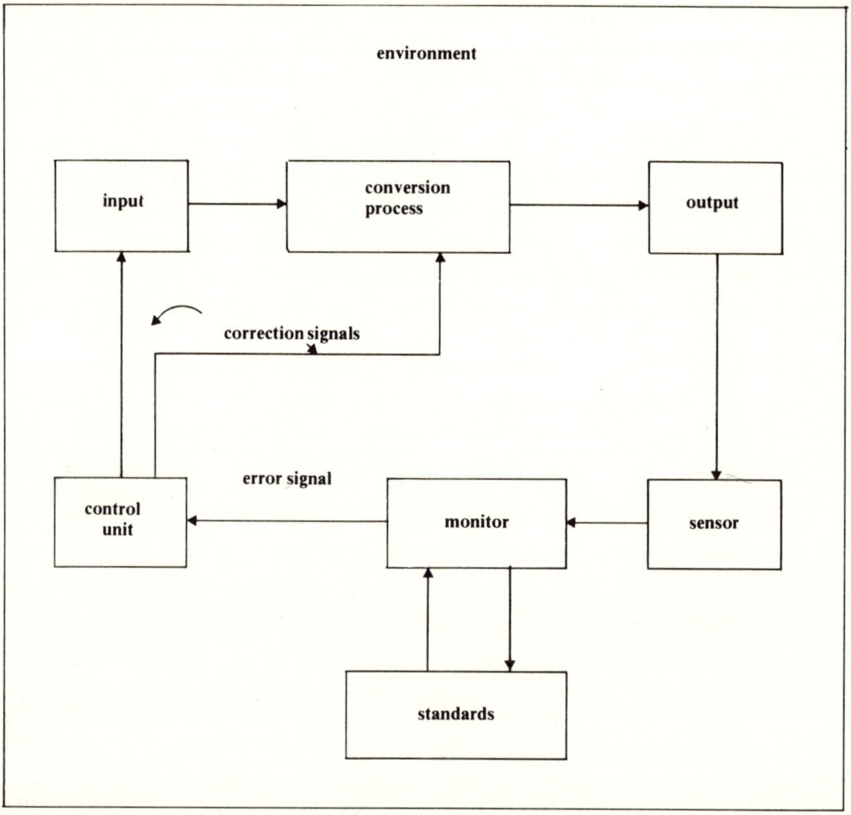

process consists of actions taken by hospital employees aided by formalized procedures, informal patterns of functioning, and supporting equipment. System outputs include services rendered to patients and the specific patient and community outcomes related to these services.

Management control is introduced in cybernetic components of the system. The sensor component continuously gathers data on the quantity of services rendered, the quality and other characteristics of these services, and the resources consumed in their provision. Data from the sensor are monitored against preestablished standards of quantity (production and service goals), quality of care, and efficiency of the service process. When standards are not met, a control process is activated to initiate necessary changes and improvements. The control process might include several ele-

FIGURE 2–7
Generalized Hospital Management Control System (Cybernetic)

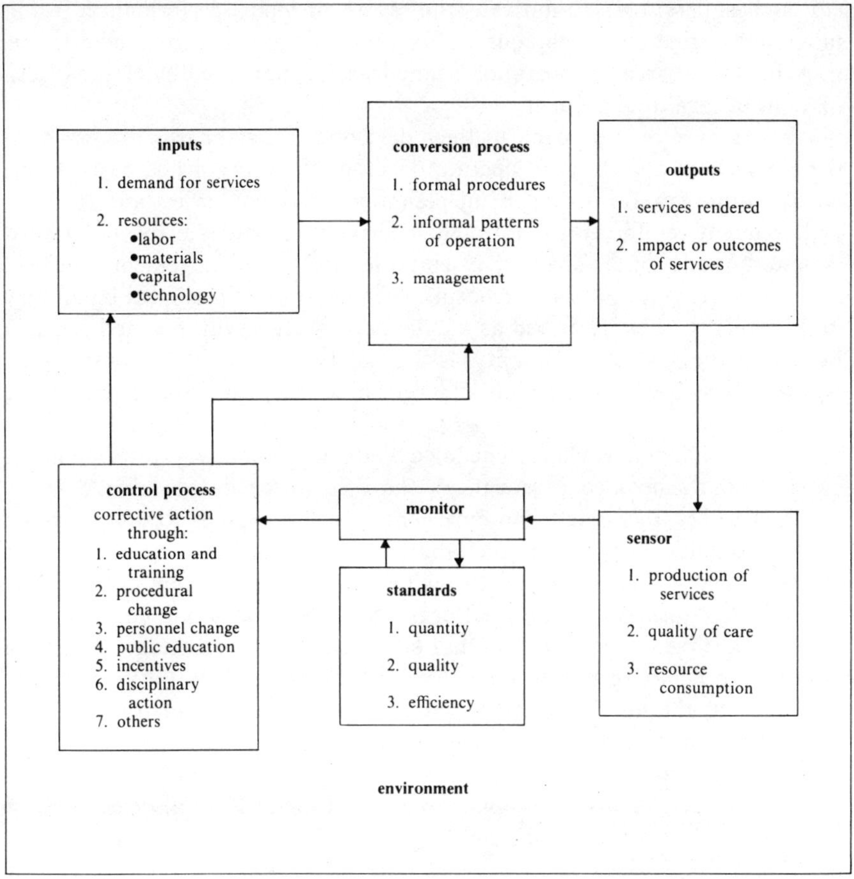

ments, including education and training of hospital personnel, community education programs, procedural changes in the process of rendering care, personnel changes in order to improve service, utilization of employee incentives, initiation of disciplinary action, and many others.

A key element in the establishment of management control in hospital systems is the establishment of standards for performance and quality control. The task of developing standards is not an easy one and requires considerable effort and thoughtful planning among hospital administrators and professional personnel practicing in or employed by the hospital. Standards can be developed in a number of ways. They can be established by administrative or medical authority in the institution. In some cases they may be developed through negotiation and subsequent agreement between employees and supervisors. Empirical studies of previous performance, using industrial engineering techniques, offer another approach to standards setting. In certain areas of operation, standards are mandated by external regulations or legal requirements.

Whatever the approach to their development, standards are essential if management control is to operate on other than an ad hoc basis. Standards require careful management planning, continual review and revision, and frequent reinforcement through incorporation into the formal reward system of the hospital. They are essential to effective management control.

As an example of these concepts, the operation of a clinical laboratory in a hospital can be described as a cybernetic system with planned controls built into the system for quality assurance and performance control purposes. Figure 2-8 is a schematic diagram describing the functioning of the laboratory in system terms.

System inputs include scheduled demand (laboratory tests planned, ordered, and scheduled in advance) and also unscheduled demand (tests required to be processed on an emergency, or stat, basis). Resource inputs include technical personnel in the laboratory, materials and equipment used in the testing process, and related technology. The conversion process consists of those formal and informal organizational actions related to collecting of specimens, conducting the lab tests, and reporting results to appropriate points in the hospital. System outputs include the test reports sent back to the nursing units or outpatient departments, charges for services rendered provided to the patient accounting department for billing purposes, and various statistical reports.

Cybernetic components for management control are also included in Figure 2-8. The sensor continuously gathers data on the number of tests conducted by various categories, quality control data, and records of resources consumed, including personnel time of laboratory technicians. These data are monitored against a set of predetermined standards, including those established by the Joint Commission on Accreditation of Hospitals (JCAH), professional standards of quality established by the chief pathologist and medical staff, and cost and efficiency goals (productivity) established jointly by administrative and medical personnel in the hospital. When standards are not met, corrective actions are initiated, including activation of continuing education and retraining, revision of operating policies and procedures, change in staffing patterns and scheduling, and the like. The laboratory operates overall as an open system influenced by several contextual or environmental factors, including the physical environment of the laboratory facility, current economic conditions of the hospital, social

FIGURE 2–8
Hospital Clinical Laboratory as a Cybernetic System

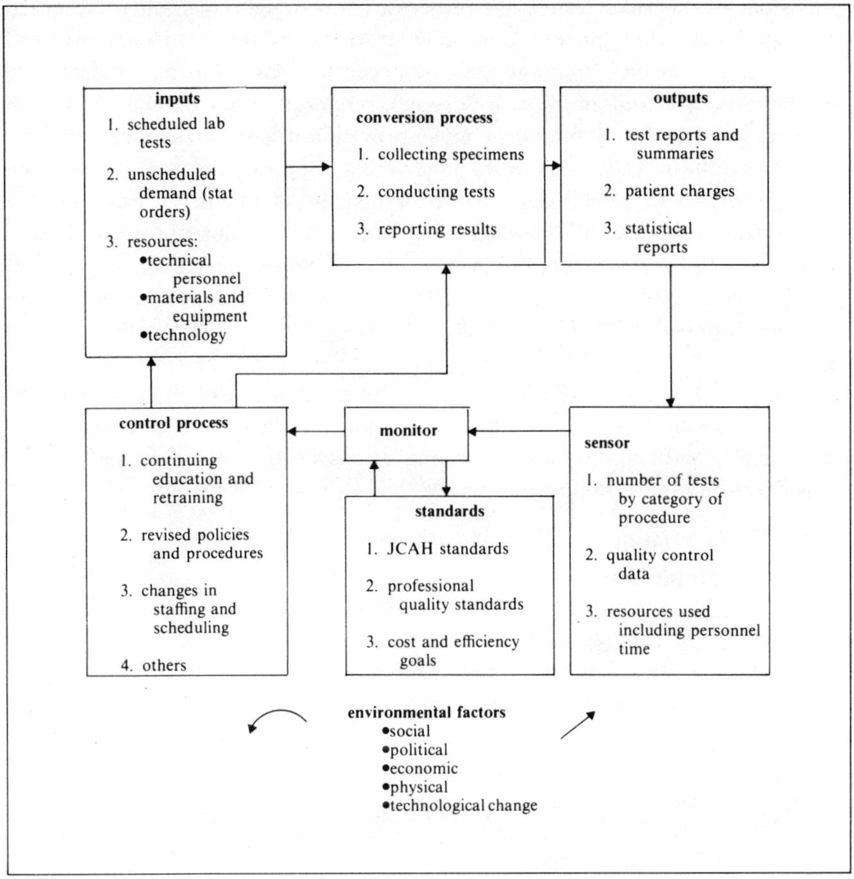

and political factors related to interaction of personnel in the department, and the advancement of technology.

INFORMATION FOR MANAGEMENT CONTROL

Any management control system in a hospital is obviously information-dependent. Information requirements permeate the system diagrams presented in the preceding parts of this chapter. In order for major hospital functions to be properly managed, information is needed about each of the major system components previously described.

Input information must be collected to continuously monitor demand, both scheduled and unscheduled, as well as the resources consumed in the provision of services. Hospital processes must be constantly observed through information on exceptions, error rates, system malfunctions, and similar measures on a management by exception basis. Output information on the quantity and quality of services rendered must be matched with information on related outcomes of the provision of specific services.

In addition, the effective manager must keep in close contact with the environment in which his department or institution functions. Environmental information is essential to this task—data such as demographic characteristics of the service population, previous utilization patterns, and recent changes in community values. An effective information system in a hospital will be designed with these kinds of management information needs in mind.

What, then, are the attributes of information useful for management control in hospitals? Some of the more important characteristics of effective management information are listed and discussed briefly below and will be considered in greater detail in Part IV.

Characteristics of Useful Management Information

- information—not data
- relevant
- sensitive
- unbiased
- comprehensive
- timely
- action-oriented
- uniform (for comparative purposes)
- performance-targeted
- cost-effective

The first, and perhaps most essential, characteristic is that information, to be useful, must be *information, not just raw data*. That is, data must be intelligently processed in accordance with predesigned plans before they become information useful to hospital management or operating personnel.

Hospital information must be *relevant* to the purposes for which it is to be used. It must be sufficiently *sensitive* to provide discrimination and meaningful comparisons for operating managers. Many information systems provide data which are so aggregated as to provide no meaningful indicators for management planning or control purposes. Overall hospital cost per patient day is a good example. By contrast, separating costs into fixed and variable components and allocating variable costs by diagnostic groupings and level of care would provide more useful information to management.

Useful information must be *unbiased* and not collected or analyzed in such a way as to meet self-fulfilling prophecies of hospital personnel. Information should be *comprehensive*, so that all elements or components of a system are visible to those responsible for administering that system.

Information must be *timely*, presented to users in advance of the time when decisions or actions are required. Many information systems produce beautiful reports which are completely useless because of failure to meet operational time requirements. Information should be *action-oriented*, designed to aid the manager directly in the decision process rather than just presenting passive facts about current operations. For example, information from an inventory control and materials management system should include direct indicators of when specific items need to be reordered rather than just presenting data on current numbers in stock.

Information systems should have as their goal the production of *uniform* reports so that hospital indicators can be compared over time both internally against previous performance and externally against the experience of other hospitals. Good information will also be *performance-targeted*, that is, designed and collected in reference to predetermined goals and objectives of the hospital.

Finally, hospital information should be *cost-effective*. The anticipated benefits to be obtained from having the information available should exceed the costs of collecting and processing that same information.

Although hospital administrators are becoming increasingly sophisticated in the effective use of information, there are still many ineffective practices which are common in the hospital industry. Administrators often utilize and frequently quote statistics about their institutions which are simplistic and insensitive indicators of actual hospital performance. Overall cost per patient day was mentioned previously as an example of this. Such an indicator is meaningless until subdivided and examined in reference to the case mix and service base of the institution. And yet many hospital information systems are not capable of combining the necessary clinical and financial information to produce useful indicators of unit costs for the institution.

Hospital administrators also tend to rely on simple averages rather than considering the variation about those averages and the more meaningful frequency distribution of a given hospital indicator. Average length of stay is the classic example. Not only does this statistic need to be examined on a diagnosis-specific basis, but a distribution of the lengths of stay of patients will be much more useful than a simple average in reviewing current operations.

Another major problem in many hospital information systems is the failure to apply consistent definitions to information elements collected continuously over a period of time. This is a particular problem when analysis of trend data is an element of management planning and control.

There are many other problems in information system design which are developed in greater detail later, and Part III of this book describes ways to eliminate such problems in the design of useful information systems in hospitals.

SUMMARY

Hospital systems include mechanical systems, human systems, and man-machine systems. Most hospital information systems fall into the latter category, with computers and other data-processing equipment used by hospital personnel to assist in the storage and processing of data.

An understanding of general systems theory is useful for hospital administrators in designing and developing management control systems and in obtaining the kinds of information which are required to enable such systems to function effectively.

A system is a set of objects together with the relationships between the objects and their attributes. Systems are characterized by unity of purpose, complexity, hierarchical relationships with other systems, and a need for stability in the face of a dynamic environment. Most hospital systems are probabilistic, in that relationships cannot be perfectly predicted or described in the design of the systems.

A simple system consists of one or more elements of input, a conversion process, and one or more outputs which flow from that process. Most systems also include feedback, by which system outputs influence future inputs and processes. Open systems are influenced by the environment in which they function, and they exchange information and energy with that environment. Environmental factors include political, social, and economic variables which influence system performance, as well as the physical environment in which the system functions.

Cybernetic systems include formally planned components which introduce automatic control into the systems. Cybernetic components include sensors to gather data on current system functioning, monitors to compare these data against predetermined standards, and control elements to change inputs or process, or both, when system functioning is out of control. Management control systems in hospitals can be designed according to principles of cybernetic system theory.

Hospital functions viewed in a systems context are information-dependent. Effective information for management control purposes has several important characteristics, including relevance, timeliness, sensitivity, comprehensiveness, objectivity, action-orientation, uniformity, performance-targeting, and cost-effectiveness. Good information systems will be developed with these characteristics constantly in view of those charged with design and implementation.

DISCUSSION QUESTIONS

2-1 Define the term *system*. What are the three general kinds of systems that will be found in hospitals?

2-2 What is the difference between an open and a closed system?

2-3 What are some of the environmental factors which will influence open systems in hospitals? How important are these factors in systems design?

2-4 What is a cybernetic system? Explain how cybernetic theory can be utilized in the development of management systems in hospitals.

2-5 Why is stability an important characteristic of a system? How can system stability be achieved in the dynamic environment of a modern hospital?

2-6 Explain how hospital systems fit together in hierarchical structures.

2-7 Why are most hospital systems described as probabilistic rather than deterministic?

2-8 Why are hospital management and operating systems said to be information-dependent?

2-9 What are some of the attributes of information that make it useful in management control systems in hospitals?

PROBLEMS

2-1 For the hospital functions listed below, use cybernetic theory to describe the operation and management control of each in systems terms:

a. the emergency room of an acute care general hospital

b. the radiology department of a hospital

c. one nursing unit on a medical floor

d. the operating suite of a general hospital

e. the admitting process of a general hospital

f. an outpatient rehabilitation and physical therapy program

g. a community hospital public relations program

h. a diploma nursing program operated by a hospital

2-2 For each of the systems listed in Problem 2-1, develop a list of information elements that would be needed for each system to operate effectively.

2-3 Prepare a brief report to a hospital's board of trustees commenting on the general characteristics of useful information for assisting in the policymaking and administrative processes of the hospital.

NOTES

1. See, for example, Walter Buckley, ed., *Modern Systems Research for the Behavioral Scientist* (Chicago: Aldine Publishing Co., 1968).
2. A.D. Hall and R.E. Fagen, "Definition of System," in Buckley, op. cit., pp. 81-92.
3. Several of these concepts are addressed in more detail in United Hospital Fund of New York, "An Administrator's Survey of Systems Concepts," in *A General Systems Approach to Hospital Management and Organization* (New York: United Hospital Fund, 1971).
4. The father of cybernetic systems theory is Norbert Weiner. See, for example, his classic work, *The Human Use of Human Beings: Cybernetics and Society* (Garden City, New York: Doubleday Anchor, 1954).

ADDITIONAL READINGS

Baker, Frank, ed. *Organizational Systems: General Systems Approaches to Complex Organization.* Homewood, Illinois: Richard D. Irwin, 1973.

Buckley, Walter, ed. *Modern Systems Research for the Behavioral Scientist.* Chicago: Aldine Publishing Co., 1968.

Griffith, John R. *Quantitative Techniques for Hospital Planning and Control.* Lexington, Massachusetts: Lexington Books, 1972. Note particularly Chapter 1, "Introduction," and Chapter 10, "Nature and Application of Control Systems in Hospitals."

Hancock, Walton M. "Dynamics of Hospital Operational Control Systems." *Hospital and Health Services Administration*, Summer 1976, pp. 23-42.

Lapatra, Jack W. *Health Care Delivery Systems: Evaluation Criteria.* Springfield, Illinois: Charles C. Thomas, Publisher, 1975. See particularly Chapter 1, "A Systems Approach to Health Problems."

Murdick, Robert G. and Ross, Joel E. *Introduction to Management Information Systems.* Englewood Cliffs, New Jersey: Prentice-Hall, 1977. Note particularly Chapters 2 and 3, "Management Information and the Systems Approach (Parts 1 and 2)."

Sheldon, A., Baker, F., and McLaughlin, C.P., eds. *Systems and Medical Care.* Cambridge, Massachusetts: MIT Press, 1970.

United Hospital Fund of New York. Chapter 2, "An Administrator's Survey of Systems Concepts." In *A General Systems Approach to Hospital Management and Organization.* New York: United Hospital Fund, 1971.

Warner, D. Michael and Holloway, Don C. *Decision Making and Control for Health Administration.* Ann Arbor, Michigan: Health Administration Press, 1978. Note particularly Part IV, "Cybernetic Control."

Young, John P. "A Conceptual Framework for Hospital Administrative Decision Systems." *Health Services Research*, Summer 1968, pp. 79-95.

3

Overview of Information Systems Development in Hospitals

Most information systems in hospitals have evolved in a piecemeal fashion rather than resulting from a carefully controlled planning process. Specific requirements for capturing data, storing them, and retrieving them when needed have developed on an ad hoc basis as new services are added to a hospital's offerings. The result often has been a series of problems and inefficiencies in the information processes of hospitals. The same data are captured repetitively in different areas of the hospital; files are duplicated needlessly; information is not always available when needed, often resulting in patient inconvenience; and numerous other gaps and inefficiencies are commonplace.

As hospital operations grow more complex and as data-processing technology becomes increasingly sophisticated, the need for careful planning in the development of information systems is paramount. Hospitals can no longer afford the luxury of a laissez-faire, evolutionary approach to the use of information. Hospital administrators must take responsibility for a careful, orderly process of planning to insure that hospital information requirements are satisfied.

This chapter presents an overview of the process of information systems development in hospitals as a prelude to more detailed material which follows in subsequent chapters.* Topics covered include master planning, systems integration, and alternative approaches to information system development. The master plan provides a framework for the detailed steps which follow in planning, designing, installing, and operating information

---

*Some technical terminology is introduced in this chapter. For definitions the reader is referred to Appendix A: Glossary of Technical Terms.

systems. The chapter ends with a discussion of the hospital administrator's responsibilities for overseeing the entire process.

MASTER PLAN FOR INFORMATION SYSTEMS DEVELOPMENT[1]

The development of information systems in a modern hospital is a complex task involving major capital expenditures and significant manpower commitments if the systems are to function properly. The development of an overall hospital master plan for information systems development is an essential first step in the process. To exclude this essential planning activity would be analogous to beginning a major hospital construction project without functional specifications for the new building. And yet, many hospitals have moved directly into the development of computer systems without any kind of master plan.

The hospital administrator should take direct responsibility for organizing the planning effort. A planning task force should be formed with representation from the major organizational units of the hospital including the medical staff, nursing service, controller's office, personnel office, physical plant, ancillary service departments, and hospital administration. The task force should be directed by a knowledgeable member of the administrative staff or by a senior systems analyst or industrial engineer, if the hospital employs such a person.

A suggested organizational chart for the planning effort is shown in Figure 3-1. Task force members should serve as chairmen for the committees; additional hospital personnel or technical consultants can serve as members of the specific committees and subcommittees.

Consideration also should be given to use of an outside consultant if additional technical expertise is needed, as it is in many hospitals. However, the consultant should be chosen carefully. He should possess technical knowledge of systems analysis and computer systems and should be well-informed about hospitals and their functioning. It is essential that the consultant be an independent practitioner not associated with any equipment manufacturer or firm which sells predesigned systems to hospitals. He must be familiar with the latest technological developments but must resist the temptation to push for applications that are too close to the leading edge.

The administrator also should insure that hospital staff members participating on the task force are provided sufficient released time from their normal duties so that they can participate fully in the planning efforts. Released time estimates should be drawn up in advance, and formal written notification of this should be provided to all involved. The hospital administration and board of trustees should be prepared to spend a significant amount of the institution's manpower resources on carrying out this impor-

FIGURE 3–1
Organizing the Planning Effort

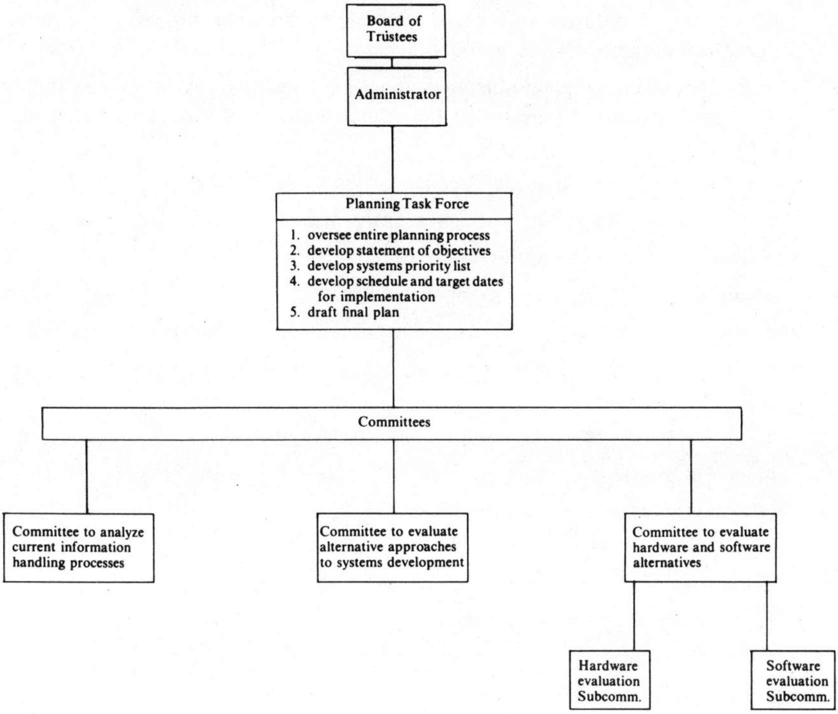

tant task. Although it is not possible to specify the time required to develop this master plan, a range of six to 12 months of intensive effort would not be at all unusual.

Figure 3-2 summarizes the major elements which should be included in the master plan, and Figure 3-3 is a flow chart showing the major steps in the planning process. The first step in the process is to carry out a general study of the hospital's current information handling activities and practices. This is sometimes referred to as a preliminary systems analysis. Before the staff can make intelligent decisions about improving information systems, it must first document the present status of the hospital. The study should document current processing steps as well as the costs of generating and using information throughout the hospital for (1) direct patient care functions, (2) supporting services, (3) administrative and financial control, and (4) quality assessment and assurance. The techniques for carrying out the study involve principles of systems analysis which are discussed in detail

FIGURE 3-2
Hospital Master Plan for Information System Development

1. General documentation of current information handling processes and practices, including costs, gaps, and deficiencies.
2. Statement of institutional objectives for the information system and establishment of a sequential priority list for implementation of the system in various areas.
3. Evaluation of alternative approaches to systems development
    a. individual systems—no attempt at integration
    b. modular approach—interchange among systems
    c. total systems approach—complete integration
    d. distributed processing approach—network of mini- and microcomputers
4. Evaluation of alternative approaches to systems analysis, design, and computer programming
    a. in-house—hire and train analysts and programmers
    b. contract services
    c. predesigned or packaged systems
    d. combinations of the above
5. Evaluation of alternatives concerning equipment
    a. acquisition of in-house equipment
    b. use of service bureau
    c. sharing services with other hospitals
    d. combinations of the above
6. Analyze costs of recommended alternatives
7. Establish a schedule and target dates for implementation of the system

in Chapter 7. Although a trained systems analyst is needed to carry out much of the work, there should also be heavy involvement of hospital operating personnel who are familiar with the functions being reviewed.

Given these baseline data on current hospital information processes, the next step for the task force is to develop a clear statement of objectives for the hospital to follow in initiating an information systems development program. These objectives should be as specific as possible and should flow from the deficiencies and gaps identified in the preliminary study just completed. Avoid general statements of objectives such as, "Information systems in Community Hospital should be designed to improve the quality of care and increase the efficiency of hospital operations." Such statements

FIGURE 3–3
Flowchart—Master Planning Process

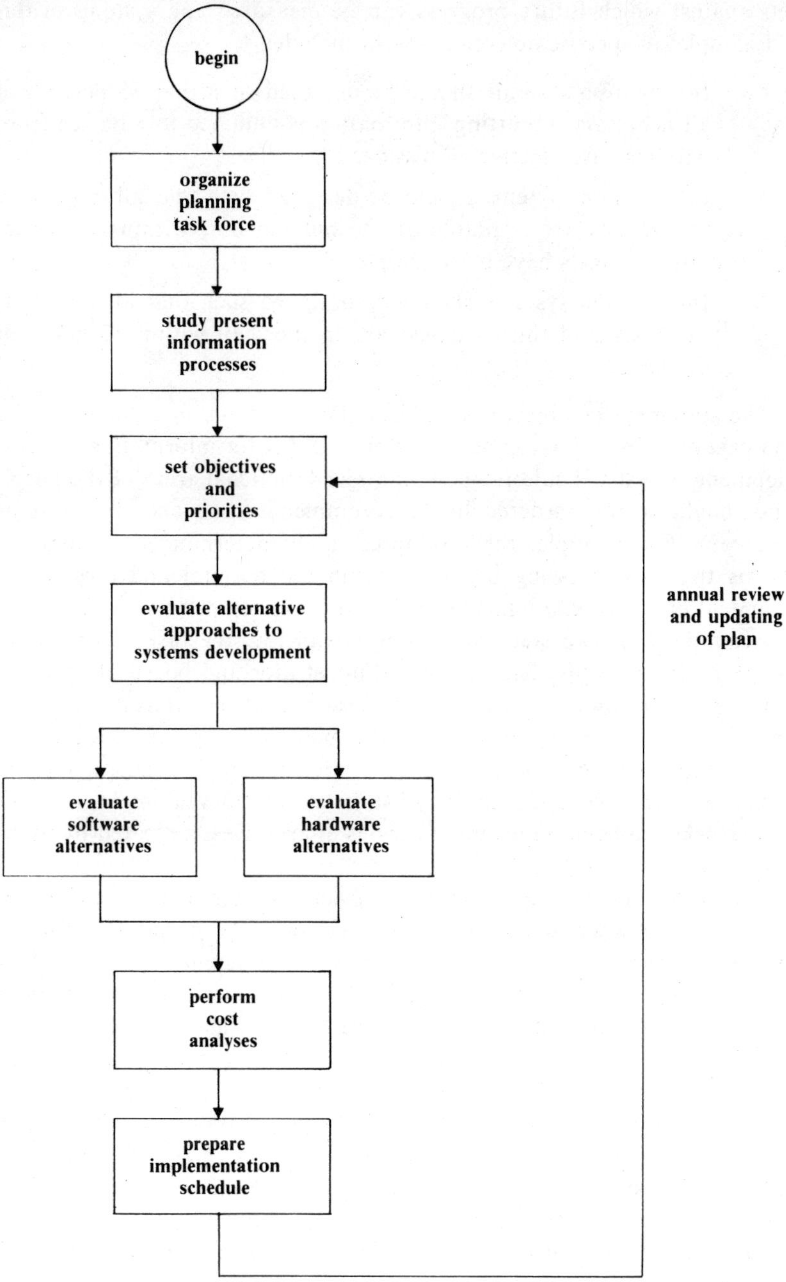

are self-evident and nonfunctional as far as planning is concerned. Rather, a detailed list of objectives should be established which will provide specific targets against which future progress can be measured and systems evaluated. Examples of specific objectives might include:

1. Information systems should be designed such that 75 percent of all necessary admitting information is obtained in advance from patients with elective admissions.
2. Information systems should be designed such that all diagnostic test results are available at the nursing unit within two hours after the tests have been completed.
3. Information systems should be designed such that all bills (patient pay and third parties) are in the mail within 72 hours of discharge.

The statement of objectives will aid the task force in completing the second part of Step 2, development of a priority list for information systems development. The list should include all major functional areas of the hospital and should be rank-ordered in the recommended sequence for systems development. For example, the task force might determine that financial control is the most pressing problem within the hospital and direct that development of a financial information system take top priority.

After the first two steps have been completed, the task force should report preliminary results back to the administrator and board of trustees. The statement of objectives and priority lists should be carefully reviewed and modified, as necessary, before the next planning steps are undertaken. Given a comprehensive analysis of current information processes, a specific statement of objectives, and a priority list for systems development, the task force now needs to begin to examine various alternatives, indicated by Steps 3, 4, and 5 in Figure 3-2.

The first (perhaps most important) set of alternatives to consider relates to various approaches to systems design in the hospital. Although many choices are available, they cluster into four groupings. First, the hospital may choose a system that has individual, "stand alone," applications and not attempt to integrate them or transfer information from one application to another. Second, it might prefer to follow the most common approach—the modular design approach, in which the system is implemented in functional units, or modules, with specifications for information interchange across modules. Third, the hospital might choose the fully integrated, or "total systems," approach, which involves one or more large central databases with communications equipment employed throughout the hospital for entry and retrieval of information. Fourth, the hospital might choose to follow a distributed processing approach with multiple minicomputers or microcomputers, or both, initiated in a network of decentralized locations throughout the institution.

The committee that is established to examine these alternatives should be staffed primarily by technical personnel—hospital information systems analysts or consultants—working with a representative of the hospital administration. This committee should review the experience in information system development of other hospitals of similar size and with similar functions. Costs are obviously an important factor. The total systems approach will require a major immediate commitment of capital, whereas the more cautious modular approach will require incremental allocations of capital. Therefore, costs and benefits should be examined for a long-range period (five to 10 years).

Once an approach to systems development has been selected, consideration must next be given to the human resources required to carry out the detailed work of systems analysis, design, and computer programming. It is important that this step be carefully planned, since major staffing commitments are required to carry out a comprehensive systems program in the hospital. Several alternatives are available. The first would be to recruit and train an in-house staff of systems analysts and programmers. A second approach would be to contract for services with firms that specialize in systems development and programming. A third would be to use predesigned or packaged programs to carry out the various functions included in the priority list. And, of course, various combinations of these approaches are possible. The hospital, for example, might choose to use contract services for development of clinical systems, to buy packaged systems for payroll and patient accounting, and to develop its own staff for systems maintenance and development of additional applications. Although the staffing decision does not have to be unalterable, initial planning of human resource requirements is an essential part of the master plan.

The final set of alternatives relates to computer and data-processing equipment choices. Once again, the hospital has several options available. It may choose to acquire and install its own equipment, either purchasing or leasing. Or it could choose to utilize outside services from organizations which sell computer time and other data-processing services. Hospitals in one community or part of a larger organization might join together in sharing the costs and services of a central computer installation. Of course, various combinations of these choices are possible. Intelligent choice among all three sets of alternatives described above obviously requires a combination of technical knowledge and knowledge of the detailed objectives of the hospital. Hence, the planning task force must be sure that both kinds of skills are available in developing its recommendations.

Once a set of alternatives has been selected, it must be subjected to a thorough cost analysis. Costs should be presented in three major categories: (1) costs of system design and implementation, (2) costs of operation, and (3) costs of system maintenance. The final element of the master plan is an overall schedule and set of target dates for implementation. Although cost estimates and target dates will be preliminary at this point, they will aid hospital administration and board members in evaluating the magnitude of institutional commitment required to implement the recommended set of alternatives.

As with any plan, the master plan for information systems development must be a dynamic instrument which is reviewed periodically and updated. At least once a year progress should be reviewed against the original criteria set forth in the plan, and the plan should be changed as necessary.

The Five Steps in Information System Development

Guided by the principles embodied in the master plan, there are well-established procedures to follow in the design and implementation of individual information systems, regardless of whether the work is being done by hospital systems personnel or through contractual services. It is the responsibility of the hospital administrator to oversee the process and to be sure that sound procedures are not bypassed or cut short in an effort to get a system implemented quickly. The five basic steps required in the complete cycle of information systems development are:

- systems analysis
- selection of design approach
- systems design
- implementation
- system maintenance

Each of these steps is examined in detail in Part III. The discussion which follows presents an overview of the entire process.

Systems analysis, the essential first step in any information systems project, is the process by which current information practices are reviewed and new or modified system requirements are established. Simply defined, *systems analysis is the process of collecting, organizing, and evaluating facts about information system requirements and the environment in which the system will operate.*[2] To use the analogy of a hospital construction project, systems analysis is comparable to the first stage of a construction program in which hospital management, working with the architect, develops functional specifications for the building. In a systems project, management should work with the head systems analyst to delineate the information requirements which the system must meet.

The second major step in the process is selection of a design approach. Guided by the master plan, which specifies the overall approach being followed by the hospital (e.g., development of compatible modules rather than the total system approach), the specific approach to design of each particular system must be delineated in advance. Choices range from minor improvements upon the existing method of obtaining the information (no automation) to complete design of an automated information system with no present constraint being placed on the new system. This point in a system project is an important transitional period in which a decision to proceed or not to proceed can and should be made. Unfortunately, too many hospitals have not been willing to make the decision not to proceed, either because of inadequate systems analysis or unwillingness to accept an analysis which indicates that the present manual system is working well.

Once a design approach has been selected, and assuming that a decision has been reached to proceed with the development of a new information system, the process of system design begins. System design is the architectural phase of the project. The results of the design effort should be a detailed set of written system specifications covering all elements of the new information system: inputs, outputs, master files, computer programs required, operating procedures, cost estimates of the new system, and other items to be discussed more fully later. In addition, plans should be included for a manual backup system to be used when the main system is down for any reason.

The system specifications should be subjected to a formal review procedure involving written sign-off by hospital administration and all operating departments involved in the new system. This represents another critical decision point at which the "go" or "no go" decision should be reviewed. The development of detailed system specifications could provide additional data showing that the new system will be too expensive or will not meet hospital requirements. If such is the case, hospital management and systems personnel must make the difficult decision not to proceed with the project.

Given a completed set of detailed system specifications approved by management, implementation of the system can proceed. Implementation involves more than just writing computer programs. It also entails ordering equipment, preparing space for the equipment, training personnel to use the system, and, above all, careful testing prior to operational use of the system. The importance of careful system testing cannot be overemphasized, and many catastrophes could have been avoided if adequate testing had been carried out in advance.

Systems maintenance is the final step in the cycle and one which is often ignored, with disastrous results. Many people, including some hospital administrators, believe that an automated information system, once operational, does not require further attention. Nothing could be further from the truth. No matter how good the system testing, operational systems are subject to occasional breakdowns, and trained personnel must be available to make quick corrections. Also, hospitals are dynamic organizations, and the requirements placed upon an information system are subject to constant changes. Hence, maintenance personnel are needed to make these required changes. Finally, all information systems should be periodically evaluated, and changes should then be made to improve the effectiveness and efficiency of each system.

Integration of Information Systems in the Hospital

Hospital information systems, to be effective, must be integrated; that is, individual systems must be able to communicate with one another and share information. For example, a computer system in the clinical laboratory designed to keep track of laboratory tests ordered must not only produce reports of test results for the patient's chart, but also this system must be able to communicate electronically with the hospital's automated patient accounting and billing system.

There are four basic approaches to integration of systems, depicted in Figures 3-4, 3-5, 3-6, and 3-7, which follow. The hospital may choose to develop individual and independent systems for each major application area with no attempt to build relationships across the several information systems to be developed (see Figure 3-4).* Note that in this alternative each system stands alone and there is no data communication across systems. Most hospitals started into the data-processing business following this approach. Although the task of systems design and programming is less complicated, the lack of integration and information transfer across systems constitutes a major disadvantage and inefficiency which often causes problems later. Almost all hospital functions, clinical and administrative, are closely interrelated, and hospitals are well advised to think seriously about the consequences of following a completely independent, nonintegrated approach to systems development.

The second approach, modular design, is the one used most frequently in hospitals. A graphic description of this approach is included in Figure 3-5. The basic concept is to design systems in functional units, or modules,

* The symbols used in Figure 3-4 are standard flow charting symbols explained in Appendix B: Key to Flowcharting Symbols.

FIGURE 3–4
Alternative Approaches to Systems Development: Individual Applications Approach

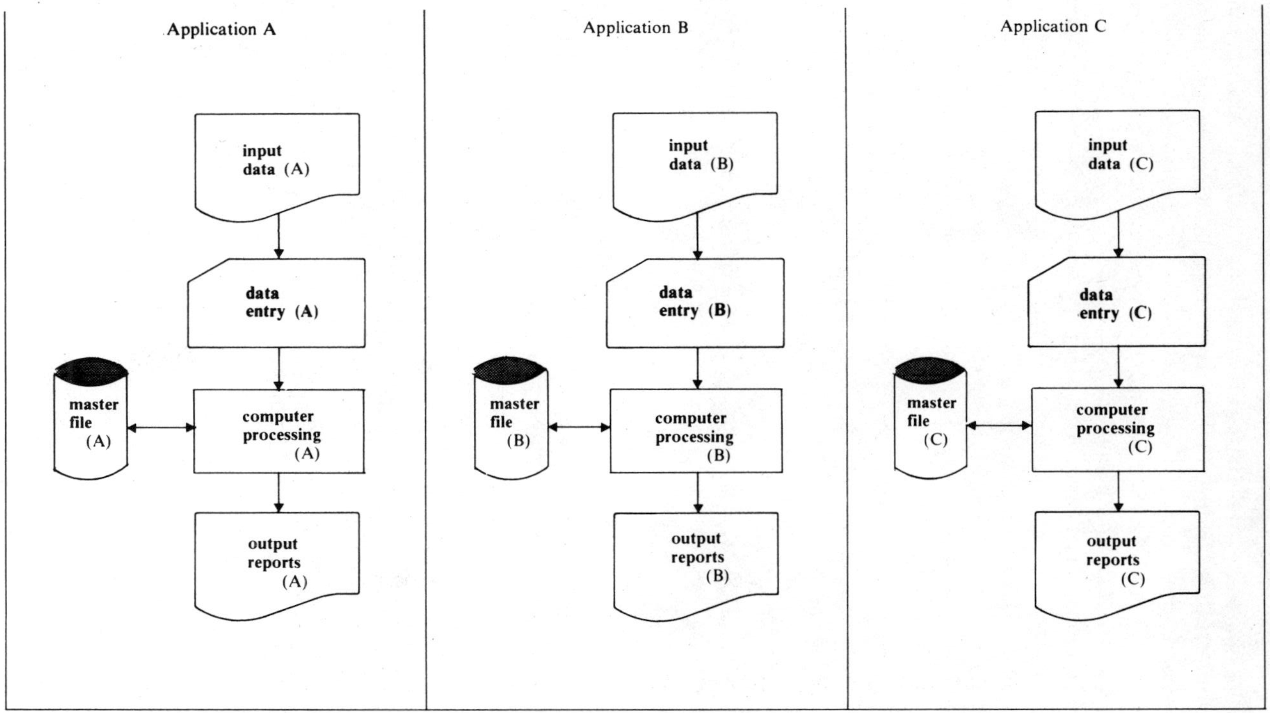

FIGURE 3–5
Alternative Approaches to Systems Development: Modular Design Approach

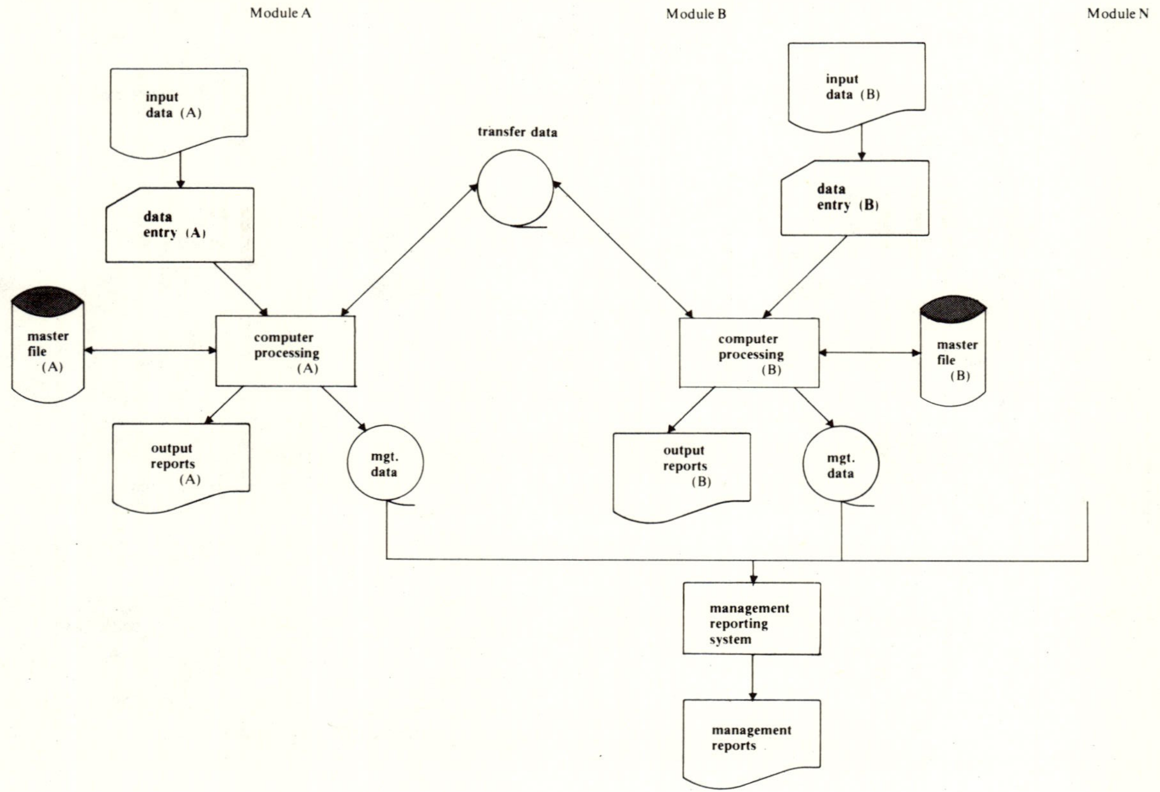

FIGURE 3–6
Alternative Approaches to Systems Development: Total Systems Approach

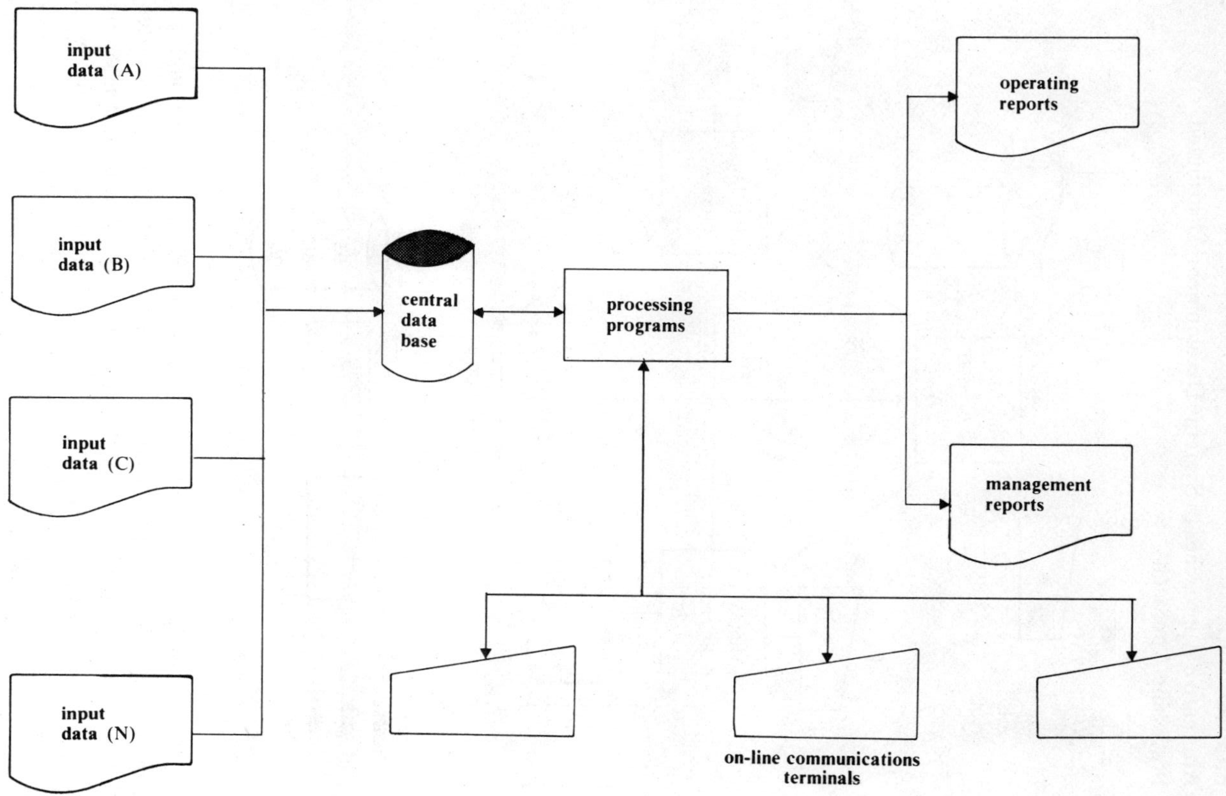

FIGURE 3-7
Alternative Approaches to Systems Development: Distributed Processing Approach

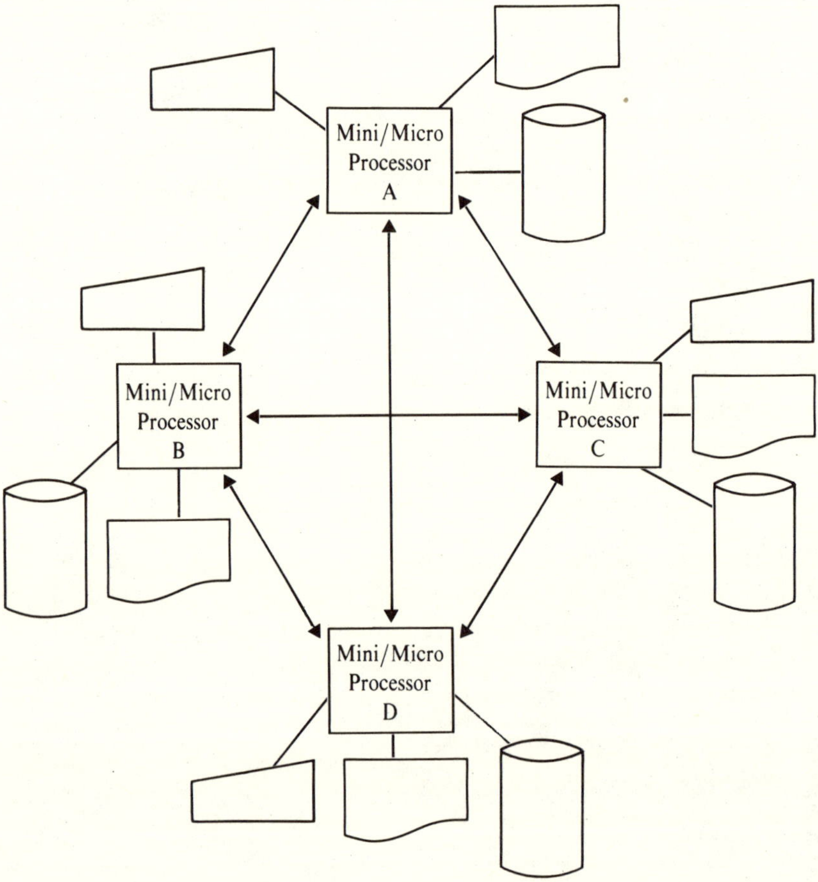

and to plan for information interchange across modules through planned data transfer techniques. Note that in Figure 3-5, Module A operates independently of Module B except in the sharing of information common to both systems. So, for example, a system might be designed for processing laboratory orders and test results (Module A), and this system could be so planned as to provide data directly to another system for processing patient charges (Module B).

The third option is the total, or fully integrated, systems approach (see Figure 3-6). In this case, one large system is designed centering around one or more central data files (referred to as a central database) which provide information to a variety of areas in the hospital.

Several prototype systems have been developed around a central file of patient information available for retrieval and automatic communication of information throughout the hospital for both clinical and administrative uses. Examples of such systems are included in Part IV. Although this alternative is an attractive one conceptually, the costs and complexity are an order of magnitude greater than the other two approaches, and the hospital would need to consider this route very carefully and be sure that there is a complete commitment to carry it out, including making sufficient capital resources available. The importance of complete integration increases with the size of the hospital, since communication breakdowns often occur in very large, complex hospital settings. Also, the resource base of a large hospital is more likely to be able to carry the expense of installing a total system, so this alternative seems to be one for serious study by larger hospitals (300 beds plus).

The fourth approach, and one of growing interest in hospitals, is the distributed processing approach (Figure 3-7). The costs of small, but powerful, mini- and microcomputers have come down substantially in recent years. Some hospitals have chosen to decentralize their information processing and install several small computers at different departmental locations throughout the hospital. Thus, the admitting department might have its own computer and do its own processing, as would the laboratory, pharmacy, outpatient department, patient accounting department, etc.

If this approach is followed, careful central planning and control must be maintained by hospital administration. Each system must be planned so that it can share information and communicate with the other systems in order for integration to be achieved. If individual hospital departments are allowed to go their own separate ways, then there is little probability that systems can be integrated, with organizational chaos the likely result.

Alternative Mechanisms for Systems Development and Implementation

Several alternatives are available to hospitals for the design and installation of information systems, including: in-house development, use of shared services, use of packaged systems, and employment of contractual services. Whatever approach is followed, decisions should be made in reference to the hospital master plan for information systems development, as discussed earlier in this chapter. If outside services are to be employed, particular attention must be paid to insuring that the resulting systems can be integrated with others in the hospital. The five-step approach to system development (analysis, selection of a design approach, design, implementation, and maintenance) should be followed regardless of whether the design work is done in-house or by contract.

There are several advantages to an in-house design effort. System requirements can be tailored to the specific needs of hospital personnel if the institution develops its own system. Control over system integration will be easier to achieve, and operational maintenance will be facilitated by having an in-house staff which is completely familiar with the system and how it functions. Disadvantages of the in-house design approach include the possibility of reinventing a system which has already been developed and tested elsewhere, as well as the relatively high costs associated with a comprehensive design and implementation effort.

Many hospitals are now employing predesigned, or "packaged," systems available from software vendors rather than entering into in-house design projects. If packaged systems can be used extensively, then fewer technical design and programming personnel will be needed, with savings accruing to the hospital's operating budget. With software packages, the developmental costs involved are shared by the multiple users of the packages.

Care must be exercised, however, in the use of packaged systems. Many predesigned packages may not meet the hospital's specific requirements and many modifications may be required. The cost of making these modifications could exceed the savings realized by using the package. System maintenance also can be a problem when packaged systems are used. The software firm may hold copyright privileges and might charge high fees for modifying the package to meet changing needs of an individual hospital. If the hospital is permitted to make its own changes, then the documentation provided by the vendor must be accurate and sufficiently detailed for use by hospital maintenance programmers.

The following factors should be considered in the evaluation of packaged systems:

1. Does the package meet the hospital's *specific* needs? If not, is the hospital willing and able to adjust to the general system specifications?
2. Who else has used the package? Careful reference checking is essential.
3. Can the packaged system be implemented on the hospital's existing computer configuration? If not, what will be the costs of hardware modifications?
4. How will the system be maintained? How good is the documentation? How difficult will it be to make changes?

5. What will be the costs to: (a) purchase the package; (b) implement it on the hospital's hardware; and (c) maintain it after it is operational?

A third alternative to in-house design or purchase of packaged systems is the use of contractual services for design and implementation of systems. Such services can be purchased from several vendors which specialize in systems analysis and programming. Contracts can range from purchase of services on an hourly basis to fixed price contracts for a total turnkey effort, in which the entire project is handled on a contractual basis. The following factors should be considered in evaluating responses to a Request for Proposals for contract services:

1. Carefully review the prior experience of the contractor. Talk to several previous hospital clients.
2. Review the credentials (experience and training) of the *specific personnel* to be assigned to the project. Insist that the contractors identify the specific individuals to be assigned to the project.
3. Check the proposal to be sure it employs well-established principles of systems analysis and design in its methodology.
4. Carefully examine the cost estimates. Be sure they are thoroughly prepared, complete, and comprehensive.
5. If necessary, use a neutral, disinterested party (independent consultant) to assist in the technical evaluation of proposals.

A fourth alternative available to some hospitals is the sharing of services with other hospitals. Shared hospital information services are available in a variety of forms, including: (1) services offered by corporate headquarters to members of hospital systems or chains; (2) voluntary affiliations of hospitals which organize to share services; and (3) contracts with service bureau organizations which sell shared services to hospitals.[3]

A 1980 report indicated that 73 nonprofit and commercial shared service organizations were providing computer services to 2,219 community hospitals in the area of financial applications.[4] Forty-four of the organizations were affiliated through formal ownership or contractual management with the hospitals they served, 18 serviced both affiliated and unaffiliated hospitals, and 29 provided services on a purely contractual basis. The author of the report concluded:

> Today, many alternatives offer the same benefits as shared services on an in-house basis. . . . While computer sharing continues to be a viable alternative, as the cost of computing power declines and software packages available for in-house computing improve, fewer hospitals will utilize shared computer hardware.[5]

Combinations of the four alternative approaches are also possible. Whatever the approach or combination of approaches to be followed, the principles of master planning, system integration, and use of well-accepted practices of systems analysis and design must be followed. Hospital management must be sufficiently involved in project oversight to insure that such is the case.

Differences in Approach Based on Hospital Size and Complexity

As with most management decisions in hospitals, decisions about the most appropriate approach to information systems development will be situational, based upon current and projected needs and the present state of development at each institution. However, certain general statements can be made about differences in approach as influenced by hospital size and complexity.

Information systems in smaller hospitals will, in general, be smaller and less complex. Potential deficiencies in system integration may possibly be overcome through direct communication among hospital personnel. Alternatives for the smaller hospital will be more limited since the budget base for capitalization of a major design and development effort will be limited. Minicomputers, particularly small business computers, are now within the price range of most small hospitals. The key to their feasibility will depend upon whether or not good software packages are available to support hospital applications. As such packages become available, small business systems will attract widespread use in small to medium-sized hospitals. Shared computing arrangements will continue to be attractive to smaller hospitals, particularly when predesigned software systems are included in the sharing agreement.

Information systems in larger hospitals are, of course, more complex and more difficult to design and implement. Integration of systems becomes particularly important in order for systems to function effectively in support of hospital operations. Predesigned packaged systems are less likely to meet the particular needs of large hospitals which tend to develop their own particular way of doing business suited to their situational environments. The budget base of the larger organization, however, makes more alternatives potentially feasible, including the relatively expensive capital costs of inhouse system development. Distributed data processing has become an attractive alternative to the cost and complexity of the total system or central database approach for large, complex facilities. However, as mentioned previously, unless careful controls are exercised by hospital management, lack of system integration and inability of systems to communicate with one another could result from the decentralized approach.

BEHAVIORAL ASPECTS OF SYSTEMS DEVELOPMENT

The major problems encountered in system development projects are human problems. Computer technology has advanced rapidly, and well ahead of our ability to employ it effectively. Consequently, attention to behavioral factors in the design of systems is essential. An understanding of these factors by management personnel will facilitate effective project oversight. Adminstrators need to understand some of the characteristics of technical personnel involved in systems analysis and programming and must also consider how personnel from user departments may respond to a new approach to doing business.

Consider first some of the concerns which user personnel often have about a systems project.[6] Fear of change is a common problem faced in many system development efforts with resultant employee anxiety and tension. Employees will have concerns about possible effects of the new system on their own jobs and possible changes in the work environment that may be required. Managers may have concerns about changes that could result in the redistribution of power, greater centralization of authority, or increased accountability as by-products of the new system. Some may have concerns that the information system will result in more rigid and less flexible patterns of operations, with resultant lack of discretion in carrying out a task. Often, these concerns are unfounded and based upon misunderstanding of the technology involved.

Whisler describes another common concern—that automated systems somehow will inhibit creativity on the part of the innovator, the entrepreneur, the organizational maverick. On the contrary, when properly designed, automated systems should open up new opportunities for creativity because of expanded information available to the innovator and decision maker.[7]

Technical personnel (programmers and analysts) also have their idiosyncracies. Characteristics of such personnel are discussed in more detail in Chapter 10. However, at the risk of overgeneralization, they tend to be technocratic, absorbed in the mechanical details of their systems, and may not be people-oriented in their approach to problem solving. And yet, analysts and programmers must work closely with personnel from the user departments in the development of system specifications. On occasion, technical staff may lack understanding of the politics of an organization and become so fascinated with the technology as to ignore the realities of the organizational setting in which the system must function.

There are several ways to deal with the human problems. Open communications are essential. Whenever possible, avoid being secretive during a systems development project. Provide a comprehensive program of staff orientation and training prior to initiating a design effort. User involvement at all stages of a project is essential. Structure the project in such a way that users will be part of the design of the system and "buy in" from the very beginning. Make top-level management support explicit and visible, and reinforce that support periodically.[8] Develop appropriate institutional rewards which encourage creativity and risk-taking, and develop procedures for resolving conflict when that becomes necessary. Above all, managers must work at understanding the needs and motivations of all the people who will be involved in the system in order to develop an effective work plan and mode of operation for the development project.

Ramsgard summarizes the need for a new kind of systems management quite well:

> When the systems analyst becomes a member of the user group and functions truly as a doctor of business, a diagnostician of business ills, the caste system will break down and we can anticipate changes in traditional roles. Administrators will begin to replace technicians as the directors of computer operations. . . . Long ago it was found that the best surgeon did not make the best hospital adminstrator, nor did a good engineer always make a good engineering manager. Now it is data processing's turn to become professionally administered.[9]

Hospital Administration's Responsibilities

What, then, is the hospital administrator's role in developing an information system? In general, the administrator's responsibilities are to oversee the entire process and to be sure that the systems development in the hospital is properly managed. It is very important that the administrator participate actively in these developmental efforts and insure that other key hospital personnel do the same. The need for careful management is self-evident given the magnitude of capital expenditures required for the development of computer systems in the hospital.

An important responsibility of the hospital administrator is to organize project teams for systems analysis, design, and implementation. Each major information systems development project should be so organized. A senior systems analyst, knowledgeable about the hospital and its idiosyncracies, should serve as team leader. At least one key person from each operating department to be included in the system should be assigned to the team, and there should be one administration representative as well. After the team has been organized and has completed a preliminary assessment of the task to be accomplished, a written schedule and time commitment for each member of the team should be drawn up and approved by the administrator. This is an important step, since the pressure of day-to-day operations and the crises which inevitably occur can stand in the way of effective participation if not formalized and agreed to in advance.

The administrator should insist upon receiving periodic progress reports and updated schedules from the project team. He should meet with the team regularly for an oral report and sharing of information. In reviewing progress, he should be certain that the five-step procedure described in the previous section is being followed. Specifically, he should insist that careful systems analysis precede any implementation decisions. The recommended design approach should be checked for compatibility with the hospital's master plan, and system specifications should be carefully prepared and formally reviewed before implementation begins.

During the implementation phase of the project, the administrator should check to see that adequate training of personnel who will be involved in the new system is conducted and that good documentation and procedures manuals are prepared. Of paramount importance, the administrator should check plans for complete system testing prior to final conversion to operational status. He should also insure that proper provisions have been made for systems maintenance after the new system goes into production.

Management responsibilities in information system projects were summarized by a national study group as follows:

> Particular emphasis in data-processing management needs to be placed on improved methods for:
> — planning for service and applications requirements, as well as for personnel and equipment requirements;
> — managing the entire applications development process;
> — managing costs and resources;
> — allocating costs for services . . .;
> — responding to changing requirements . . .;
> — assessing the contribution of data processing to the enterprise . . . [10]

SUMMARY

Information systems development in the hospital should begin with development of a master plan. The plan should include study of existing information processes, statement of objectives and priorities, examination of alternative system designs, examination of staffing approaches, analysis of equipment alternatives, cost analysis, and schedule and target dates.

Systems analysis, design selection, systems design, implementation, and maintenance are five steps essential to the development of good information systems, and none of these should be cut short in a rush to make a system operational. Decisions can and should be reached at various points in this cycle to drop the system when data show that costs may be prohibitive or that the system will not provide the anticipated benefits.

System integration, that is, the ability of information systems to communicate with one another and share information, is essential. Integration can be achieved through the modular design approach, a total systems approach employing a central database, or a carefully planned network of distributed processing centers located throughout the hospital.

Several alternatives are available to hospitals for the design and installation of information systems, including in-house development, purchase of packaged systems, employment of contractual services, use of shared services, and various combinations of these alternatives. Hospital size and complexity will influence the alternatives chosen, with in-house development more practical for larger hospitals and use of packaged systems on minicomputers becoming attractive to smaller hospitals.

Since information systems are designed, operated, and used by people, knowledge of behavioral factors and how they can affect a system is essential. Computer technology is well ahead of our human ability to employ it effectively in organizations.

It is the responsibility of hospital administration to insure that good management practices are followed in the planning and design of information systems. Management must take the lead in the development of a hospital-wide master plan and must carefully monitor specific systems development efforts which spring from the plan to be sure that good design practice is followed.

Part III of this book is a more detailed and somewhat more technical explanation of the principles and processes introduced in this chapter, and Part II presents technical information on computers. The reader who does not desire more detail on computer hardware and software, systems analysis, design, and implementation may turn to Part IV for a discussion of specific information system applications in hospitals.

DISCUSSION QUESTIONS

3-1 Why is planning so important in the development of hospital information systems?

3-2 Describe the elements of a master plan for information systems development in hospitals.

3-3 What is meant by the term *information systems integration*? Discuss some of the alternative ways in which systems integration can be achieved.

3-4 What alternatives should a hospital consider in planning for the staffing of information systems development projects?

3-5 Define *systems analysis*. Why is it so important in initiating a systems development project?

3-6 What factors should enter into a decision to proceed or not to proceed with development of a hospital information system? At what point(s) in the developmental process should such decisions be made?

3-7 Why are written system specifications important in the design phase of a project? Who should review and approve these specifications?

3-8 Is planning for the implementation phase of a project necessary? If so, why, and what elements should be considered?

3-9 How important is systems maintenance after an information system is operational? Why is maintenance required?

3-10 Describe some of the alternatives available to hospitals for system development and implementation. How are these alternatives affected by hospital size?

3-11 How important are behavioral factors in a system development project? In what ways do these factors influence a project?

3-12 Since information systems analysis and design are technical tasks, hospital administrative and operating personnel do not need to be heavily involved. Do you agree with this statement? Why or why not?

3-13 What are the responsibilities of hospital administration in providing oversight to information systems planning and development?

PROBLEMS

3-1 Develop an outline of a model master plan for hospital information systems development. State your assumptions about the hospital and its characteristics first, and then develop the outline of the plan accordingly.

3-2 As a follow-up to Problem 3-1, develop a list of 20 specific information system objectives to cover various functional areas of your hypothetical hospital.

3-3 Assume you are the administrator of a 400-bed community general hospital. To date, your hospital has not made use of computer equipment, and information systems have evolved rather than been planned. You are now ready to consider seriously the hospital's growing information needs, and you are about to initiate a planning process.

a. Describe how you would organize the planning task force. Whom would you appoint as members?
b. Write a statement charging the task force with the development of a master plan.

NOTES

1. Charles J. Austin, "Planning and Selecting an Information System," *Hospitals*, October 16, 1977, pp. 95-100, 202.
2. Based on the definition in Robert H. Gregory and Richard L. Van Horn, *Automatic Data-Processing Systems: Principles and Procedures* (Belmont, California: Wadsworth Publishing Co., 1965), p. 175.

3. Sheldon I. Dorenfest, "Computer Shared Services: Hospital Chains Become Important Providers," *Modern Healthcare*, November 1981, pp. 77-84.
4. Sheldon I. Dorenfest, "Computer Time-Sharing: 73 Groups Provide Full Financial Functions," *Modern Healthcare*, October 1980, pp. 71-78.
5. Ibid., p. 78.
6. Ada Demb, *Computer Systems for Human Systems* (New York: Pergamon Press, 1979), pp. 3-5.
7. Thomas L. Whisler, *Information Technology and Organizational Change* (Belmont, California: Wadsworth Publishing Co., 1970), pp. 126-128.
8. Ada Demb, op. cit., p. 14.
9. William C. Ramsgard, *Making Systems Work: The Psychology of Business Systems* (New York: John Wiley & Sons, 1977), p. 227.
10. T.A. Dollotta et al., *Data Processing in 1980-1985: A Study of Potential Limitations to Progress* (New York: John Wiley & Sons, 1976), p. 159.

ADDITIONAL READINGS

Bingham, J.E. and Davies, G.W.P. Part I, "The Six Steps of Systems Analysis." In *A Handbook of Systems Analysis*. New York: John Wiley & Sons, 1976.

Doyle, Owen. "Database: New Management Power." *Modern Healthcare*, May 1980, pp. 88-90.

Gore, Marvin and Stubbe, John. *Elements of Systems Analysis for Business Data Processing* (Second Edition). Dubuque, Iowa: Wm. C. Brown Co., 1979.

Hammon, Gary S. "Planning and Involvement Are the Words to Remember for an In-house Computer System." *Hospital Financial Management*, February 1974, pp. 38-42.

Howlett, P.J., Kenyon, N.G., and Kinder, N.J. "Information Handling in the Hospital: A Flexible Minicomputer Approach." *Journal of Medical Engineering & Technology*, January 1981, pp. 36-39.

Kennedy, O. George. "Smooth Implementation Depends on Planning Input from System's Users." *Modern Healthcare*, May 1980, pp. 92-94.

Lucas, Henry C. *The Analysis, Design and Implementation of Information Systems* (Second Edition). New York: McGraw-Hill, 1981.

Ramsgard, William C. *Making Systems Work: The Psychology of Business Systems*. New York: John Wiley & Sons, 1977.

Taggart, William M. *Information Systems: An Introduction to Computers in Organizations*. Boston: Allyn & Bacon, Inc., 1980. Note particularly Chapter 9, "Project Planning and Management."

II

Computing Concepts

4

Hardware Concepts

William J. Harvey

Familiarity with fundamental concepts and terminology of computer hardware is useful for individuals who must make decisions on computer system acquisition. This chapter describes the major categories of computer hardware and their functions.

Introduction

Tracing the development of computers from their beginnings to today's complex systems provides insights into their fundamental design. Electronic computers bring together a variety of clerical functions that have been performed since the earliest permanent settlements required records on trade, goods stored in warehouses, tribute, and taxes. Modern computer hardware incorporates features of a number of ancestor devices: mechanical and electronic calculators; mechanical keyboard devices, such as typewriters, for document preparation; magnetic recording technology used originally for sound recording; telegraph, telephone, and wireless communication; television displays; and early computers based on vacuum tubes.

Computers in health care environments fulfill much the same functions as those in other specialized contexts. Information is entered, stored, and retrieved; calculations are performed; messages are accepted or generated and displayed; errors are detected; files are updated; control signals are transmitted to climate-control and other devices; and reports are printed. The nature of the hospital environment requires that: (1) systems be available at all times; (2) errors be reduced to a minimum; (3) persons who are neither computer experts nor adept at keyboard skills utilize the computer facilities; and (4) certain functions be performed rapidly. In addition, there are legal requirements for detailed information on actions taken with regard to patient care. These specialized needs have led to an emphasis on the acquisition of reliable hardware and appropriate input–output equipment.

Evolution of Hardware

This discussion of the evolution of hardware covers the following topics: computing devices in general; data storage technology; input–output devices; and data transmission.

Computing devices have existed for centuries. Their development has been traced from the abacus, Napier's "bones," and the slide rule to the early mechanical calculators. Two of the first calculating machines were constructed in the seventeenth century by Blaise Pascal and Wilhelm Leibnitz. During the eighteenth century, Benjamin Franklin, Luigi Galvani, and Alessandro Volta improved our understanding of electricity, and experimentation began on punched-card and paper-tape control of processes in the weaving industry. In the early nineteenth century, Joseph Jacquard perfected the punched-card control of looms, perceptions about electricity and magnetism matured, and the law of electromagnetic induction was formulated by Michael Faraday.

The first design commonly acknowledged to incorporate essential features of a computer in the modern sense was Charles Babbage's plan for an analytical engine. This proposed device not only was to perform calculations, but was to offer decision-making capabilities. Further technological advances were required before Babbage's concept could be implemented. A major step forward came in the 1890 U.S. census, with electric card reading and processing of data stored on cards. Herman Hollerith designed the electric tabulating system used in that census. After the demonstrated success of Hollerith's system, card-based data processing expanded worldwide during the twentieth century and laid the basis for data input and off-line data storage of the first electronic computer systems.

John V. Atanasoff is credited with designing and building, in 1939, the first computer to incorporate the concepts of serial calculation, regenerative memory, and logic circuits.[1] Improved electronic computers were successfully constructed in the 1940s. By 1946, John von Neumann and others had formulated the principles of modern computers: use of binary data representation and storage of the program in the computer. The von Neumann computer stored programming instructions in memory in the same way that it stored data files. This advance eliminated the need for physical modification of the system for each new task: before then, computers required rewiring and resetting of switches to obtain a new program. Computers designed in accordance with the stored-program concept are true general-purpose computers. The standard components of modern computer architecture are an arithmetic and logic unit, a control unit, central memory for storing data (including programming), input–output facilities, and signal connection lines, called *buses*. Buses link the central processing unit (arithmetic, logic, and control) with primary memory and with input–output facilities.

Three *generations* of computers are commonly acknowledged. The primary memory of the first generation of computers (1946–1959) relied initially on vacuum tubes. The early computers were physically very large and somewhat unreliable, and they produced considerable heat. Magnetic core primary memory, using ferrite rings strung on intersecting wires, provided random-access capability for some first-generation computers and improved speed of access to data stored in main memory. Another type of high-speed storage device introduced during the first generation of computers was the magnetic drum, which had fixed read–write heads. The invention and refinement of the transistor led to the second generation of computers (1959–1964). Transistors made it possible to reduce size and increase reliability.

The third generation is generally considered to have begun in 1964, when integrated circuit components had an impact on the design of computers available for purchase. Integrated circuits reduced the size of the central processing unit, increased the speed of performance, increased reliability, and reduced the costs of processing and main storage. A multiplicity of changes in hardware and software and the complexity of the continued evolution of computers make it difficult to identify succeeding generations. There have been many attempts to define a fourth generation for the period from 1972 through the beginning of the 1980s and a fifth generation for new developments that have appeared since 1980, but there is no general agreement on criteria.

Input to the computer was made available first by switches, card readers, and paper-tape readers. The use of magnetic tape gave increased speed and flexibility. Keyboard terminals (both those with *hard copy,* or paper copy, and those with cathode-ray tube displays) enabled interaction between the computer and the user, or operator. Mark sense and optical scanners allowed input from sheets marked in predetermined locations. Calculators, computing devices, and typewriters advanced from mechanical forms through electromechanical versions to electronic systems. The keyboards of such devices resemble portions of keyboards of modern computer terminals and microcomputers.

The standard QWERTY keyboard is obviously a descendant of the typewriter keyboard, while the ten-key data-entry cluster on many terminals and microcomputers is a descendant of adding machine and calculator keyboards. Of course, special function keys have been added to serve the purposes of computer systems. Three characteristics of keyboards are apparent: the QWERTY keyboard is retained because so many people are familiar with it, even though the key arrangement is not efficient; the numeral 1 key is standard, and the use of that key rather than a lower case letter l must be learned by those familiar with older American keyboards (the numeral 1 remained standard, however, on European typewriter keyboards); there is, unfortunately, no standard location for many of the new special symbols used for computer data entry, programming, or word processing. Many computer keyboards contain two numeric *keypad* arrangements: one descended from ten-key adding machines, and one descended from the configuration used on keypunch machines.

Hospital data-entry needs led to the use of a variety of designs for computer terminals. The main aim was to reduce the amount of typing, and thus the potential for error and delay, in use of a terminal. One strategy was to assign special functions to individual keys in order to avoid typing entire words. This strategy can be effective where there is a limited number of well-defined functions in a normal transaction. The IBM 1050 terminal attempted to provide function capabilities for keys by the use of replaceable mats that could be laid over the keyboard to identify the functions in different contexts. Later developments that were found practical for hospital applications included function buttons next to the screen, optical scanner wands for reading bar codes or characters, light pens, and touch-sensitive screens.

Printed output and off-line storage of data at first borrowed from existing data-processing and office technologies. Typewriters, adding machines, and calculators developed the single-key impact printing technology as well as typewriter printing elements. The earliest output printing devices were adapted from typewriter technology in various forms—typewriters, teletypes, adding machines. Light-based output devices evolved from light bulbs to the cathode-ray technology that made television broadcasting possible. Cathode-ray tubes are an excellent means of displaying text and graphic data in computer information systems. Important modes of computer output are provided by *light-emitting diode* (LED) and *liquid crystal display* (LCD) devices.

Punched-hole data storage technology (punched cards and paper tape) was important in the early years of computer development and is still extensively used in many countries. Punched-card systems began with automatic looms in the early 1800s and matured through the work of Herman Hollerith and the U.S. Census Bureau. A well-known use of paper tape for noncomputer data storage was the punched-paper roll used in player pianos.

Paper-tape systems provided a versatile form of data storage and input for early computers and are still used in specialized applications today. The progress of magnetic recording technology from early wire recorders to tapes with oxide surfaces was important in providing storage capacity for computers. Today, high-speed disks provide great storage capacity and high rates of data access. To achieve greater reliability in storage of data, the Winchester disk technology provides a sealed, protected environment for disk surfaces and heads.

Modern data transmission between terminals and computers and between different computer systems evolved from telephone and telegraph technologies. Telegraph systems contributed experience in electrical transmission of codes. Telephone systems required progress in mechanical and electromechanical switching of circuits and provided a network later exploited for transmission of data between computers. In both cases, advances in propagation and recognition of signals were eventually vital to later computer networks. Wireless transmission of code and voice preceded the use of microwaves for transmission between stations on the Earth's surface and satellite stations in orbit.

Central Processing Unit

The *central processing unit* (CPU, Figure 4-1) is the hardware that carries out high-speed arithmetic, logic, and control operations. The term is sometimes carelessly applied to the cabinet that contains the CPU.

Electric current states are exploited as signals within the computer and for communication between processors. Each state signals a binary value of 1 or 0. Binary values are commonly referred to as *bits*, a contraction of *binary digits*. For example, five volts (+5 v) can be used to signify the value of 1, and no voltage (0 v) can be used to signify the value of 0. Each value is represented by a range of voltage values. The term *nominal* is applied to the approximate voltage levels: 1 is said to be represented by a nominal +5 v and 0 by a nominal 0 v. In reality, 1 is communicated by approximately five volts and 0 is communicated by a very low voltage (close to none) or no voltage. A time framework is then necessary to interpret the current state at any given instant as a 1 or 0. Successive 1s between 0 states (0110), for example, would be represented by change of state from 0 to 1 followed by maintaining the 1 state for two time units and then a return to the 0 state. (See Figure 4-2.)

Under actual operating conditions there are not only fluctuations in voltage but unavoidable losses in transmission. The ranges of voltages used to detect 1 or 0 values must be slightly greater than the range used in sending a transmission. The most reliable system is one that must distinguish only between two values.[2]

FIGURE 4-1
Diagram of a Computer Showing Hardware Components and Relationships to Peripherals

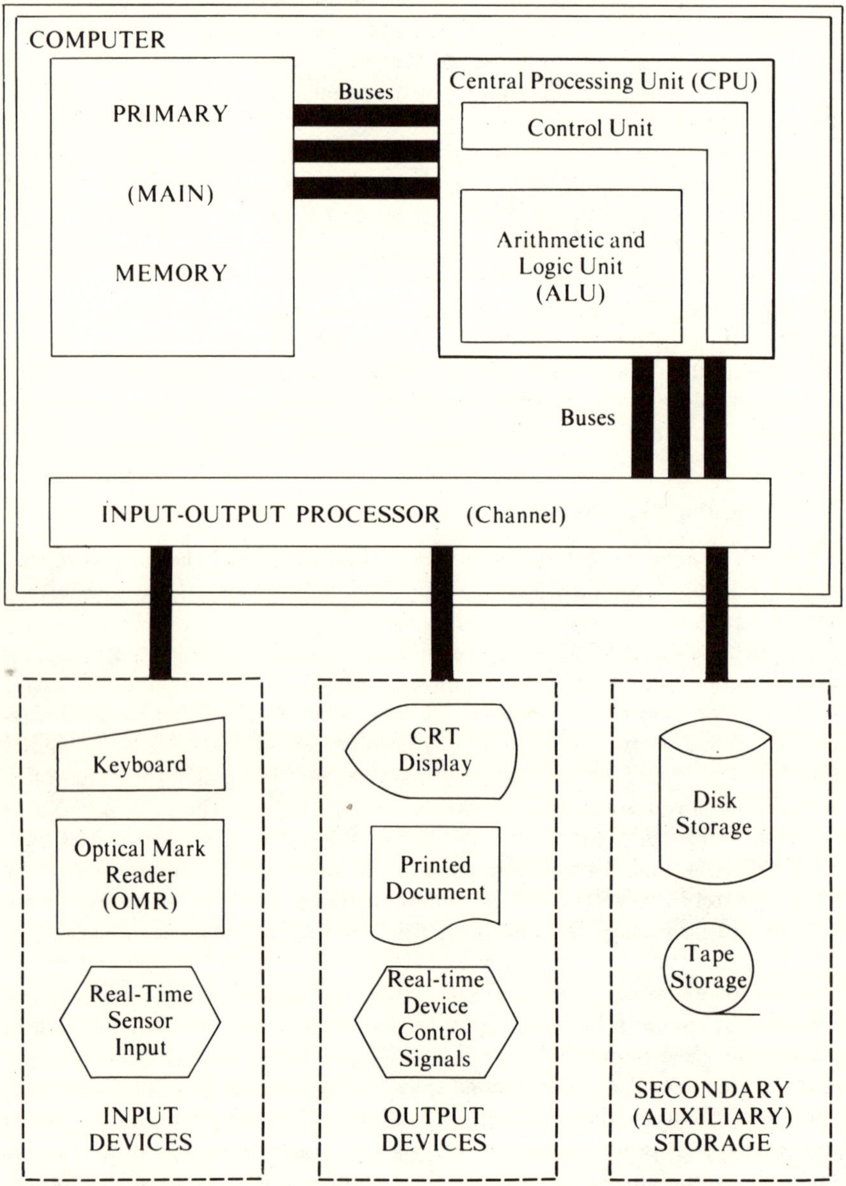

Peripherals

FIGURE 4-2
Electric Pulses as Binary Values

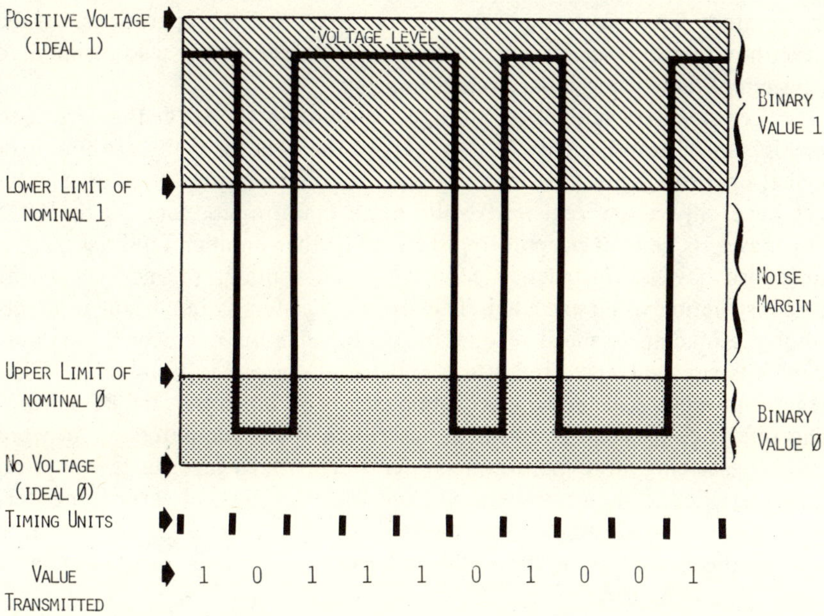

The *arithmetic and logic unit* (ALU) can perform operations on numbers and pairs of numbers. Arithmetic operations include addition, subtraction, multiplication, and division. Some computers use a combination of adding and shifting numbers to perform multiplication. Instead of *borrowing* to do subtraction as we are taught to do in school, computers can perform subtraction by converting negative numbers into complements and then adding. Some computers have only adding and shifting capabilities, which are used to perform all arithmetic operations.

Comparisons and tests are functions of the ALU. In order to make automatic decisions in a computer program, it is often necessary to compare two values. Six relationships are possible: greater than, less than, equal to, greater than or equal to, less than or equal to, not equal to. A useful operation is to test a given value for its relationship to zero (greater than zero, equal to zero, less than zero). To exploit this capability of the ALU, some operations produce condition codes in terms of relationship to zero.

Logical operations involve electronic equivalents of the logical terms *and*, *or*, and *not*. Although we do not think about it very often in everyday transactions, there are two variations of the logical connector *or*: the *inclusive or* means at least one and possibly both, while the *exclusive or* means at least one but not both. Figure 4-3 shows the use of the logical connectors, or operators. These operations are referred to as *Boolean* operations, named after the nineteenth-century mathematician George Boole, who formulated a system of logic using binary representation.

Registers are temporary storage locations in the CPU that are used for high-speed transactions. At least part of the data for many arithmetic or logical operations must be in a register. Microprocessors for microcomputers have only a few registers, while large mainframes, such as the IBM 370, have 16 general-purpose registers and other similiar facilities. CPUs must also have an instruction counter, which contains the address of the next instruction to be executed. The size of registers is important in determining a machine's speed of operations. In an 8-bit microcomputer, only eight bits can be transferred into a register at one time. In an IBM 370, a general-purpose register will accommodate a 32-bit entity, called a *word*. The reference to 8-bit or 16-bit in describing small computers, or to word size in describing large mainframe systems, essentially involves two physical characteristics of the computers: (1) the width, in bits, of certain registers or entities being transferred into and out of registers and (2) the width, in bits, of the buses inside the CPU and thus the number of parallel wire paths connecting parts of the CPU.

The purpose of the CPU is to execute the instructions it receives in the form of programs. Some programming in the CPU is protected from normal access by programmers; the control section today normally contains *microcode* to provide built-in instructions for control purposes. Microcode is read-only code and cannot be altered by programming.

One of the ways of measuring the performance of a computer is in millions of instructions per second (MIPS). Computers can be compared on the basis of their respective MIPS ratings. In comparing the capacities of IBM mainframe computers, David Mishelovich and Bonnie Teufel utilize the MIPS ratings of ten IBM models.[3] In comparing systems used primarily for scientific research, millions of floating-point arithmetic operations carried out in a second (megaFLOPS) are often used. The speed with which a CPU carries out instructions is related to the rate of clock pulse cycles of the CPU. The rate of a CPU clock signal is normally expressed in million pulses per second or *megahertz* (MHz).

Data Representation

All computer programs and data are represented as sequences of numbers. The binary number system (two-state number system) is used

FIGURE 4-3
Logical Operators as Used in Computer Evaluation of Data

(a) *and* means *both*

One Truth Value	*Logical Operator*	*Other Truth Value*	*Resulting Truth Value*
true	and	true	true (both are true)
true	and	false	false (at least
false	and	true	false one is
false	and	false	false false)

For example, imagine this statement:
Systole > 200 mm Hg *and* diastole > 100 mm Hg

Systole Value	*Diastole Value*	*Value of Whole Statement*
205	105	true
205	90	false
190	105	false
190	90	false

On the top line, where the systole is 205 and the diastole is 105, both conditions in the statement are satisfied; it is true that the systole is greater than 200 and it is true that the diastole is greater than 100.

(b) *or* means *at least one and possibly both* (inclusive *or*)

One Truth Value	*Logical Operator*	*Other Truth Value*	*Resulting Truth Value*
true	or	true	true (at least
true	or	false	true one is
false	or	true	true true)
false	or	false	false (not even one is true)

For example, imagine the following statement:
cost > $3.50 per inpatient-day *or* reliability < 97.5%

Cost per Inpatient-Day ($)	*Reliability Figure (%)*	*Value of Whole Statement*
4.00	96.4	true
4.00	98.9	true
2.75	96.4	true
2.75	98.9	false

In everyday English, this statement might be used in the following context: *If the cost*

—continued

FIGURE 4-3—*continued*
Logical Operators as Used in Computer Evaluation of Data

per inpatient-day is greater than $3.50 or if the reliability of the system is less than 97.5 percent then we will not consider this vendor one of the finalists.

(c) *xor* means *at least one but not both* (exclusive *or*)

One Truth Value	*Logical Operator*	*Other Truth Value*	*Resulting Truth Value*
true	xor	true	false (both not allowed)
true	xor	false	true (at least one
false	xor	true	true and not both)
false	xor	false	false (not even one is true)

because of its reliability and versatility of representation. In this system there are only two numbers: 0 and 1. All numbers in the computer (and, therefore, all programs and data) can be thought of as sequences of 1s and 0s. The binary 1s and 0s can also be used to represent logical truth values (1 for true and 0 for false).

The hexadecimal (16-base) number system is also used extensively in computers. While computers use the binary system for data representation, the hexadecimal system serves as a kind of shorthand for binary digit patterns. Since 16 is 2^4, each hexadecimal digit can represent a 4-bit pattern. Figure 4-4 shows the equivalents in the binary, hexadecimal, and decimal number systems through the number 15.

The additional six numerals for the hexadecimal system are obtained by using the first six letters of the alphabet (A-F) to represent 10 through 15. Notice that from 0 through 15, each 4-bit binary pattern can be represented by a single hexadecimal digit. Conversion from binary to hexadecimal or from hexadecimal to binary is simple. Hexadecimal equivalents of the contents of memory (called dumps) or of memory locations are easier to read than binary versions of the same numbers. For example:

Binary 01010101111010101010101011000001010101011000110101101010

Hexa-decimal 5 5 E A A A C 1 5 5 8 D 6 A

There would also be greater likelihood of error in using the binary representation exactly as it occurs in the computer's registers and storage locations.

References to two coding systems are frequently encountered in working with computers: ASCII (American Standard Code for Information Interchange) and EBCDIC (Extended Binary Coded Decimal Interchange Code). In each coding system, a binary pattern called a *byte* is chosen to

FIGURE 4-4
Number Systems Used in Computers

Binary (Bit Patterns)	*Hexadecimal (Numbers)*	*Decimal (Numbers)*
0000	0	0
0001	1	1
0010	2	2
0011	3	3
0100	4	4
0101	5	5
0110	6	6
0111	7	7
1000	8	8
1001	9	9
1010	A	10
1011	B	11
1100	C	12
1101	D	13
1110	E	14
1111	F	15

represent each letter of the alphabet, with different patterns for the uppercase and lowercase of the same letter; numbers; special characters, including punctuation marks; and control signals. To provide all of these, at least a 7-bit code is required. The 7-bit ASCII code is used in most computers and commonly in data communications; the 8-bit EBCDIC code is standard for IBM systems. Thus a byte can consist of seven or eight bits, depending on the code used. Figure 4-5 shows the actual code used to represent the English word "hospital" in the ASCII system.

Other codes are used in computers and data transmission. The Hollerith code is used for punched cards. Optical scanners may use the bit patterns in the ASCII code to represent marking patterns on survey form sheets. Microcomputers use some of the code patterns to represent graphics display characters or as space compression characters. Data entry systems using touch-tone telephone facilities use three-character codes for letters of the alphabet (the character *, the number of the key on which the letter appears, and the number of the letter in sequence on the key).

Without the context of a program, where instructions follow in sequence and according to conditions, there is no way to tell binary numbers stored in the computer from codes used to represent characters. For example:

010110111111001011110101

FIGURE 4-5
The Byte as Character and as Code

Uppercase Letter (Byte Outside Computer)	*Binary Code (Byte in Computer)*	*Hexadecimal Equivalent*
H	1001000	48
O	1001111	4F
S	1010011	53
P	1010000	50
I	1001001	49
T	1010100	54
A	1000001	41
L	1001100	4C

could mean $25 in EBCDIC code, or it could mean 6,025,973 as a binary number. It could even represent machine language commands.

STORAGE DEVICES

Computer storage can be classified as on-line or as off-line. On-line storage is immediately accessible through programming; that is, a program is able to specify an address (storage location) for any data stored on-line. Data stored off-line must be entered into the system before they can be used. If a program requires off-line data, the data must be loaded in with the program (as with a deck of punched cards or a spool of paper tape) or else the computer system will stop the program and wait for the off-line data to be supplied (by mounting a spool of magnetic tape on a tape drive).

There are many types of storage that can be accessed by the computer system while it is operating (that is, while it is on-line), two of which are main storage, which is instantly accessible to the central processing unit, and auxiliary storage. The main storage in a computer can be imagined, from the standpoint of bytes or words, as organized like a single, long street, with addresses from zero to the capacity (in bytes or words) of the system. A 64K microcomputer has main memory addresses from 0 to 65535 (*K* means 1024 or 2^{10} rather than 1000). Today, the main storage portion of the computer system consists of chips (semiconductor integrated circuits) with the appropriate connections and addressing facilities. Such storage is traditionally called *core memory* because of its function in the CPU, although magnetic core technology is no longer used in new systems. From a physical standpoint, the locations of individual bits in the memory are accessed according to which chip they are on and where they are on that chip; a decoder converts memory addresses into physical addresses in the bank of memory chips. This type of storage, which permits instant access to the bit pattern stored at a particular address, is called *random-access memory* (RAM). Semiconductor RAM cannot be maintained if there is an interruption of power; it is therefore called *volatile memory*.

RAM can be augmented by *read-only memory* (ROM), which contains permanent instructions that cannot be altered by ordinary programming. ROM facilities provide storage that is not affected by loss of power and is, therefore, immediately available when the system is powered up. ROM is *nonvolatile memory*.

The most commonly used auxiliary storage devices in hospital computer systems today are tape drives and disk drives. As magnetic disk storage technology has improved, magnetic drum storage has become less attractive for new systems. More recently developed mass storage technologies, such as data cartridges and bubble memory, are not typically used in hospital systems. At present, attention is focusing on the improvement of laser storage methods, which would employ a technology related to that of laser videodiscs. While magnetic disk technology allows complete reusability, present-day videodiscs cannot be reused. If certain practical problems can be solved by research, laser disk storage may offer important cost advantages to offset some of the limitations in use.

Tape-based memory is referred to as *sequential-access memory*, while disk-based memory is referred to as *direct-access memory*. Since the data stored on a tape are arranged sequentially, the tape read-head must pass over all records in sequence between one record and another. The constraints of sequentially accessed data cause tape access to be slow compared to disk access. Disks are divided into concentric tracks and radiating sectors. A directory stored on a portion of the disk indicates what is stored where on the disk. Related data items do not have to be located physically next to each other on the disk. Since the disk rotates at a high rate of speed, there is little delay in reaching any point on its surface. Large programs or collections of data may be divided into noncontiguously stored fragments, with the starting address of each fragment stored in order in the directory. Linked lists provide another option for noncontiguous storage of data. A linked list operates like a treasure hunt: each item in the list has a pointer pointing to the next item or to the end of the list.

Disk drives, or *spindles*, provide on-line storage to augment the direct-access main memory. Today's operating systems make it possible for a program to consult files stored on disk quickly and with considerable flexibility. *Virtual* memory systems exploit the capabilities of disk storage to expand the effective working space of main memory. Portions of programs are moved into main memory from storage on disk as needed. At any given moment, some portions of a large program being processed are actually in the main memory of the computer and some are on disk, but the entire program can be addressed as if it were all in main memory. Virtual memory systems thus operate with more storage addresses than would be possible on the basis of physical main memory alone.

Tape drives (see Figure 4-6) provide a means to read data stored off-line. Normally a modern system has only two tape drives. Some activities require two drives, such as reading from and writing to two tapes during a single operation or copying tapes. The presence of two drives provides minimal redundancy in case of failure of a disk drive. The number of disk drives will depend on the amount of on-line storage required by the hospital. Disk drive capacity must accommodate the following: (1) virtual storage requirements of the operating system; (2) data sets used by the hospital database in routine transactions; and (3) total capacity in excess of anticipated peak requirements.

Factors that affect access time of a disk drive and storage capacity of a disk pack are speed of rotation, density of recording, and type of head mechanism. Density of recording is attained by decreasing the space between the read-write head and the disk surface. Disk drives require air cooling, since the high-speed rotation devices produce considerable heat, and regular maintenance to prevent mechanical failure. Because of the high speed of rotation and the close tolerance between the read-write head and the disk surface, contact between the head and the surface is catastrophic. Providing a fixed head for each track instead of a single head that must move from track to track permits faster access and eliminates the mechanical moving parts needed for positioning, but it is more expensive. One of the advantages of magnetic drums was fixed read-write heads. Sealing the disk off from open air, which may contain small particles of dust or smoke, improves reliability.

Input, Output, and Data Communications

As computerized hospital systems complete the trend away from batch processing and toward predominantly on-line processing, cathode-ray tube (CRT) terminals (Figure 4-7) have become the standard device for data entry. Computer input is accomplished by means of terminals with video display or an array of other types of terminals. The punched-card reader becomes a specialized device that is used infrequently.

CRT terminals in hospitals often are equipped with a typewriter-style keyboard; a calculator-style data entry keypad; and a data-entry aid such as a light pen, a set of function buttons, or an optical scanner wand. The keyboard serves for entry of numbers and names. To reduce the need for

FIGURE 4-6
Disk Drives and Tape Drives

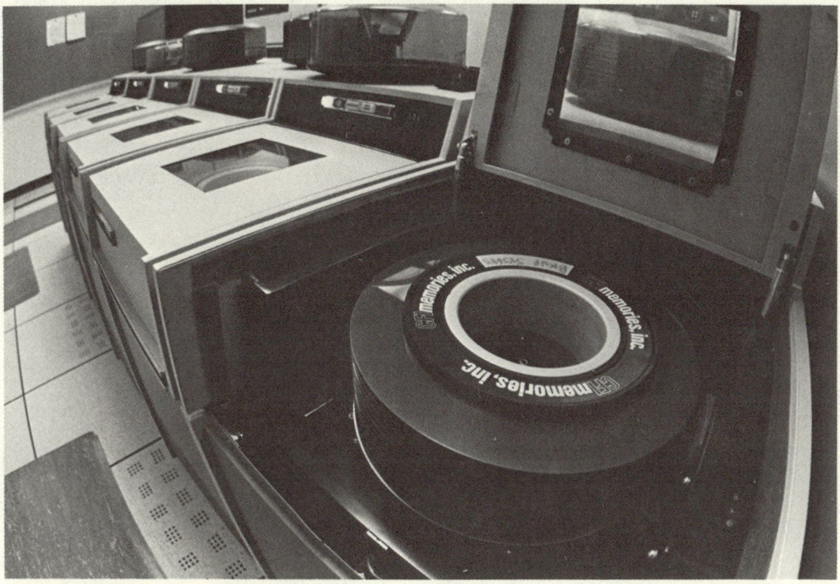

Disk Drives (East Texas State University)

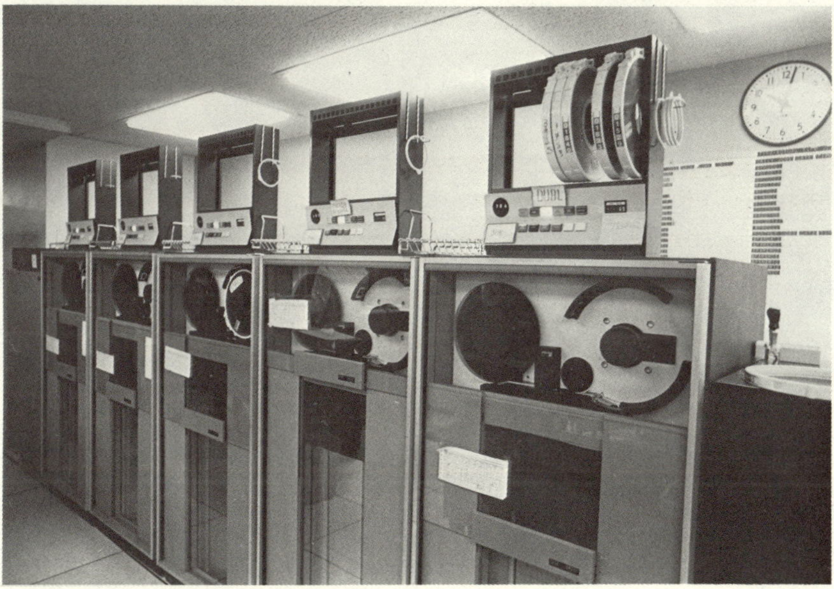

Tape Drives (Parkland Memorial Hospital, Dallas)

FIGURE 4-7
Computer Display Terminals

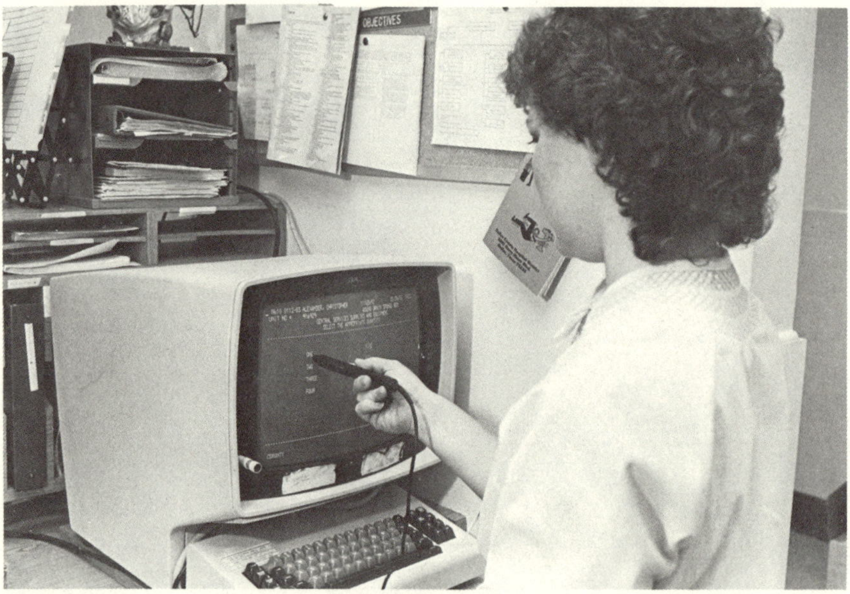

IBM with Light Pen (Parkland Memorial Hospital, Dallas)

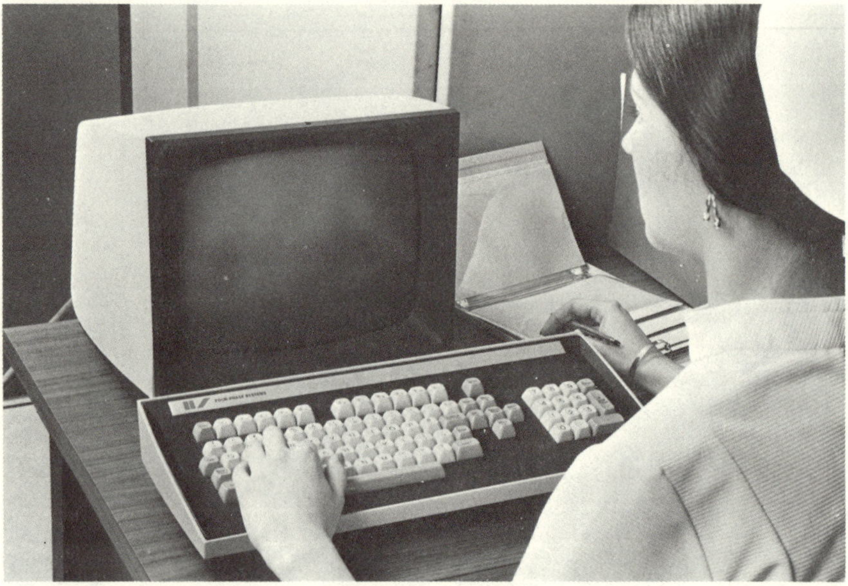

Four Phase (Four Phase Systems, courtesy of Shared Medical Services)

FIGURE 4-7—*continued*
Computer Display Terminals

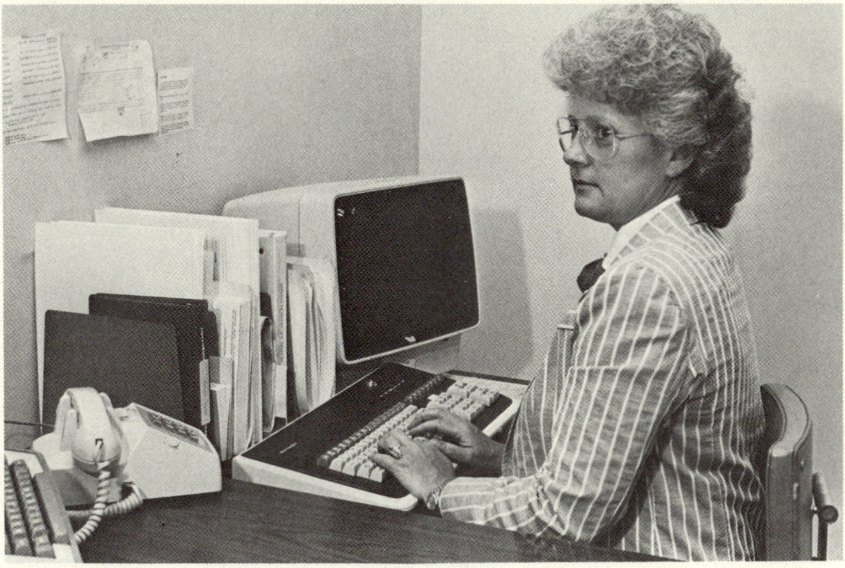

Burroughs (Presbyterian Medical Center, Dallas)

professional medical personnel to use the keyboard, light-pen data entry is used as much as possible in modern installations. A *menu* (list of options) with positions for various selections by light pen is displayed on the screen of the terminal to speed up selection of services and options. The user selects one option by (1) touching a position on the screen with a light pen; (2) touching a position on the screen with a finger (touch-sensitive screen); (3) pressing a button to the left of the screen and next to the item selected; (4) moving an optical scanner wand over a character, word, or bar code in a manual available at the terminal; or (5) typing in the first letter of the option selected or a number code given on the screen with the option.

Several strategies can be employed to facilitate data entry. In a hospital environment, it is vital to make simple procedures available at on-line work stations so that transactions can be conducted rapidly and accurately under diverse conditions. The majority of persons using on-line facilities in a hospital have limited experience with computers. Professional personnel, such as physicians and nurses, expect to be able to enter orders or retrieve information with a minimum of delay. Extensive computer applications in a hospital will require a variety of persons to use computer work stations, so procedures must be straightforward. Considerable effort has been put into

FIGURE 4-7—*continued*
Computer Display Terminals

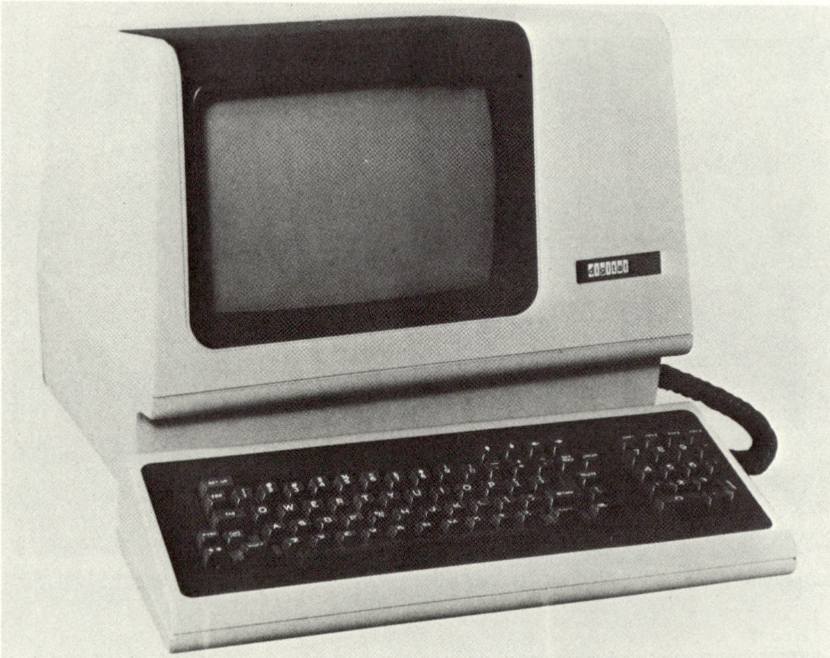

Digital (Courtesy of Digital) **See Figure 13-2 for NADACOM terminal.**

the design of data-entry aids. The main advantage of light pens is ease in selecting an option; a disadvantage in systems requiring the alternate use of light pen and keyboard (alphanumeric text) entries is that the user will have to keep picking the light pen up and laying it back down again. Data-entry strategies that require an *ancillary device*, or appendage to the terminal, such as a light pen or optical wand, are subject to greater maintenance problems than terminals with buttons at the side of the screen or no special data-entry aids. Examples of specialized terminals are IBM terminals 3277 through 3279 equipped with light pen; NADACOM 80-3285 terminals, equipped with 20 function touch-points to the left of the screen; and Four-Phase FASTRAK work stations with touch-sensitive displays. Formatted screens help assure that textual and numeric data, such as order numbers, patient identification, personnel identification, text messages, and text observations, are entered properly.

Intelligent terminals, which have the capabilities of microcomputers to process data independently of the main system, reduce the load on the main system by storing currently used screen formats for local recall. Intelligent terminals can also store valid data ranges and instructions adequate to perform some checking of data entered at the terminal. Obvious errors, such as entry of values that are outside pre-established ranges can be ignored, and the terminal will prompt the user to enter the data again. Such processing in the terminal improves response time for the user, conserves main system resources by relieving the main system of the need to check data entered, and prevents the processing of unusable or erroneous data. Examples of intelligent terminals are the Burroughs MT 1541, with 64K of RAM, designed for the Burroughs Hospital Information System (BHIS); and the Four-Phase FASTRAK work station, with 64K of RAM and diskette drives.

Physical measuring or sensing devices provide the input of continual, or *real-time*, data. Examples are monitoring systems for patients in intensive care, energy management systems for buildings, and emergency warning systems (such as fire and smoke alarm systems and water detection systems for computer rooms). Devices that measure physical conditions on a continuous scale are called *analog devices*, in contrast to *digital devices*, which measure according to discrete increments. Data such as heart rate, blood pressure, central venous pressure, intracranial pressure, pulmonary artery pressure, temperature, and respiration rate may be gathered on a real-time basis.[4]

Badge-reading devices connected to terminals are a convenient way of checking the identity of persons using a hospital information system. Badges and other key devices may operate on the basis of a magnetic strip, an embedded processor, an optically read bar code, optically read characters, or holes punched in the device.

Other means of data entry are touch-tone entry and voice entry. Touch-tone data entry is done by means of an ordinary telephone and requires a convention regarding entry of letters of the alphabet. An advantage of touch-tone methods is that any telephone can be used; a disadvantage is that the codes are cumbersome: for example, the letter k requires three tones, **52*. Voice data entry remains of limited use because, with the present state of the art, the vocabulary of recognizable words and phrases must be limited, each user must *tune* the recognition procedure each day, and words must be pronounced as distinct, separate entities, rather than in the manner of continuous speech. An important advantage of voice data entry is that the user does not need to touch the computer or look at it to input data. Voice recognition systems can be quite effective as security devices: characteristic voice patterns can be stored in digital form and matched against pronunciation of certain words.

Optical scanner systems offer another data-entry technology. Modern

FIGURE 4-8
Optical Mark Reader Form for a Radiology Laboratory

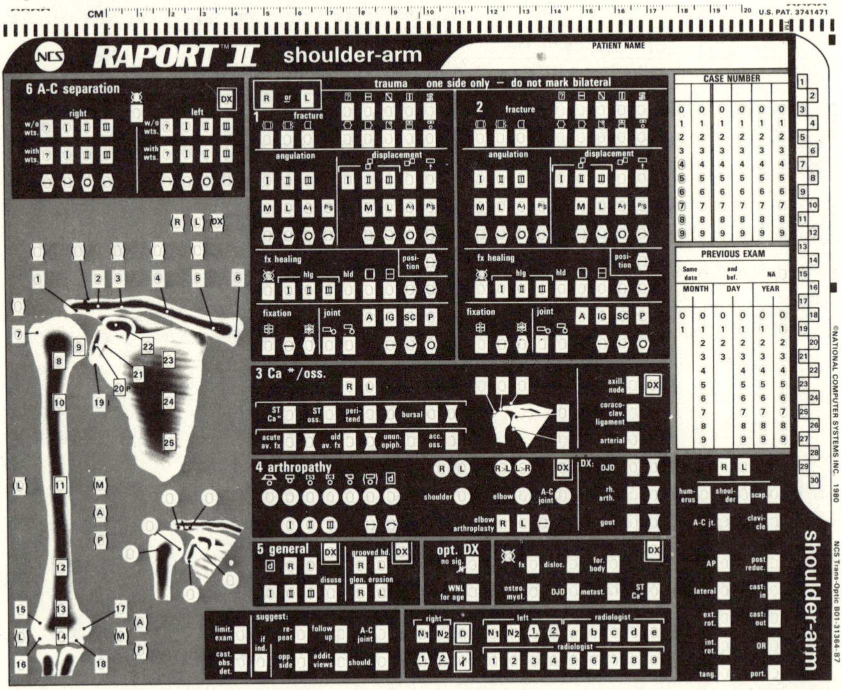

(Courtesy of National Computer Systems)

scanner-reader devices are much more flexible than traditional punched-card technology. Forms used in optical mark scanner terminals range in size from small cards to full letter-size sheets (Figure 4-8). Some compact, modern devices can read either marked forms or punched cards. Careful design of input sheets for specialized applications, such as in laboratories or radiology departments, can simplify and speed up data entry. The strategy is similar to that of menus and screen formats for CRT display: the scanner input form presents all the options to be dealt with and the user marks appropriate locations. Some optical scanner equipment can interpret typewritten copy. For most such systems, specially designed typewriter elements or printwheels must be used in preparing the copy to assure error-free interpretation. Other scanners, however, accept normal typewriter type styles within certain specifications. Optical interpretation of bar codes can serve for applications ranging from inventory to security.

Tapes are commonly used to enter data into modern computer systems and to store data to which immediate access is not normally required.

Tapes provide a number of advantages: convenience of transport, convenience of storage, and off-line status. Data stored on tapes do not require expensive on-line resources, and the tapes can be moved to and from remote security locations to satisfy backup and security requirements of the system. Tapes of data that will not need to be available in the on-line database under normal conditions can be stored relatively inexpensively. When hospitals are converting from one system to another, tapes may be used to transfer data or to provide test data bases and transactions for testing and simulation of operations.

Batch input in the form of cards or tape files, or a combination of these, is used in the newest hospital systems only under such unusual conditions as conversion to a new system, transfer of data from one system to another, or special operations requiring a higher level of security or approval than daily transactions. In most cases, data for batch operations will come from files stored on disks rather than on tapes.

Low-speed, small diskettes, normally called *floppy diskettes*, are common for microcomputer and small business systems. Most floppy diskettes are 5.25 or 8 inches in diameter. Because of limited storage capacity and some reliability problems, such diskettes are rarely used with large systems. In some large systems, a floppy diskette may be used for loading initial instructions to reset and restart the system after a full failure.

Computer output comes in several forms: (1) display on a CRT screen; (2) print on paper; (3) alarm signals of monitoring systems; (4) display on an LCD or LED readout; (5) graphics plotted on paper; (6) synthesized speech; (7) recording on tape for removal to archives; (8) image recorded on microfilm or microfiche; and (9) punched cards.

Printers (Figure 4-9) are classified according to image formation (as either impact or nonimpact) and according to how the output process is organized (as character, line, or page printers). All *impact printers* involve physical contact with the paper, normally with an inked ribbon placed between the part of the printer that forms the character and the paper. In the case of large chain printers, hammers behind the paper push the paper against the ribbon and character link in the chain. The hammer blows must be timed to strike precisely when the character to be printed is passing on the opposite side of the paper. Because the timing of events is designed in terms of the line of print as a whole, this type of printer is called a line printer. Line printers can deliver from 300 to 1,800 lines of print per minute.

Dot-matrix impact printers use a print head that contains small wires. The wires advance, in the proper pattern to form a character, and push the inked ribbon against the paper. As with a typewriter, the paper is between the inked ribbon and a platen (roller) behind it; the print head pushes the

FIGURE 4-9
Printers and COM

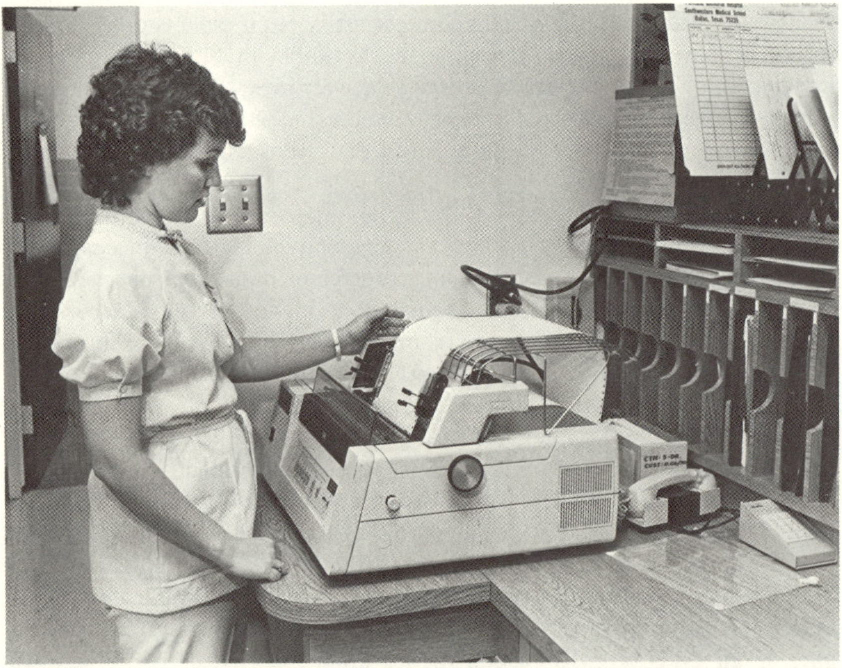

Character Printer, Dot Matrix (Parkland Memorial Hospital, Dallas)

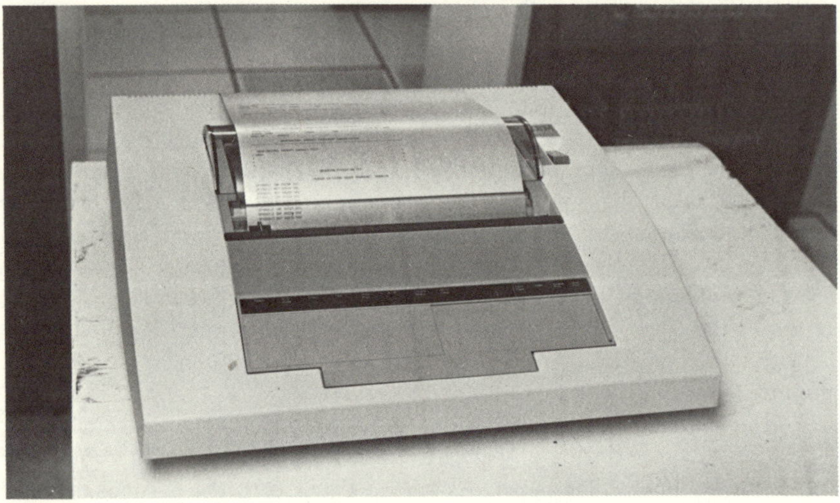

Character Printer, Dot Matrix, Foil Paper (Parkland Memorial Hospital, Dallas)

FIGURE 4-9—*continued*
Printers and COM

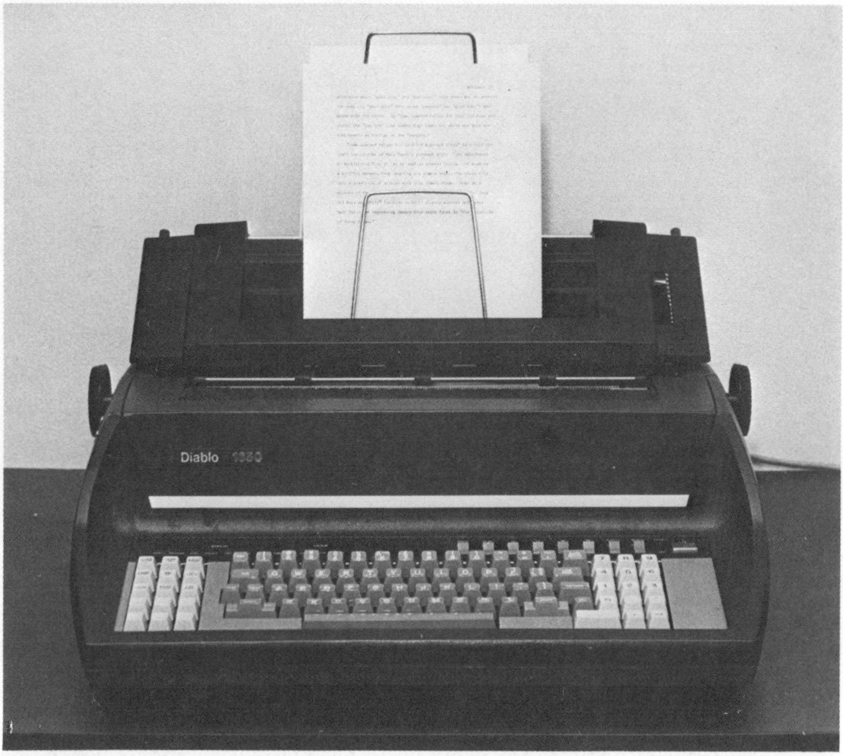

Character Printer, Daisy Wheel (East Texas State University)

ribbon and paper against the platen to obtain enough pressure to form the character image. Such printers deliver from 40 to 200 characters per second. Impact printers are typically high-maintenance devices because of the number of moving parts and the precision required in positioning and timing.

Nonimpact printers include laser page printers, which print at very high speeds. Laser printers have the advantage that line images can be placed on the paper along with the character text, thus eliminating the use of preprinted forms. The resulting appearance will be superior to that obtained by using the characters of impact printers (dashes, dots, equal signs, asterisks, and others) to give the impression of a form. Where output volume requirements are extremely high, the output rate of a laser printer (2,000-3,000 pages per minute) offers a substantial advantage. Laser print-

FIGURE 4-9—*continued*
Printers and COM

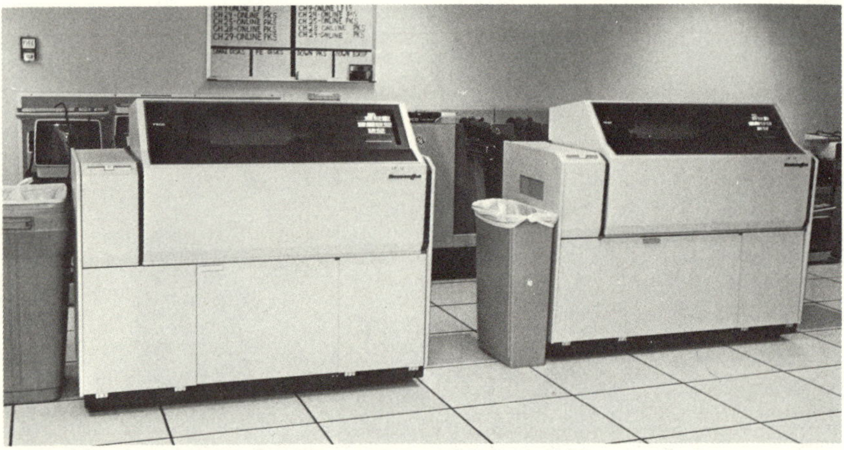

Line Printers (Presbyterian Medical Center, Dallas)

ers are expensive, not only in terms of purchase cost, but also in system resources needed to support the printing operation. Hospital requirements are such that even new systems tend to prefer the established impact printer technology for most batch processing. As costs of laser printers decline, however, hospitals may be expected to adopt them more often. Other high-speed page printers are based on xerographic and ink-jet technologies.

Two types of printers are common in hospital environments: large line printers, which use a high-speed print chain, or train; and small dot-matrix character printers, which use a moving print head. Line printers are normally located in the hospital's computer center, while dot-matrix printers or printer-terminals are located at various sites throughout the hospital, such as nursing stations and laboratories.

A light-based output procedure commonly used in hospitals is imaging on film. This type of capability produces *computer output microfilm* (COM) and provides permanent records on microfilm or microfiche. Because of legal requirements for some hospital records and storage advantages of microfiche, COM technology is practical for hospital information systems.

Many different kinds of technology can be exploited in storing and transmitting data when the binary number system is used: paper tape, punched cards, transistor-transistor logic (TTL) signals (pulses) as used inside a computer, signals as used for transmission over distances, modu-

FIGURE 4-9—*continued*
Printers and COM

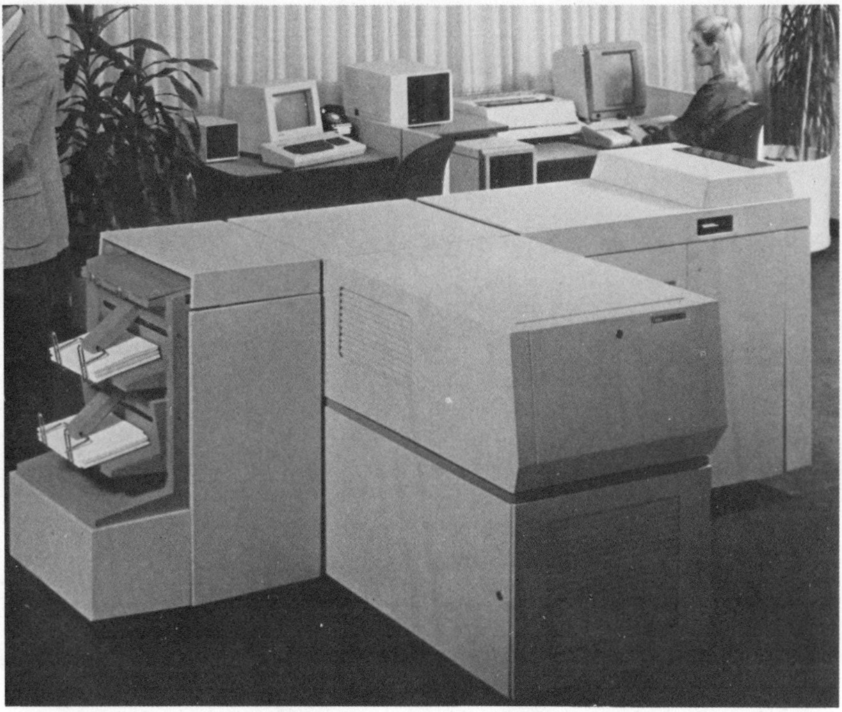

Page Printer (Courtesy of Xerox Corporation, Office Products Division)

lated signals used in microwave or acoustic telephone signals, displays on control panels, and laser-read videodiscs. Here are different ways of representing two states in the environments cited:

hole in paper tape	vs.	no hole in paper tape
hole in card	vs.	no hole in card
some voltage (+5 v) (current on)	vs.	no voltage (0 v) (current off)
positive voltage (+15 v)	vs.	negative voltage (−15 v)
north magnetic polarity	vs.	south magnetic polarity
high frequency signal	vs.	low frequency signal

FIGURE 4-9—*continued*
Printers and COM

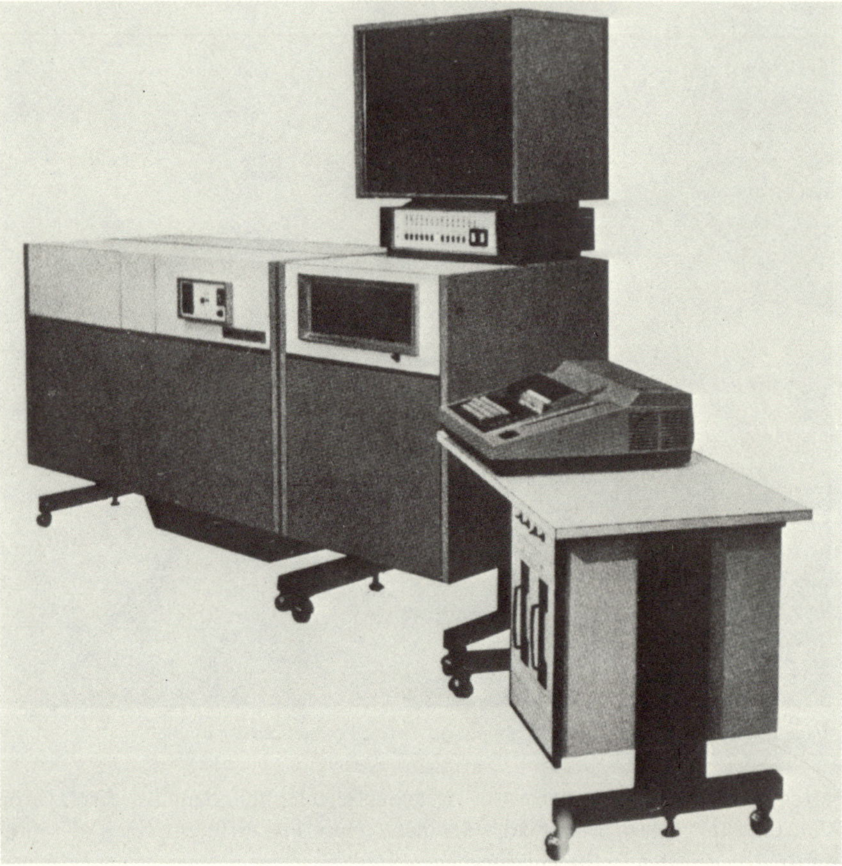

Computer Output Microfilm (Courtesy of Datagrafix Corporation and Zytron)

light on	vs.	light off
pit in surface of disk	vs.	level surface

Card readers, for example, must determine what data are stored on a card by determining whether or not a hole is in a certain position. It is relatively easy to keep a card reader functioning correctly when its sole task is to decide whether or not a hole is present. Similarly, optical mark readers must determine whether or not a mark is present in a given position on a sheet of paper. Thus two-state systems are preferred for reliability.

Messages between computers and terminals or messages that are sent from one computer to another require certain conditions. There must be a proper communication path, usually a direct wire connection or a leased telephone wire, and proper conventions of message exchange. The rate of transfer of data over a communication link is normally given as the *baud rate*, which usually means the number of bits sent per second. Common baud rates are 110, 300, 600, 1,200, 4,800, and 9,600. There must also be a convention as to how a computer and a terminal or two computers can communicate with each other about practical problems of data transmission. For example, when a device such as a printer consumes data at rate slower than that at which the sending device is supplying it, there must be some way for the printer to signal to the computer that it can receive no more data or is ready for more data. These conventions are referred to as *handshaking*, or *protocols*. Other terms used commonly in describing computer communications have to do with assuring that two devices agree on timing and interpretation of signals: asynchronous, synchronous, and binary synchronous. *Asynchronous* transmissions do not have to be continuous: a *framing* procedure tells the other device when a transmission is coming. Thus, for example, computer terminals that send characters to the computer intermittently can use asynchronous transmission. On *synchronous* transmission lines, signals are transmitted continuously. In *binary synchronous* transmission, blocks of data are transmitted, framed by appropriately formatted messages that identify the transmission.

Communication pathways in the central processing unit and to adjacent facilities are parallel connections, with each bit position having its own *traffic lane* (Figure 4-10). For longer distances, serial transmission is used; the individual bits of a byte or word being transmitted are arranged one after the other in order and proceed single file to the destination. Obviously, parallel connections permit high rates of data transmission and are essential to the inner functioning of the CPU. Since the physical conditions of circuit pathways in a parallel connection are not identical, corresponding bits transmitted more than a short distance cannot be kept lined up parallel with each other; this produces a condition called *skew*. Serial connections are practical, therefore, for devices located at a distance from the CPU. Serial connection facilities are referred to by a standard called RS-232C. A standard, 25-pin connector is normally used for RS-232C connections.

The nature of signal transmission is such that signal quality decays over distance. Errors and timing synchronization problems increase with distance. Signals that must travel greater distances require amplification or, in cases where commercial, sound-carrying telephone lines are used, conversion to modulated status for transmission and then conversion back to digital status for use at the destination. Devices used to connect computer

FIGURE 4-10
Parallel and Serial Transmission of Data

SERIAL — DIRECTION OF TRANSMISSION ➔ ➔

11010100	11000101	11100011	11100010	11101000	11100010
M	E	T	S	Y	S

PARALLEL — DIRECTION OF TRANSMISSION ➔ ➔

1	1	1	1	1	1
1	1	1	1	1	1
0	0	1	1	1	1
1	0	0	0	0	0
0	0	0	0	1	0
1	1	0	0	0	0
0	0	1	1	0	1
0	1	1	0	0	0
M	E	T	S	Y	S

equipment to lines carrying modulated signals are called *modems (modulator-demodulator)*. The baud rate affects the potential for error: the faster signals are sent, the greater the likelihood that signal distinctions will diminish and that the signal will not be interpreted correctly on the receiving end of the link. High baud rates require excellent communication facilities and rapid processing. Communication links which are limited to a particular use, such as high-speed computer transmissions, are called *dedicated* links. A common baud rate for computer transmissions over normal telephone lines is 300 baud, which is low enough to obtain excellent reliability of transmissions. There are various strategies for detecting and even correcting errors in transmission, but such techniques require additional bits for each character sent or sophisticated coding and interpretation. Baud rates over dedicated lines in a hospital will be from 1,200 baud to 9,600 baud.

Since dedicated lines are expensive to install or lease, there is an incentive to send multiple computer signals over single transmission paths. The process of combining two or more signals into a single signal, transmitting it, and then sorting the original signals out again at the destination is called *multiplexing.* A practical use of multiplexing in a hospital installation is the simultaneous sending of separate signals to a CRT terminal and to a small printer located at the same nursing station. In such cases, the printer will be attached to the CRT, and the CRT must be specially equipped with a microprocessor capable of separating incoming printer and CRT messages and of combining outgoing messages for transmission to the CPU. Independent use of two devices dependent on a single line is far superior to making the printer a *slave* to the CRT terminal. When printing is slower than the presentation of output on a CRT display, for example, the control messages that must be sent to the CPU make CRT terminal operations uneven and slow. Another use of multiplexing is to increase the number of on-line facilities that can be connected to a given computer system (each computer system will have a limited number of ports to which devices can be connected).

Typical Hardware Configurations for Hospitals

Computer hardware in hospitals includes the following:

- Large mainframe systems with extensive on-line facilities
- Combinations of mainframes supporting on-line facilities and mainframes supporting batch services
- Small mainframe systems (minicomputers)
- Distributed processing systems (networks supported by mainframe systems)
- Small single-user systems (small business computers or microcomputers), sometimes networked
- Communications installations for large systems or networks

Although the trend is toward on-line capabilities and away from batch processing, many installations add on-line capabilities and retain some batch processing. A network may link specialized computer systems (laboratory, pharmacy) with the main system used for communication and database management. According to Tanenbaum, a *computer network* is an interconnected collection of autonomous computers.[5] Computers in a network can be connected by a variety of means: wire circuits, optical fibers, and microwaves routed near the Earth's surface or by way of satellites in orbit. Networking of computers will become increasingly important in the future. Schultz and David describe the use of a Sperry-Univac V77-600 minicomputer for the PROMIS network,[6] and Schwartz describes the use of a DEC PDP VAX-11/780 as the host computer for a network in a discussion of simulation of queuing in computer networks.[7]

Under some circumstances, networks can provide several advantages:

1. Greater reliability, since all the autonomous computers in a network are unlikely to be disabled simultaneously;
2. Lower overall expenditures, assuming the particular configuration of computers, networking facilities, and peripherals costs less than a single-computer system and performs comparably;
3. Improved operational speed in cases where simultaneous functioning of several small, networked computers can outpace a single, large computer.

Megargle et al. describe the strategies used in a microcomputer-based laboratory network (LABNET) to achieve these advantages through redundancy, flexibility, and efficiency.[8] A cable television channel is used to link LABNET microcomputers.

Configurations depend upon the cycle of system replacement or upgrading. As a hospital completes a five-year or other extended period of use of its main computer system, it then has an opportunity to take advantage of the latest technology in on-line services and distributed processing. Smaller hospitals with limited resources are likely to begin with small business or minicomputer systems or even with microcomputers.

Among the tasks performed by computer systems in hospitals are the following:

— On-line electronic mail system
  - Messages and orders
  - Messages generated automatically as a result of orders
  - Confirmations of orders and services
  - Reports of test results
  - Automatically generated reminders for scheduling, medication, and transfer of patients

— On-line data entry and record updating
  - Registration of patients (admission, discharge)
  - Identification of patients to be scheduled for laboratory tests, appointments, therapy, or surgery
  - Supply transactions
  - Laboratory procedures

Pharmacy procedures
Insurance data-entry

— On-line access to stored data

Patient location (current room assignment or current location where the patient can be found)

Medications

Allergies, special needs (blind, language other than English)

Patients assigned to nursing station

Physicians assigned to patient

Blood bank rare donor list

Blood bank inventory

Organ recipient list

Inventory of beds

Diagnosis information on patients

— Verification of authorized status of system user

— Real-time sensing or control applications, or Intensive care monitoring

Emergency warning systems

Energy management systems

— Batch processing of reports

Daily schedules for surgery, therapy, and outpatient appointments

Periodic management reports for departments and hospital payroll, personnel actions, and purchase procedures

— Audit trail for patient care

Hospital hardware configurations must sustain this variety of processing tasks, maintain the extent of the on-line database required, support numerous on-line terminals, and interface with special facilities. Because of the nature of the services provided, virtually absolute reliability is required, as interruption of computer processing could degrade the delivery of health care services.

Large hospital computer installations are therefore characterized by the following features:

— Redundancy of CPUs to assure reliability

— Access of multiple or networked CPUs (where installed) to database

— Large main memory and mass storage requirements because of the size of the database, the amount of text processing, and the extent of on-line services

— Closely coupled or mirrored file storage to safeguard database

— Power supply protection to assure graceful shutdown in case of power emergency so that the database is protected

— Communications facilities capable of supporting appropriate terminals in nursing stations, laboratories, pharmacy, specialized examination or therapy facilities, departments, and offices

— Redundant main printers (chain printers or equivalent)

— Air conditioning provisions

— Controllers for printers, mass storage, terminals

An example of a large, integrated configuration with extensive on-line capabilities is the following: Presbyterian Medical Center, Dallas, Texas: two Burroughs 7800 CPUs, three MB main storage per CPU, 22 spindles of disk storage with a capacity of 3.6 billion bytes, two chain printers, and approximately 250 terminals when full installation is completed. This is a multi-unit complex (hospitals, professional facility, special care facilities for elderly) with over 600 beds in the principal hospital facilities.[9]

Review of the *Component Catalog* of the *Automated Hospital Information System Survey*[10] provides the following information about hospital information systems as of the data collected and presented in 1980:

— Nearly 18 percent of the hospitals surveyed used shared services rather than independent in-house data-processing.

— Over 35 percent of the hospitals with independent in-house data-processing facilities also used shared services (involving one or more vendors, one or more other hospitals, or both).

— Over 46 percent of all hospitals in the survey used shared services.

— The average period elapsed since acquisition of a leased computer was 1.3 years.

— The average period elapsed since acquisition of a purchased computer was 3.2 years.

— Certain manufacturers accounted for over 90 percent of the computers reported in use: IBM, Four-Phase, NCR, Digital, Burroughs, Data General, Hewlett-Packard, Honeywell, and Sperry-Univac.

— In those cases where survey information indicated whether computers were leased or purchased, about 62 percent of the acquisitions were by the lease method and about 38 percent were by the purchase method.

— Over 28 percent of the hospitals with independent in-house data-processing reported multiple-computer installations.

SUMMARY

Computer hardware falls into these main categories: central processing unit, main memory, auxiliary memory, input–output devices, and communications links. The central processing unit relies on circuits and electric pulse signals to perform its work. High-speed semiconductor random-access memory serves the CPU as storage for data and programs. All data and programs are represented in the computer in binary form, which we think of as 1s and 0s.

Hospitals generally use standard computer technology, although some hardware is specialized or particularly suitable for the hospital environment. Today's hospital computer systems are oriented toward on-line services, but routine batch operations and facilities remain. Hardware characteristics important for evaluation and selection procedures are reliability, speed of processing, and capacity for data storage. Data transmission facilities are important to modern hospital computer systems, which must provide on-line access and services at points of use throughout the hospital and must provide for automated communication between departments and patient care sites in the hospital. Computer networking may be used to improve performance and reduce costs.

DISCUSSION QUESTIONS

4-1 Why is binary representation of data used in computers? What advantages does this convention provide?

4-2 Give examples of different types of storage or transmission of binary data.

4-3 What advantages are gained by storing the program (as well as the data to be processed) in the computer?

4-4 Explain the role of codes in computer input and output and in data transmission.

4-5 How can a modern computer system eliminate the need for preprinted forms?

4-6 Describe strategies of terminal design intended to meet the needs of hospital environments.

4-7 In what ways can computer hardware meet the needs of a hospital information system for reliability? What level of hardware reliability is required by a hospital information system?

4-8 How is attention to multiplexing important to hospital computer systems?

4-9 Explain the term *byte* in two ways: how is the term used in describing internal computer functions and capacities; what does the term mean outside the computer?

4-10 Describe and contrast direct-access and sequential-access auxiliary storage.

4-11 What is baud rate and how is it related to the reliability of a computer system?

4-12 What advantages can a computer network provide over a system based on a single main computer?

PROBLEM

4-1 State your philosophy on the extent to which you would require redundancy (more than one piece of equipment of the same type) to assure system reliability and availability. Justify your position. Recommend practical ways of avoiding excessive costs in systems that have dual CPUs.

NOTES

1. W. David Gardner, "The Independent Inventor," *Datamation*, September 1982, p. 14.
2. Elizabeth A. Nichols, Joseph C. Nichols, and Keith R. Munson, *Data Communications for Microcomputers with Practical Applications and Experiments* (New York: McGraw-Hill, 1982), pp. 57-59.
3. David J. Mishelevich et al., "Capacity Planning Guide for Mainframes Running the IBM Patient Care System (PCS)," *Computers in Hospitals*, September-October 1981, p. 19. A chart on p. 22 shows procedure volumes for hospital on-line functions.
4. Elizabeth Beckmann, "Observation on Computers in an Intensive Care Unit," *Heart & Lung*, November-December, 1981, p. 1055.
5. Andrew S. Tanenbaum, *Computer Networks* (Englewood Cliffs, New Jersey: Prentice-Hall, 1981), p. 2.
6. Morton D. Schwartz, "Analysis of Hospital Computer Networks," *Journal of Clinical Engineering*, October-December, 1980, pp. 311-320.
7. Jan R. Schultz and Layton Davis, "The Technology of PROMIS," *Proceedings of the IEEE*, September, 1979, p. 1237.
8. Robert Megargle et al., "LABNET—A Microcomputer Network for Clinical Laboratories," *Proceedings of the Fifth Annual Symposium of Computer Applications in Medical Care*, New York: Institute of Electrical and Electronics Engineers, 1981, p. 500.
9. Interview with Carroll J. Innmon, Director of Information Systems, Presbyterian Medical Center, Dallas, Texas. See also Donald A. B. Lindberg, *The Growth of Medical Information Systems in the United States* (Lexington, Massachusetts: Lexington Books, 1979), p. 37. Chapter 4 (pp. 37-58) contains several detailed descriptions of medical information systems.

10. University of Missouri Health Services Research Center/Health Care Technology Center, *Automated Hospital Information System: AHIS Component Catalog*, Vol. 3 (Columbia, Missouri: University of Missouri, 1980).

ADDITIONAL READINGS

Cole, Robert. *Computer Communications*. New York: Springer-Verlag, 1982.

Covvey, H. Dominic and McAlister, Neil Harding. *Introduction to Computing Concepts. Computers in the Practice of Medicine*, Vol. 1. Reading, Massachusetts: Addison-Wesley, 1980.

Giarratano, Joseph G. *Foundations of Computer Technology*. Indianapolis: Howard W. Sams, 1982.

Lu, Cary. "Microcomputers: The Second Wave." *High Technology*, September-October 1982, p. 36.

Peterson, H.E. and Isaksson, A. I., eds. *Communication Networks in Health Care*. Amsterdam: North-Holland, 1982.

Sauter, Steven L. "Job and Health Implications of VDT Use: Initial Results of the Wisconsin-NIOSH Study." *Communications of the ACM 26*, April 1983, p. 284.

Tolchin, S. G. et al. "Implementation of a Prototype Generalized Network Technology for Hospitals." In *Proceedings, The Fifth Annual Symposium on Computer Applications in Medical Care*, pp. 942-948. Henry G. Heffernan, ed. Los Angeles: IEEE Computer Society, 1981.

Walsh, Myles E. *Understanding Computers: What Managers and Users Need to Know*. New York: Wiley, 1981.

5

Software Concepts

William J. Harvey

Software includes sets of instructions for the computer hardware. These instructions are grouped in programs. The fundamental logic used by the programs is the same logic used by human beings and used in the design of hardware circuits. In a broader sense, software also includes documentation of hardware and software in printed form such as manuals and books. Since the user has access to the capabilities of computers through software, he or she has the impression of using a machine quite different from the actual hardware (see Figure 5-1). Computer hardware responds to instructions in binary form; the apparent machine the user interacts with accepts decimal numbers and responds to specialized commands in a form similar to English or the notation of algebra. The function of software is to present a machine that can be used effectively in data processing, technical, health care, research, academic, or other environments.

PROGRAMS

A program is a set of instructions to the computer. Each instruction is stored in the computer as a sequence of binary numbers (1s and 0s). When a program is *executed*, the computer receives directions on how to get to the first instruction in the program and then proceeds to follow the sequence of instructions where it leads. Programs either terminate, or stop executing, and then pass control on to other programs or arrive at a waiting state where data must be received from outside the program in order for further instructions to be executed.

The written program is referred to as *code*, since a program is written in a special structure that can be automatically translated into instructions

FIGURE 5-1
From Machine to User—The Levels of Software

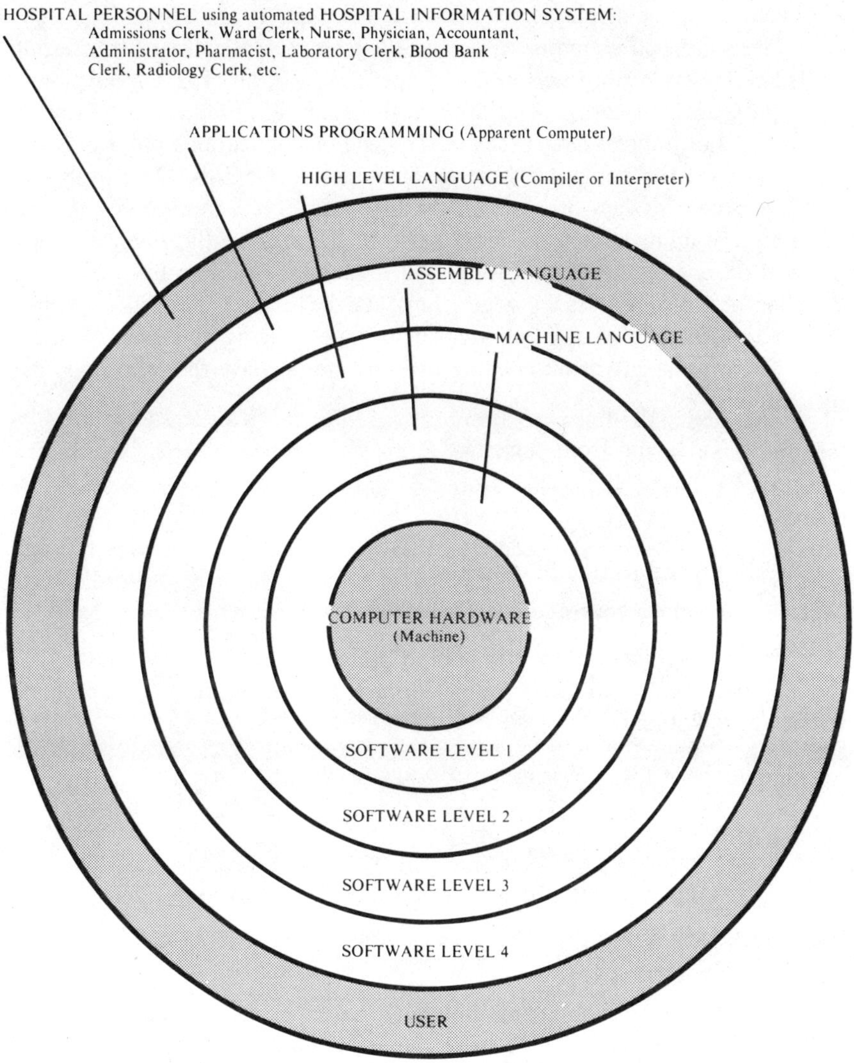

for the computer. Code is organized into individual *statements* that have a prescribed form. Different programming languages have different specifications as to what a statement can consist of, how long it can be, how many statements can appear on a given 80-column line, and, in some cases, in what column of the display screen or card a statement can begin.

There are three major types of programs: applications, translation (called compilers or interpreters), and operating system programs. Applications programs perform a desired task, such as producing a report. Compilers and interpreters translate the code of applications programs into code that uses the computer's set of machine instructions. Operating systems are programs that manage all the functions of a computer system and allow a large number of tasks to be performed concurrently. Each program is based on one or more algorithms. An *algorithm* is a step-by-step procedure for performing a task. Algorithms can be used to describe common daily activities, such as starting a car or using a vending machine. An algorithm for using a soft-drink vending machine might have the following constituent acts:

— Take coin from pocket,
— Insert coin in coin slot,
— Select beverage,
— Press selection button, and
— Remove beverage container from machine.

Programs organize algorithms and present them to computers so that the intended task or tasks can be performed. Programs are made up of the following constituents:

— Declaration of program storage needs
— Evaluation of expressions
— Assignment of values
— Sequential order of instructions and specifications
— Testing
— Branching
— Commands for communication with peripherals (mass storage, such as disk or tape drive; input facilities, such as the keyboard; and output facilities, such as a CRT display or printer)

Declaration of storage needs is something like buying a lot if you want to build a house or acquiring the right-of-way for a highway. Adequate space must be reserved for storing values needed for a program. Programs use variable names, such as X or B2 or ROOM-RATE, to label storage locations reserved for use in a program. Variable names are linked by the program with storage addresses in the computer. The programmer keeps track of values stored by referring to variable names; it is the responsibility of the program to assure that the correct address is used when data are obtained from or placed into storage. Each program must set up a directory, or symbol table, to use as a reference in handling variable names.

Storage reservations are important for programming for the same reasons that various kinds of reservations are needed in other environments.

1. Storage requirements are different: consider the different parking needs of a car, large truck, and motorcycle.
2. Storage space is limited: land, building floor space and parking capacity are all limited, and some allocation system is needed to assure availability to many users.
3. Use of space must be protected: conflicts over use of space need to be avoided; misunderstandings about ownership of buildings could lead to destruction of one person's structure by another.

The principles implicit in the analogies given above are vital for use of computer storage by a program that is in the process of execution.

1. Different values require different storage: among the variety of values to be stored are integer numbers, numbers with fractions, and alphanumeric data such as text.
2. Limited storage needs to be used efficiently: locations associated with variable names should be set up so that space allotted to a program is not wasted.
3. Program space in a computer's memory should be protected against encroachment by other programs: there must be assurance that the activities of one program will not obliterate data or instructions belonging to another program or, worse yet, to the operating system.

The different storage and processing requirements of different categories of data lead to the concept of *data types*. The most common data types are *numeric* and *alphanumeric*. Numeric data fundamentally require adequate space for storage of a binary number. Since storage of integers is not as complex as storage of numbers with fractional parts, a distinction is usually made between *integer* and *real* data types. Variables declared as of the integer type cannot accommodate the storage of fractions, whereas variables declared as real can. In some scientific calculations it is necessary to provide for storage of more fractional digits than for common calculations; such enhanced storage capability may be referred to as *double precision*.

Numbers can also be stored in the form of the ASCII or EBCDIC byte-length codes. A somewhat more efficient storage of these display-oriented codes is referred to as *packed decimal* storage. Text data are referred to as alphanumeric, or *string*, data. In storing strings, the most important considerations are the order of the characters and the length of the string. Portions of strings are referred to as *substrings*.

Through the conventions of the programming language used, each computer program declares its storage requirements. Some languages, such as COBOL or Pascal, require that all such declarations be grouped at the beginning of the program. In other languages, such as FORTRAN, BASIC, or MUMPS, variables are established as they are encountered in compiling or interpreting the program.

A particularly useful storage structure is the *array*, an organized grouping of storage locations of the same type. An array is to a single variable what an apartment building is to a single-family dwelling. Just as in an apartment building apartments are indexed by a numbering system revealing floor and location on a floor, arrays are indexed by one or more subscripts. A numbering system for a single apartment building (rooms 1 through 50) would be similar to a one-dimensional array requiring a single subscript. Numbering systems for apartment buildings with several floors (for example, rooms 101 through 340) are organized according to two dimensions: floor and location on a floor. This type of organization is found in the two-dimensional grid used for maps; two subscripts are needed to find a given location. Apartment complexes or motels with several buildings use a three-dimensional numbering system: a building designator and then a room number revealing floor and location on the floor (A-101 through D-340).

Evaluation of expressions occurs throughout computer programs. An *expression* may contain a sequence of variables, numbers, arithmetic operators, and alphanumeric strings. Arithmetic operators, such as the familiar plus and minus for addition and subtraction, slash for division, and asterisk for multiplication, are actually instructions to the computer to perform a given arithmetic operation. The values to be processed according to the arithmetic instruction are called *operands*. In order to evaluate an expression, there must be a convention as to which parts of the expression are evaluated first. Copies of the values stored in each location referred to by a variable must be obtained and substituted for the variables in performing arithmetic. Assuming that variables contain values as shown:

TOTAL-BEDS contains 455

BEDS-OCCUPIED contains 402

the expression (BEDS-OCCUPIED/TOTAL-BEDS)*100 is evaluated as follows:

> the value of BEDS-OCCUPIED is fetched as 402
>
> the value of TOTAL-BEDS is fetched as 455
>
> BEDS-OCCUPIED is divided by TOTAL-BEDS
>
> the result of the division is multiplied by 100

Once an expression has been evaluated, the resulting value may be stored in a new location. A command to the computer to store a value is called *assignment*. Thus the entire statement:

```
OCCUPANCY-RATE := (BEDS-OCCUPIED/
                   TOTAL-BEDS)*100
```

calls for the expression on the right of the assignment operator (that is, :=) to be evaluated and for the resulting value to be stored in the location designated by the variable name OCCUPANCY-RATE.

Statements in computer programs resemble algebraic statements, but the two should not be confused: statements in computer programs are sets of instructions for the computer to perform specified operations, not statements of the equality of two expressions. A common assignment statement used to add some amount to an existing value stored under a variable name illustrates the point. Assume that BEDS-OCCUPIED-COUNT contains a value of one and that the amount stored in BEDS-OCCUPIED-COUNT is to be increased by one of the following statements in a program:

```
BEDS-OCCUPIED-COUNT := BEDS-OCCUPIED-COUNT + 1
```

Such a statement would be impossible as an algebraic statement. Many computer languages use a modified equals sign for assignment to underscore the distinction. BASIC interpreters permit or require LET for assignment:

```
LET X = 5
```

Pascal, ADA, and ALGOL use a combination of a colon and equal sign for assignment.

Only the simplest computer programs consist of a linear sequence of statements. Most contain statements providing for testing and branching. In the example of an algorithm for the use of a soft-drink vending machine, the coin return feature is an example of a test. If a coin is tested by the machine and released through the coin-return slot, then the machine user has received information from the test—namely, that the coin was not acceptable. At this point in the algorithm, provision needs to be made for branching back to insert a different coin. Other tests that might cause branching would be the machine's testing of its stock of change coins and of its supply of a particular kind of soft drink. This test information is made available to the user by indicators that specify "use quarters only" or "do not select if light is on." In a computer program, there must be statements commanding that a test be conducted so that a decision can be made as to whether to continue to follow the linear sequence of instructions or to branch to another instruction. The IF statement serves this purpose:

> If WARD-BEDS-OCCUPIED-COUNT is greater than or
> equal to WARD-BED-COUNT then
> Do ALTERNATIVE-ASSIGNMENT procedure.

Obviously, in order to execute such a program statement, the computer must:

1. Evaluate variables used (find current values of WARD-BEDS-OCCUPIED-COUNT and WARD-BED-COUNT);
2. Compare the two values;
3. Signal the result of the comparison; and
4. Test the signal.

If the test of the signal or code resulting from the comparison shows that the condition (WARD-BEDS-OCCUPIED-COUNT is greater than or equal to WARD-BED-COUNT) is true, then the procedure ALTERNATE-ASSIGNMENT will be executed instead of the next statement in sequence after the IF statement. If the condition is false, the statement immediately following the IF statement will be executed.

Subroutines and subprograms are valuable to program design. Subprograms can be reused from any number of locations in the main program, thus saving repeated code. Use of subprograms contributes to the modular construction of a program. The main program *calls* subroutines or subprograms through an established convention. In order to invoke the subprogram, the status of the calling program must be saved in memory, so that execution of the calling program can resume after the subprogram is completed. Except in BASIC and COBOL, use of subprograms and subroutines involves an interaction between the calling program and the called subprogram called *parameter passing.* Through parameter passing, the values stored in certain variables in the main program are stored or referred to by certain variables in the subprogram. The parameter-passing convention amounts to a kind of membrane, or insulation, between the main program and a subprogram. Some variables in the subprogram may not have any role in the main program. Variables restricted to the subprogram are called *local variables*; variables in effect for the entire program are called *global variables* in most programming languages. In COBOL and Pascal, subprograms are referred to as procedures.

The receiving and sending of data is essential for the use of computer programs in implementing algorithms. Input–output commands permit management of communications. Instructions in a program can cause code to be transmitted to a device such as a CRT or printer for display or for control of the device.

The form in which programs are entered for a compiler is called *source code*. When a program has been successfully tested, the compiled version is cataloged and stored on-line in the system so that the compilation does not need to occur every time the program is run. The stored version is called *object code*. Object code is ready to run as machine code in every respect except the designation of specific addresses in the computer. The locations to be used by the object code are not known until execution of the program. Such code is called *relocatable code*. A diagram of the programming process is shown in Figure 5-2.

Operating Systems

Operating systems are programs that manage the computer's resources. The operating system mediates conflicts among programs competing for use of memory space, use of the printer and use of the processor.

The applications programs (programs that perform tasks for the user of the computer) run as subprograms of the operating system. Since at any given moment in a modern system a number of programs may be in a runnable state in different *partitions* of the computer's memory, the operating system must determine which program gets to use the main processor. One solution to the need to provide at least some progress to each program admitted to a partition is to give each program a predetermined *slice* of time. When the time allotment has been used, the program is interrupted and another program is allowed to use the processor.

Beginning with the *bare machine*, the operating system provides additional levels of control over the computing environment: management and scheduling of the use of the processor, management of the use of memory, management, or *traffic control*, of input–output devices, and management of the file or database system or both.[1] Early computers, which did not have operating systems, could process only one job at a time. When one job was using the processor but not the printer, a second job did not have access to the printer. Operating systems have been designed to assure the most efficient possible use of computer resources.

FIGURE 5-2
Programming in a High Level Language (COBOL)

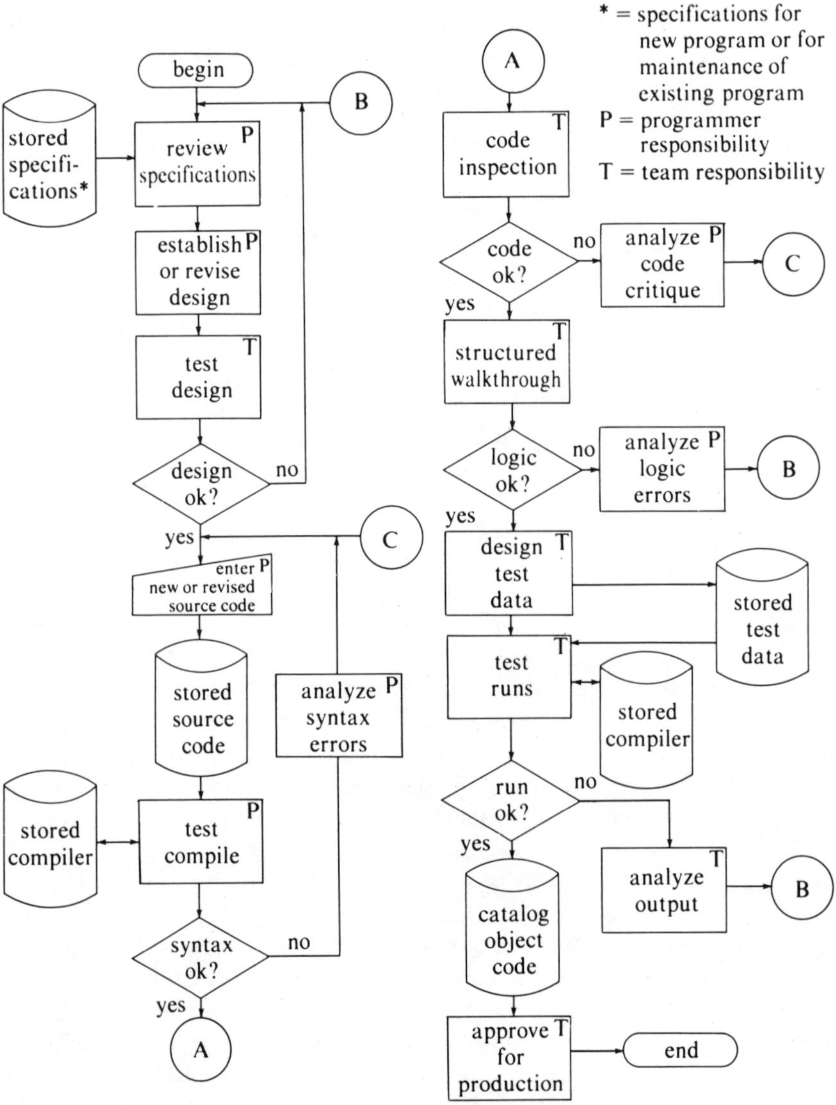

Several conditions contribute to the complexity of operating systems.

1. Devices function at greatly different speeds; printers and data-entry equipment are relatively slow, compared to the main processor; disk access is faster than tape access; direct access to main memory is faster than disk access.
2. Programs have different requirements: some require extensive use of the main processor but relatively little input–output time, while other programs process quickly but produce prodigious printed output; some programs require little memory and some have substantial memory needs.
3. Deadlock must be avoided: situations in which each of two programs has control over a resource which the other requires to proceed will degrade or halt performance.
4. Programs must be protected from each other: the bounds of memory space allotted to each program must be controlled so that an error in one program cannot enable it to write over the data or instructions of another program waiting to continue execution.
5. There must be communication in the system regarding states of devices and programs; synchronization of events is provided by message systems of various types.
6. There must be conventions and a process for transfer of control of the processor from a program no longer in a runnable state to one that is.
7. Queues must be maintained for programs in various waiting states: waiting for initial reading, waiting for a memory partition, waiting for use of the processor, or waiting for use of an output device; queues are also used in transaction processing systems in the polling of interactive terminals connected to the system.
8. Memory must be managed: records must be kept of what portions of memory are occupied by program uses, what portions of programs can be accessed where on disks in virtual memory systems, and where free memory is available for the next use.
9. Files must be managed: pointers from one part of the file to another or from a directory to entities in the file must be maintained, and the integrity of data in the file must be protected from simultaneous attempts to access the same data.

In considering the memory management responsibilities of the operating system, it is important to realize that *logically* related data, such as parts of the same program, may not necessarily be located in *physically* adjacent storage in main memory or on disks. Many analogies can be used to gain a sense of how memory management must function. For example, imagine a bank of six elevators at a large, crowded hotel with a convention in progress. Among the *logical* groupings present waiting to use an elevator might be a sales team, a group going to a party, some couples, and so forth. As long as the destinations are communicated within the various groups, it is not necessary that each member of a logical grouping travel in the same elevator as the other members of the group.

An important concept in today's operating systems is *SPOOLing.* SPOOL is an acronym for simultaneous peripheral operations on-line. In a computer system that serves a number of users simultaneously, the vastly different speeds of input and output, on one hand, and internal processing, on the other hand, lead to a requirement for special management and temporary storage facilities. For example, although two jobs calling for printer output might deliver their output ready for the printer at about the same time, only one job at a time can use the printer. SPOOLing provides temporary storage on disk for jobs waiting in a queue to use the printer. When any job is ready for printer output, it is effectively dispatched to the printer by being transmitted to the SPOOLing software, although actually the output may remain stored for a period of time until the printer is available. The SPOOLing software thus presents a *virtual* printer to the system. This virtual printer can absorb output at a rate not directly related to the speed of the physical printing device. SPOOLing allows use of the main processor to proceed without the delays that might be imposed if jobs could only be processed when the physical printer was available.

Operating system programs are normally written in the appropriate assembler for the system or the microprocessor or in a high-level language suitable for systems programming, such as ALGOL, PL/I, or concurrent Pascal. The programming language used for the operating system is normally different from the language or report generation system used for applications programming.

The vastly enhanced capacities of today's computer systems are due not only to the technological advances in storage and in processing speed, but also to the sophistication and efficiency of operating system software.

Programming Languages

Most programming languages are *assembly languages*, or *high-level languages*. Assembly language programs have a direct relationship to the machine instruction set of the processor. High-level languages are designed for greater ease of programming and in most cases resemble the structures of English and algebra. Programs written in high-level language code are translated into assembly language or machine language programs or both for execution.

Assembly languages are designated according to the system (IBM 370 assembler or PDP-11 assembler, for example) or the processor (6502 assembler or Z-80 assembler, for example). Each instruction in an assembler program represents a specific instruction or group of instructions available on the processor for which the assembler is intended. Assemblers establish lists of symbols (called symbol tables) to keep track of names of storage locations used in the programs; thus they can determine exactly where instructions and data are located.

Every programming language is made available by a program called a *compiler*, or *interpreter*. A compiler analyzes an application program (source code) written in the given language in order to translate it into code the machine can execute (object code). The compiler program inspects the application program to make sure that the forms of the statements can be analyzed. When the compiler finds a statement in a form it does not recognize, it announces (in an error message) the discovery of a *syntax error*. Obviously the compiler has *syntax rules* to use in checking program statements. Compilers can check for certain obvious mistakes in program structure and issue warnings or error messages. When the compiler finds any serious error (such as a syntax error), it may refuse to allow the program to be executed. If the program has detectable errors, then it might not be possible to predict the results of using that program. It is normally assumed that a program with unpredictable results must be revised before it enters production or on-line status.

Compilers translate entire programs from source code into object code. The translated program can then be executed. Interpreters convert programs by utilizing pre-established subroutines as translations of the lines of code. Compilers offer the advantage of efficient translation of an entire program and are best suited to batch processing and repeated processing. Interpreters are best suited to interactive environments and applications.

Programming languages in common use include FORTRAN, COBOL, BASIC, Pascal, PL/I, and RPG II. MUMPS is extensively used in hospital environments. APL is used in some environments. A relatively new language, ADA, is expected to gain widespread use. Artificial intelligence projects, including some medical diagnostic applications, are written in LISP. BASIC, APL, MUMPS, and LISP are designed for interactive use as interpreters. FORTRAN, COBOL, PL/I, and Pascal are normally compiled, although interactive editors can enable them to be used in on-line environments. Except for RPG II and LISP, the languages mentioned

FIGURE 5-3
Coding of a Statement in Various Programming Languages

The following indicates how a statement is coded in various programming languages to let the value of C be the same as the total of the value of A added to the value of B (evaluate A, evaluate B, calculate the sum of the two values, and store the sum in the location represented by C):

ADA:
```
C := A + B;
```

APL:
```
C ← A + B
```

ALGOL:
```
C := A + B;
```

Pascal:
```
C := A + B;
```

MUMPS:
```
SET C = A + B
```

BASIC:
```
LET C = A + B
```

FORTRAN:
```
C = A + B
```

COBOL:
```
ADD A TO B GIVING C.
```

Assembler (IBM 370):
```
L    5,A
L    6,B
AR   5,6
ST   5,C
```

RPG II:
```
A    ADD    B       C
```

PL/I:
```
C = A + B;
```

above are classified as *procedural languages*. Procedural languages follow a sequence of steps in executing a program which resembles the sequence of steps executed by the computer. RPG II is classified as a nonprocedural or problem-oriented language; programming is restricted to a description of files according to specified formats and a listing of arithmetic and logic operations to be performed.[2] LISP is classified as a list-processing language. Figure 5-3 shows examples of statement form for widely used programming languages.

Standard versions exist for most languages, but there are varieties of implementations for commonly used languages. The designator *ANS* is applied to versions of programming languages approved by the American National Standards Institute (ANSI). There are ANS versions of COBOL, FORTRAN, and MUMPS. Information on the individual languages follows.

1. ADA (named after Ada Babbage; originated in the 1980s) offers a structure suitable for a wide range of applications from business data processing to real-time operations. It is sponsored

by the U.S. Department of Defense and is based to a large degree on Pascal.

2. ALGOL (algorithmic language; originated in the 1950s) contains specialized functions for loops, multiway branching, and string handling. It offers *recursion* (program structures that can successively call themselves) and exists in a number of implementations.
3. APL (a programming language; originated in 1962), an interpretive language designed to exploit the manipulation of arrays and a unique character set, is preferred for some mathematical applications. It is limited by the character set and input–output characteristics of standard APL, although modified versions are adequate for business applications. Programs are condensed in appearance and require very little code for sophisticated programming.
4. BASIC (beginner's all-purpose symbolic instruction code; originated in the 1960s) was designed initially to make computer technology accessible to all students and faculty at Dartmouth College. The form of assignment statements resembles that of FORTRAN, and it is normally implemented as an interpreter. BASIC contains automatic features to avoid contact of learners with problems of data type distinctions or output formatting and offers enhanced string-handling capabilities. It is used in education, business and various other environments.
5. COBOL (common business oriented language; originated in the 1950s) is characterized by its division of programs into four parts, called divisions—identification, environment, data, and procedure. It represents an attempt to make programming independent of particular machine or system environment and less subject to software development problems inherent in team projects, changes of personnel, and maintenance requirements. A number of implementations are in use; COBOL offers numeric processing and data types especially suited to business data processing.
6. FORTRAN (formula translator; originated in 1957) is used in scientific and technical applications because of its straightforward, efficient execution and strong tradition of use in research, industry, and other environments. There are several versions (FORTRAN IV, FORTRAN 77) available, as well as specialized versions for instruction (WATFIV) and certain industrial applications.

7. LISP (list processing language; originated in 1950s) is the best-known list-processing language; it is used for most artificial intelligence research and applications. Two major *dialects*, or implementations, are in use: Eval and Evalquote.
8. MUMPS (Massachusetts General Hospital utility multi-programming system; originated in 1966) is described as a general-purpose, interpretative, high-level programming language designed for interactive data management applications. It offers enhanced string handling, hierarchically structured database functions, and built-in operating system features.[3]
9. Pascal (named after Blaise Pascal; originated in the 1960s) was originally designed to serve as an initial language for computer science instruction. It is characterized by requiring that all variables, data types and structures, and procedures be declared before the main body of the program. It is considered to be especially suited to structured programming techniques. Pascal provides for user-defined data types and exists in several mainframe and microcomputer implementations.
10. PL/I (programming language one; designed in the 1960s) was developed to combine the best features of the earlier major languages (FORTRAN, COBOL, and ALGOL) and to offer features suitable for a wide variety of applications. It is intended to be equally appropriate for scientific and technical applications on one hand and business data processing on the other.
11. RPG (report program generator; developed in the 1950s) is an applications-oriented or problem-oriented language for intermediate-sized systems designed to provide preparation of business reports. It is widely used; the most recent version, RPG III for IBM System/38, features database capabilities.

Careful inspection of vendors' specifications and standard acquisition guides for data-processing managers will reveal the programming languages offered. Changing systems or applications language will, of course, necessitate the retraining of in-house programming personnel and extensive software conversion.

Program Design and Development

The first job in program development is analysis of the problem. The term *structured*, when used in designing computer programs, refers to (1) the top-down approach to refinement of the task; (2) development of modules to perform parts of the task; and (3) restriction of logical structures used in programming.

Although programs could be based on bottom-up analysis (that is, beginning with individual tasks and later integrating these into a whole program), top-down analysis assures that individual tasks and subtasks will function well together and will not have to be completely redesigned as work proceeds on the project.

Programs should be general solutions to problems. Assumptions about operating conditions should be recognized so that the program can be designed to respond to variations and unanticipated conditions. For example, the algorithm described above regarding use of a soft-drink vending machine contains a number of assumptions:

1. The price of a container of the beverage is predetermined,
2. Only one coin will be adequate for purchase,
3. The coin will be accepted,
4. No one will use slugs, defective coins, or noncoins,
5. Only one container of beverage will be purchased, and
6. No change will be returned.

The original algorithm requires extensive modification and amplification to avoid narrowness of implementation. In order to account for all possible transactions, the algorithm design would have to deal with the following:

1. Evaluation of price and coins available and deposit of coin(s) based on testing of circumstances,
2. Repetition of procedure for each container of beverage to be purchased until all desired purchases have occurred or no more complete sets of coins can be assembled to meet the price requirements,
3. Possibility that noncoins or defective coins will be deposited,
4. Possibility that the amount deposited will exceed the price for a single purchase, causing coins to be returned that would be added to the set of available coins,
5. Possibility that the supply of a category of beverage will be exhausted,
6. Possibility that appropriate coin supply will be exhausted before all intended purchasing is completed, and
7. Possibility that the coin supply could be replenished by exchanging unusable coins (such as pennies) and paper money for usable coins.

The treatment of various special cases could be presented in individual *modules*, or procedures. A complete algorithm, ready for general use and stated with the level of detail required for computer program design, would have to take all of these function specifications into account.

Algorithms are converted from design into program through the process of coding. Some testing of the program can begin during the coding phase. The design and development of complex programs is approached systematically by implementing and testing portions of a program, beginning with the main program; thus difficulties are identified as soon as a new module is implemented. In COBOL programming this strategy is referred to as *stub testing.*

Programs should be designed to review incoming data to determine whether they are within guidelines for acceptable and usable values. Among the criteria for such built-in testing are range checks for numeric data and spelling checks for textual data. Within the program, there should be safeguards against values that would cause division by zero, an attempt to access a position in an array that does not exist, or an infinite repetition of a portion of code. Repeating a portion of code is called *looping*, and the failure of a program or part of a program to terminate execution can be extremely wasteful of computing resources.

Data and procedures should be devised to test the new program thoroughly. While it is impossible to test all possible situations in a complex program, careful test planning can take into account branching and looping in the program. Program malfunctions often occur due to unforeseen changes in the way a program is used.

Applications programming normally takes place in the context of teamwork. Communication is essential to successful team programming and is furthered by (1) design of program specifications in terms of input, processing, and output; (2) review of specifications to exploit insights gained during the process of design and development; and (3) *documentation.* Documentation, in the form of comments embedded in the program, enables a team of persons, the original programmer, or a person other than the original programmer to understand the intent of a section of code. It records the functions of variables and program structures and narrates a *play-by-play* account of what the portions of a program accomplish.

The final phase of program development, normally referred to as program *maintenance*, incorporates continued design and testing. As improved performance is requested or changed conditions for use of the program occur, redesign will be required. Testing and debugging, or removal of errors, continues as previously undetected errors surface, new conditions of use lead to malfunctions, or revisions must be tested. Program maintenance costs must be taken into account in evaluating the impact of software costs on an organization.

PROGRAM FLOWCHARTS AND OTHER PROGRAMMING AIDS

A simple computer program can be quickly designed, coded, and tested. The programs used for routine operation of a hospital information system are far from simple. Applications and systems programs consist of large numbers of procedures and involve complex relationships between variables; such programs cannot be designed and coded efficiently without organizing the work carefully. In order to develop programs of substantial complexity and extensive detail, an intermediate stage of representation and design permits programmers to visualize the operation of the program apart from attention to the type of detail involved in writing code in a specific programming language. Just as outlining is often useful preparation for writing a long essay, various methods of preliminary analysis contribute to logical design of computer programs. Charts and diagrams frequently help programmers and teams of programmers in the program design process.

A *flowchart* consists of what steps are to be programmed and the sequence in which they are to be performed.[4] Flowcharts are based on the following symbols:

- Rectangle = process
- Parallelogram = input–output
- Diamond = decision (for branching)
- Small circle = connector (between parts of the diagram)
- Oblong = terminal (for beginning or end of the program)

Entries are written inside the symbols to specify input-output operations, assignments or calculations, and conditions for branching decisions. Arrows, called *flowlines*, connect the symbols. Additional symbols are used to indicate the beginning and end of the program, initialization procedures, and connections between portions of the program. Recently a symbol has been devised for the multiway branch, or *case*, situation. Flowcharts are helpful in analyzing the program and in designing the appropriate algorithm.

Figure 5-4 gives a flowchart for the computer processing necessary to locate the smallest number in an array containing 20 values. This task requires that:

1. Variables exist for the 20 positions of the array, a counter that serves as an index in looking in successive positions in the array, and a place exist to store the smallest number found so far;
2. The smallest-number-found variable be set equal to the first value in the array;
3. The index counter be set properly;

FIGURE 5-4
Flowcharts and Other Programming Aids

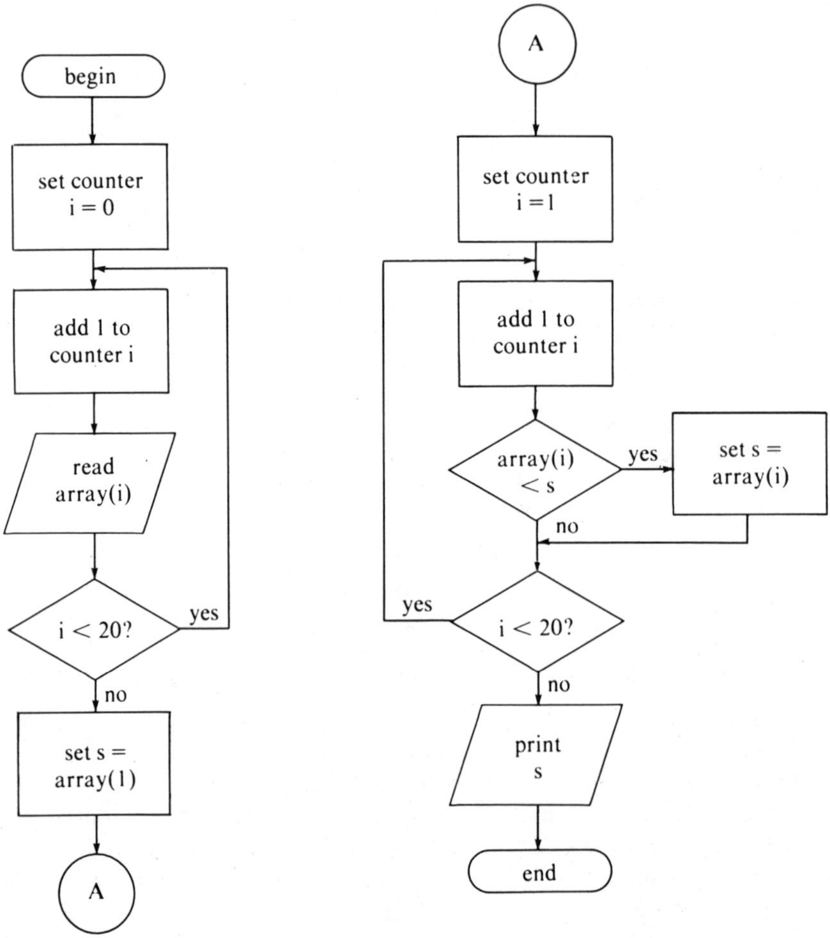

FIGURE 5-4—*continued*
Flowcharts and Other Programming Aids

NASSI-SHNEIDERMAN CHART

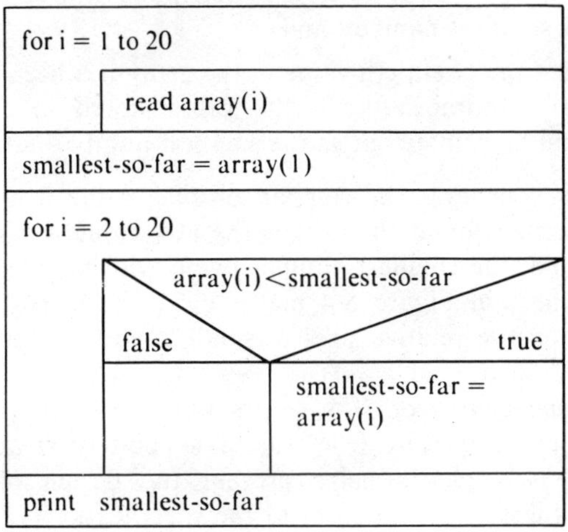

DECISION TABLE

Detect smallest number						
Conditions	Rule					
	1	2	3	4	5	
1 array(i)<s	Y	N				
2						
3						
4						
Actions						
1 s =array(i)	X					
2						
3						
4						

4. A process be repeated in which successive values in the array are compared to the value stored in smallest-number-found;
5. Any time a number smaller than the smallest-number-found is discovered, the smallest-number-found will be set equal to that new smallest number; and
6. When the twentieth value in the array has been compared to the smallest-number-found, the value stored in smallest-number-found be printed out as the smallest number in the array.

Obviously, whenever the comparison of a value from the array with the smallest-number-found shows that the new value is bigger than smallest-number-found, the smallest-number-found will be left as is. The corresponding flowchart in Figure 5-4 makes clear the loop structure and the decision based on the relative sizes of smallest-number-found and the new array value examined.

Nassi-Shneiderman or *N-S* charts were designed to represent program logic more adequately from the standpoint of structured programming. Use of N-S charts helps prevent the design of program flow configurations that do not conform to the specifications of structured programming. Figure 5-4 shows the same algorithm for finding the smallest number in an array as is displayed in flowchart form. Among the advantages of N-S charts are more adequate space to write in variable names and other information, as well as clear treatment of the effects of evaluating conditions for branching. Among the disadvantages is greater difficulty in revision.

Shelly and Cashman recommend that a *hierarchy chart* be drawn to show the relationship between modules of a COBOL program.[5] A kind of tree structure illustrates which modules of the program control which other modules. In accordance with control relationships, modules are placed on different levels. At the topmost level will be the main control module for the report or other task. The components activated by instructions in the main control module appear on the second level. Any modules controlled by modules on the second level will appear on a third level.

Various types of simplified or outline code procedures have been proposed: according to Shelly and Cashman, *pseudocode* specifies the detailed steps required in solving a problem, and lists the required files, records, and fields to be referenced in the program.[6] Pseudocode is generally written in simplified English, with some conventions of standardized references to repeated segments of the proposed program and the use of indentation to clarify program structure. Complete lists of files, records, and fields of records amount to a preliminary form of declaration of all variables. At the stage of writing pseudocode, attention is focused on making the list complete; at the stage of coding, attention shifts to coding each entry correctly.

Decision tables present logical relationships in two-dimensional fashion, as *truth tables* do. Decision tables and *decision trees* are especially useful in representing decision strategies of programs dealing with medical diagnosis and analysis of symptoms. Decision tables can be used in analyzing any task to be performed by a computer program. Welland cites the two main weaknesses of narrative and flowchart presentation of complex logic structures as weaknesses in precision and relevance.[7] He characterizes the flowchart as failing in defining program logic because it can be understood only by tracing through the relationships displayed in a serial fashion. Welland points out that it is difficult to check a complex flowchart thoroughly. Decision tables, on the other hand, can be checked for omissions and inconsistencies. Proponents of the use of decision tables see the tabular presentation of program structure as a "viable alternative to conventional 'algorithmic' languages."[8]

Data-processing installations can adopt whatever programming aids and procedures are suitable in view of local circumstances and preferences. The principal advantage of adopting and using customary techniques lies in a standardized approach which (1) enables an individual or team to attack a complex problem effectively; and (2) gives different team members or maintenance programmers a common basis for analysis of program structure.

Alternative Sources of Software

Once a hospital has installed a basic system, there are several options for further software development: (1) new software can be designed by the hospital data-processing staff; (2) commercial or public domain software that approximates hospital needs can be bought and then revised by the local data-processing staff; or (3) a contract can be made with a facilities management firm to supply and maintain software.

Careful cost-benefit analysis should precede any decision to develop software internally: the time and expense involved in producing a fully tested and documented system may be prohibitive. Where several hospitals share services and can support a substantial programming staff, capabilities for independent software development obviously increase.

A hospital or group of hospitals can establish a programming staff adequate for modification of software obtained from commercial or public domain sources. Modification can range from minor revisions to enable self-contained packages to run in the local environment to substantial upgrading of current packages to meet new or altered needs. In-house programming capabilities also permit the development of special reports when required and the extension of functions of existing software packages.

Facilities management firms either recommend software to the hospital or supply their own proprietary software. In addition, they usually offer some programming capability. Shared computer organizations, and service bureaus in particular, have ongoing software development activities. New programs are either supplied to customers as improvements to the installed systems or are sold as new products. As shared computer organizations grow larger, they become less able to develop programs that meet the needs of any specific organization. Instead, their new products are a response to the changing needs of their entire customer population.

The productivity of existing programming resources can be enhanced through (1) well-organized cooperation of users and programmers in the application program development process; (2) well-designed database management systems that permit new reporting procedures to benefit from data presently stored in the system; and (3) automated program or report generation systems. Although the progress of application program development from design specifications to coding and testing is in the hands of data-processing specialists, users in the hospital environment can contribute actively to the design process. McLean describes the prerequisites for achieving a cooperative development process: recognition that needs change over time, user understanding of the scope of the system, and user refinement of specifications.[9] McLean points out that personal applications access to computer resources expands the use of data processing without increasing demands on data-processing professionals to support these applications. Examples include a variety of data access and interactive facilities that do not normally require highly detailed protocols. Among the services that may directly aid users is word processing. Ivers reports on a MUMPS-based system that offers end users word-processing services such as list processing and sort-merge capabilities, and development of user-defined databases.[10] Extensive user involvement in interactive systems can lead to demand for greater storage capacity, which can also produce systems programming demands.

Criteria for acquisition of commercially available software packages must be set up carefully. Expected advantages from saving on costs and productivity can be offset by unanticipated needs for modification. Externally produced software must be reviewed with regard to file access methods, documentation, and modularity of structure. Since today's integrated hospital information systems involve extensive use of database management systems and on-line transactions, software that is acquired and is found not to be suitable in some important respect, and yet must be implemented for a period, can degrade system performance. The development philosophies of the host system and the acquired software package must be in harmony.[11]

Sources of information on software in the public domain are reports on projects sponsored through federal grants and contracts. Such software may be available for the cost of tape duplication, but it may also require extensive modification and adaptation to function in the local environment. Public domain software is cost-efficient when development costs are avoided and modification costs turn out to be low.[12] System and language user groups provide much valuable information on software.

GUIDELINES FOR ACQUIRING SOFTWARE

Establishing the functional requirements of software is the first step in preparing for acquisition. Requirements should be organized and presented according to departments in the hospital to be served and should include the following:

1. Statement of functions and responsibilities of the department;
2. Outline of communication functions (messages, requisitions, orders) including interaction with other software or departments, or both, resolution of conflicting or redundant order situations, security measures, and message priority categories;
3. Printed reports with frequency of each report specified;
4. Database specifications in the form of data elements needed to support the work of the department; and
5. Any special features.

An outline of the standard content of orders should be provided for each type of order.

Evaluation criteria for software, including database management software, should be established and included in the Request for Proposal (RFP) to be disseminated. The Request for Proposal is discussed in more detail in Chapter 6.

Information on sources of software can be acquired from directories, vendors of systems and software, publications of users' groups and other organizations, other hospitals, and specialized consultants.

In order to make the final selection process practical, it is necessary to identify the software sources that will be regarded as finalists. Once this has been done, the software available from the finalist should be subjected to thorough evaluation and comparison. When a best source has been identified, the negotiation of the contract is the next step. Terms and conditions must be appropriate to the purchaser as well as to the vendor.

Installation and testing for acceptance are the final stages of the acquisition process. Because of the extensive on-line facilities and services typical of modern hospital information systems, testing of system components and determining that the system is functioning acceptably are challenging tasks. Rusnak describes the preparation and implementation of test packages for validating hospital information systems programs.[13] Sophisticated testing is vital to assure adequate performance after full implementation, to identify problems before implementation, and to reduce costs associated with implementation of new software.

SPECIFIC SOFTWARE PACKAGES FOR HOSPITALS

The *AHIS Component Catalog*, published by the Health Services Research Center of the University of Missouri-Columbia, identifies over 200 different information functions or applications which are grouped in the following categories:

- Administration
- Admissions
- Business office, accounting, financial management
- Blood bank
- Central supply, purchasing, materials management
- Clinical laboratory
- Computer center
- Courier, patient transfer
- Dietary-food service
- Laundry-linen
- Maintenance, housekeeping, physical plant
- Management engineering, productivity anaylsis
- General medical-clinical functions
- Specialized medical-clinical functions
- Medical records
- Nursing service
- Outpatient-ambulatory services
- Payroll, personnel
- Pharmacy
- Radiologic services
- Social services

The 1980 edition of the catalog described 112 examples of software from 70 vendors or sources.[14] The catalog lists for each software component the applications functions performed, date of first installation, application and system languages, core memory requirements, and the number of installations using the component.

Two widely used standard data-processing resources, DataPro[15] and Auerbach,[16] include detailed listings of software currently available for installation in hospitals and health care environments. Jacobs describes the hospital information system market, providing an historical perspective on major vendors.[17] The following are examples of information systems software specifically intended for the hospital environment:

- Burroughs Hospital Information System (BHIS), Burroughs
- MEDPRO hospital information system, HBO and Company
- TECHNICON hospital information system, Technicon Data Systems Corporation
- DATACARE hospital information system, Datacare, Inc.
- NADACOM hospital information system, National Data Communications, Inc.
- Patient Care System (PCS), IBM
- Medical Information and Communication System (MEDICS), NCR

Considerable software has been developed for use in systems that run the MUMPS programming language and operating system:

- Meditech Interpretative Information System (MIIS), a general purpose minicomputer operating system that is a refinement of ANS MUMPS;[18]
- EPIC, a time-oriented database management system, written in the MIIS dialect of MUMPS[19]
- MEDUS/A, a database management system[20]
- Computer-Assisted Pathology Encoding and Reporting System (CAPER), written in MUMPS[21]
- MEDINFO, a general-purpose computer-based medical information storage, retrieval, and analysis system written in MUMPS[22]
- Computer-Stored Ambulatory Record (COSTAR), a comprehensive centralized, and integrated information system for patient medical records written in MUMPS[23]
- VA File Manager, an applications programming tool.[24]

Examples of software not based on MUMPS include:

— Problem Oriented Medical Information System (PROMIS), a problem-oriented medical guidance system written in a specially designed programming language (PPL or PROMIS programming language);[25]

— DIASTU, a computerized database system for medical diagnostic studies written in FORTRAN and assembly language database handler;[26]

— PHACTS, a computerized pharmacy information system designed to automate drug distribution, clinical services, and administrative activities[27]

Specialized software has been developed for networking and distributed data processing such as:

— FOCUS, a nonprocedural language for management information system development[28]

— VAPID minicomputer network software[29]

Such networking and distributed data-processing software may not be designed specifically for hospital environments, but it is valuable for single-hospital and multihospital systems with mainframe systems of different types or with distributed use of microcomputers with mainframe systems. A description of the application of such software packages will be found in Section IV of this book.

SUMMARY

The apparent machine the user sees consists of bare computer hardware enhanced by several levels of computer software. Between the machine itself and the applications programming activity or interactive use of a database are the operating system, assemblers, database management facilities, compilers, interpreters, and additional programs. The design of computer programs is based on algorithms, or step-by-step descriptions of how to carry out the desired task. Designing and developing computer programs requires a careful analysis of the problem and good communication among team members. Programming begins with specifications, which must faithfully reflect the needs of the end user. Programming aids, such as pseudocode and various types of charts, can facilitate analysis of the problem and communication among the members of the team. Program test data are derived from program specifications and program structure. Testing begins with an incremental checking of the program at each stage of development and proceeds to testing of the fully formed program. Test data are derived from program specifications and take program structure into account.

Hospital information systems obtain software from a variety of sources. In-house programming resources are normally used to modify commercial software packages, rather than to write complete new packages. Among the considerations that must be explored in planning for new software acquisitions are the extent to which the package meets local needs, its compatibility with local database management facilities, the programming language used, documentation, and prospects for cost-effective maintenance of the software.

DISCUSSION QUESTIONS

5-1 Give specific examples of the three major types of computer programs.

5-2 Explain what an algorithm is and give examples, using tasks with which you are familiar.

5-3 What are the functions of declarations of variables in some computer languages? What is the purpose of having variable names in computer programs?

5-4 Why are data types needed in computer languages?

5-5 What is the significance of the concept *byte* for operations inside the computer? What does the concept *byte* usually mean to people when they are discussing computer acquisitions?

5-6 Why is the array structure important in computer programming?

5-7 Explain the difference between x = b + 2 as an algebraic equation and x := x + 2 as a statement in a computer program. What is the difference between the left-hand side of an assignment statement and the right-hand side?

5-8 How is *testing* related to *branching* in computer programs?

5-9 Cite the major responsibilities of an operating system.

5-10 What is the advantage of having a *SPOOL* facility in a computer system?

5-11 Explain the difference between assembly languages and high-level languages.

5-12 Name three high-level languages used in hospital information systems.

5-13 How are programming aids useful? Give examples of three programming aids.

5-14 What are the major alternative sources of software for a hospital information system? Cite advantages and disadvantages of each source mentioned.

5-15 Outline the process of acquiring software for a hospital information system.

5-16 What functions must be fulfilled by software in a hospital information system?

PROBLEMS

5-1 Outline the function requirements for software for the following departments:
— Blood bank
— Food service
— Radiology
Refer to the recommendations given in the section on guidelines for acquiring software.

5-2 Establish evaluation criteria to select the best software proposals for a payroll and personnel system. Refer to standard guides, such as Datapro and Auerbach, or alternative sources of specific information on appropriate software.

NOTES

1. Stuart E. Madnick and John J. Donovan, *Operating Systems* (New York: McGraw-Hill, 1974), p. 19.
2. D. A. Fletcher, "Nonprocedural Languages," in *Encyclopedia of Computer Science*, A. Ralston, ed. (New York: Van Nostrand Reinhold, 1976), p. 962.
3. *MUMPS—Questions and Answers*, published by the MUMPS Users' Group, 4321 Hartwick Road, #308, College Park, Maryland 20740.
4. N. B. Stern, *Flowcharting: A Tool for Understanding Computer Logic* (New York: Wiley, 1975), p. 42.
5. Gary B. Shelly and Thomas J. Cashman, *Introduction to Computer Programming: Structured COBOL* (Fullerton, California: Anaheim Publishing, 1977), p. 6.18.
6. Shelly and Cashman, op. cit., p. 3.3.
7. R. Welland, *Decision Tables and Computer Programming* (London: Heyden, 1981), p. 1.
8. A. Lew, "On the Emulation of Flowcharts by Decision Tables," *Communications of the ACM 25*, December 1982, p. 904.
9. E. R. McLean, "End User Application Development," in *Proceedings of the Fifth Annual Symposium of Computer Applications in Medical Care* (New York: Institute of Electrical and Electronics Engineers, 1981), pp. 48-52.
10. M. T. Ivers, "End User Application Development—Observations in VA Medical Centers," in *Proceedings of the Fifth Annual Symposium of Computer Applications in Medical Care* (New York: Institute of Electrical and Electronic Engineers, 1981), p. 50.
11. D. Schmeetz et al., "Implementation und Einsatz von Industrie-software im administrativen Bereich eines Universitaetskrankenhauses," in *Informationsverarbeitung in der Medizin, Medizinische Informatik und Statistik*, vol. 16 (Berlin: Springer-Verlag, 1979), p. 288-290; T. Munnecke, "Software Portability Considerations for Multiple Applications of Multiple Sites," in *Proceedings of the Fifth Annual Symposium of Computer Applications in Medical Care* (New York: Institute of Electrical and Electronics Engineers, 1981), pp. 38-42.
12. Suzanne LaViolette, "Public Domain Computer Software Can Save Many Hospitals up to 20%," *Modern Healthcare*, August 1980, p. 26.

13. James E. Rusnak, "A Method of Conducting Controlled Testing of Hospital Information System Components," in *Proceedings of the Fifth Annual Symposium of Computer Applications in Medical Care* (New York: Institute of Electrical and Electronics Engineers, 1981), p. 917.
14. University of Missouri Health Services Research Center/Health Care Technology Center, *Automated Hospital Information System: AHIS Component Catalog*, vol. 2 (Columbia, Missouri: University of Missouri, 1980).
15. The following publications from the Datapro Research Corporation, Delran, New Jersey 08075: *Directory of Software, Directory of Microcomputer Software.*
16. Auerbach Publishers, Pennsauken, New Jersey.
17. Stanley E. Jacobs, "Hospital-Wide Computer Systems: The Market and the Vendors," *MUG Quarterly*, Fall 1982, pp. 1-12.
18. "MIIS," in *Datapro Reports on Minicomputers*, (Delran, New Jersey: Datapro Research Corporation, 1981), pp. M12-620-101 through M12-620-103.
19. J. R. Faulkner and M. J. Gorodezky, "EPIC—A Time-Oriented Approach to Data Base Management," *MUG Quarterly*, Winter 1981-82, p. 27.
20. David J. Marcus, "Medical Applications in MUMPS on Micros—A Survey," *MUG Quarterly*, Winter 1981-82, p. 45.
21. S. J. Robboy et al., "Retrieval in a Computer-Assisted Pathology Encoding and Reporting System (CAPER)," *American Journal of Clinical Pathology*, May 1981, p. 654.
22. D. C. Johnson and G. O. Barnett, "MEDINFO—A Medical Information System," *Computer Programs in Biomedicine*, 1977, p. 191.
23. G. O. Barnett et al., "COSTAR—A Computer-Based Medical Information System for Ambulatory Care," *Proceedings of the IEEE*, September 1979, p. 226.
24. Martin E. Johnson, "Overview of the File Manager," in *Proceedings of the Fifth Annual Symposium of Computer Applications in Medical Care* (New York: Institute of Electrical and Electronics Engineers, 1981), p. 56.
25. Jan R. Schultz and Layton Davis, "The Technology of PROMIS," in *Proceedings of the IEEE*, September 1976, p. 1237.
26. L. I. Rosen et al., "A Computerized Database System for Medical Diagnostic Studies (DIASTU)," *Computer Programs in Biomedicine*, 1980, p. 249.
27. G. I. Simon et al., "Computerized Pharmacy Services in a Large Community Hospital," *American Journal of Hospital Pharmacy*, May 1976, p. 459.
28. N. S. Read and D. L. Harmon, "Assuring MIS Success," *Datamation*, February 1981, p. 109.
29. Paul D. Keltz et al., "A Minicomputer Network for Diverse Operating Systems and Languages," *Journal of Medical Systems*, 1980, p. 305.

ADDITIONAL READINGS

"Applications-Oriented AI Research: Medicine." In *The Handbook of Artificial Intelligence*, vol. 2, pp. 175-222. Avron Barr and Edward A. Feigenbaum, eds. Stanford, California: HeuisTech Press, 1982.

Aron, Joel D. *The Program Development Process*, Parts I and II. Reading, Massachusetts: Addison-Wesley, 1974. Part I deals with the individual programmer and Part II with the programming team.

Auerbach Publishers, ed. *Practical Data Base Management*. Reston, Virginia: Reston Publishing, 1981.

Barnett, G. Octo et al. "MUMPS—An Evolutionary Commentary." *Computers and Biomedical Research*, 1981, pp. 112-118.

Beizer, Boris. *Software Testing Techniques*. New York: Van Nostrand, 1983.

Bowie, J. and Barnett, G. O. "MUMPS—An Economical and Efficient Time-Sharing System for Information Management." *Computer Programs in Biomedicine*, 1976, pp. 11-22.

Davis, William S. *Operating Systems: A Systematic View*. Reading, Massachusetts: Addison-Wesley, 1978.

Glass, Robert L. *Modern Programming Practices—A Report from Industry*. Englewood Cliffs, New Jersey: Prentice-Hall, 1982.

Greenes, R. A. "MUMPS: Second Decade Design Considerations." *Computers and Biomedical Research*, 1981, pp. 104-111.

Krieg, Arthur F. and Shearer, Lucille K. *Computer Programming in ANS MUMPS, An Instructional Manual for Non-Programmers*. College Park, Maryland: MUMPS Users' Group, 1981.

London, Keith R. *Decision Tables*. Princeton: Auerbach, 1972.

Martin, James. *An End-User Guide to Data Base*. Englewood Cliffs, New Jersey: Prentice-Hall, 1981.

Martin, James. *Application Development Without Programmers*. Englewood Cliffs, New Jersey: Prentice-Hall, 1982.

Mishelovich, David J. et al. "The POIS (Parkland On-line Information System) Implementation of the IBM Health Care Support/Patient Care System." *IEEE Computer*, 1980, pp. 19-33.

Patterson, David A. "Microprogramming." *Scientific American*, 1983, pp. 50-57.

Van Tassel, Dennie. *Program Style, Design, Efficiency, Debugging, and Testing*, 2nd ed. Englewood Cliffs, New Jersey: Prentice-Hall, 1978.

Walters, Richard F. "Is MUMPS the Cure?" *Kilobaud Microcomputing*, 1982, pp. 54-61.

Wickizer, C. R. "The Missouri Automated Radiology System: Its Past and Future," *MUG Quarterly*, Winter 1981-82, p. 30.

Wingert, F. *Medical Informatics: An Introduction*, Lecture Notes in Medical Informatics, vol 14. D.A.B. Lindberg and P. L. Reichertz, eds. Berlin: Springer-Verlag, 1979.

Wirth, Niklaus. *Systematic Programming*. Englewood Cliffs, New Jersey: Prentice-Hall, 1973.

6

Computer Systems

William J. Harvey

Computing resources consist of hardware and software functioning together in the form of a system. A system includes the central processing unit, mass storage facilities, input–output facilities, control equipment, communications equipment and lines, and all software required for operation.

CLASSES OF COMPUTER SYSTEMS

Computer systems are classified by size or attributes of the central processing unit, by mode of operation, or by degree of centralization of database or facilities. They are further classified by the size of certain facilities or operations as 8-bit, 16-bit, or 32-bit systems. Business computer systems are equipped for decimal arithmetic operations, while scientific and technical computers are rated according to the speed of floating point operations, which use special hardware.

The largest computers are called *supercomputers* and are used for national data-processing and database networks, defense installations, and other situations calling for rapid processing of large volumes of data. Most multi-user systems are referred to as *mainframes*. Large mainframe computers are also called *maxicomputers*; small mainframes are usually called *minicomputers*. A group of computers between the two is represented by the large minicomputers, which are called *superminis*. The classification of small business computers ranges from minicomputers to multi-user microcomputer systems. The term *microcomputer* usually refers to a single-user system. Figure 6-1 shows examples of three commonly used classifications by size: large mainframe computers, minicomputers, and microcomputers.

FIGURE 6-1
Examples of Computer Classifications

Classification	*Vendor*	*Model or Series*
Large Mainframe Computers	Burroughs	B7700
	Burroughs	B7900
	Digital	DECsystem-20
	Honeywell	Level 64
	IBM	System/370
	IBM	4331 Series
	IBM	3031 Series
	NCR	Century Series
	NCR	8400 Series
	Singer	System 10
	Sperry-Univac	System 80
Minicomputers, Superminis	Burroughs	B 80
	Burroughs	B1800 Series
	Data General	NOVA 4
	Data General	Eclipse
	Datapoint	8600
	Digital	PDP-11
	Digital	VAX-11
	Four-Phase	IV/60
	Four-Phase	IV/80
	Harris	500
	Hewlett-Packard	1000
	Honeywell	Level 6 DPS
	IBM	Series 1
	IBM	System/3
	MAI/Basic Four	610
	Microdata	4000 Series
	Modcomp	Classic 7840
	NCR	I 8000
	Nixdorf	8870/1
	Perkin-Elmer	Series 3200
	Prime	300
	Point 4	Mark 3
	Sperry-Univac	V 77-400
	Tandem	NonStop Systems
	Texas Instruments	990 Series
	Wang	VS
Microcomputers	Apple	Apple III
	AVL	Eagle III
	Commodore	CBM 8096
	IBM	Personal Computer

FIGURE 6-1—*continued*
Examples of Computer Classifications

Classification	*Vendor*	*Model or Series*
	North Star	Advantage
	Osborne	Osborne I
	Tandy	TRS-80 Model 4
	Xerox	Xerox 820-II
	Zenith	Z-100

Systems that are designed to emulate the function of computers manufactured by another vendor are called *plug-compatible machines*, or *PCMs*.

Traditionally, computer systems have been classified as *batch processing* systems or as *interactive, on-line* systems. Today's automated hospital information systems provide on-line and batch services. A batch is a set of data or transaction records of the same type. Typical of batch processing are daily, weekly, and other periodically generated reports. The data processed in batch programs normally originate from interactive data entry or from data generated automatically by interactive transactions, such as orders or laboratory reports. Batch processing utilizes a master file and a file of currently needed update transactions. The peak time for batch processing each day is usually in the middle of the night, when on-line demands are lower. Many daily hospital reports must be ready for use early in the morning, when offices open and day shifts go on duty. (See Figure 6-2 for flow of data in batch processing.) Monitoring the flow of information is crucial in running a batch system. Adequate processing controls should exist to assure that all data collected are entered, processed, and accurately reported. To avoid errors, change request procedures are used to document requests for revision of applications programs and to assure proper implementation of the changes needed.

Interactive processing of records on line is a form of *real-time* processing and makes virtually immediate response available to the user. Terminals in wards and data entry stations in offices provide access to on-line services. The interactive features of hospital order processing include online viewing of charts, transfers, orders, reminders, and doctors' or nurses' notes. Demand reports are also examples of interactive processing. Order processing in integrated hospital information systems combines batch and interactive services, as shown in Figure 6-3.

Distributed Processing Systems

Distributed systems have multiple processing units that are intercon-

FIGURE 6-2
Flow of Data in a Batch Computer System

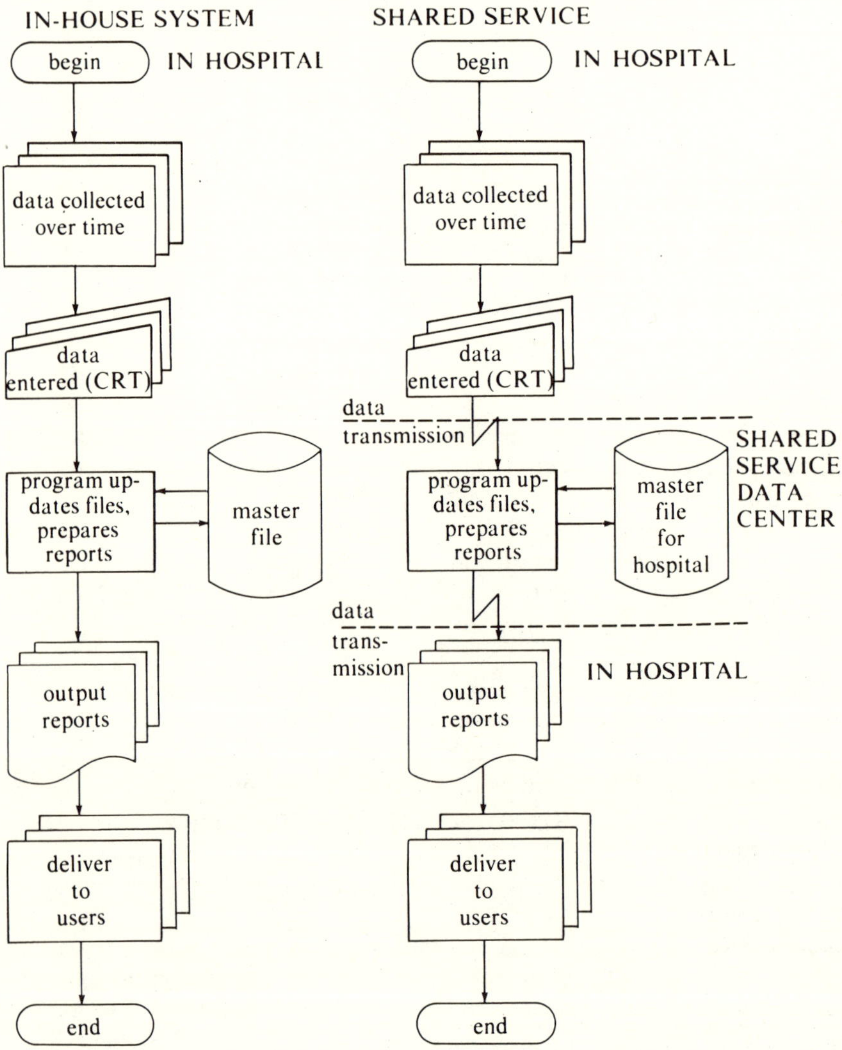

FIGURE 6-2—*continued*
Flow of Data in a Batch Computer System

Examples of Batch Reports in a Hospital Information System

	ACCOUNTS PAYABLE	PATIENT CENSUS	PATIENT BILLING	PAYROLL	INVENTORY
ON DEMAND AS INQUIRIES RECEIVED		Admission Report	Discharged Patient Account		Bin Labels
DAILY OR AS UPDATED		Room and Bed Report	Activity Journals		General Ledger Entries
WEEKLY	Unpaid Vouchers		Medicare Revenue Logs	Timecard Activity Journal	Purchase Orders
MONTHLY	Register of Checks Written	Occupancy Report	General Ledger		Stock Status
QUARTERLY	Vendor Catalog		Trial Balance	Turnover Analysis	
ANNUALLY OR AT FISCAL YEAR END	Liability by Vendor		Year End Audit	W-2 Form Wage and Tax Statement	Use History

FIGURE 6-3
Flow of Information in Hospital Order Processing

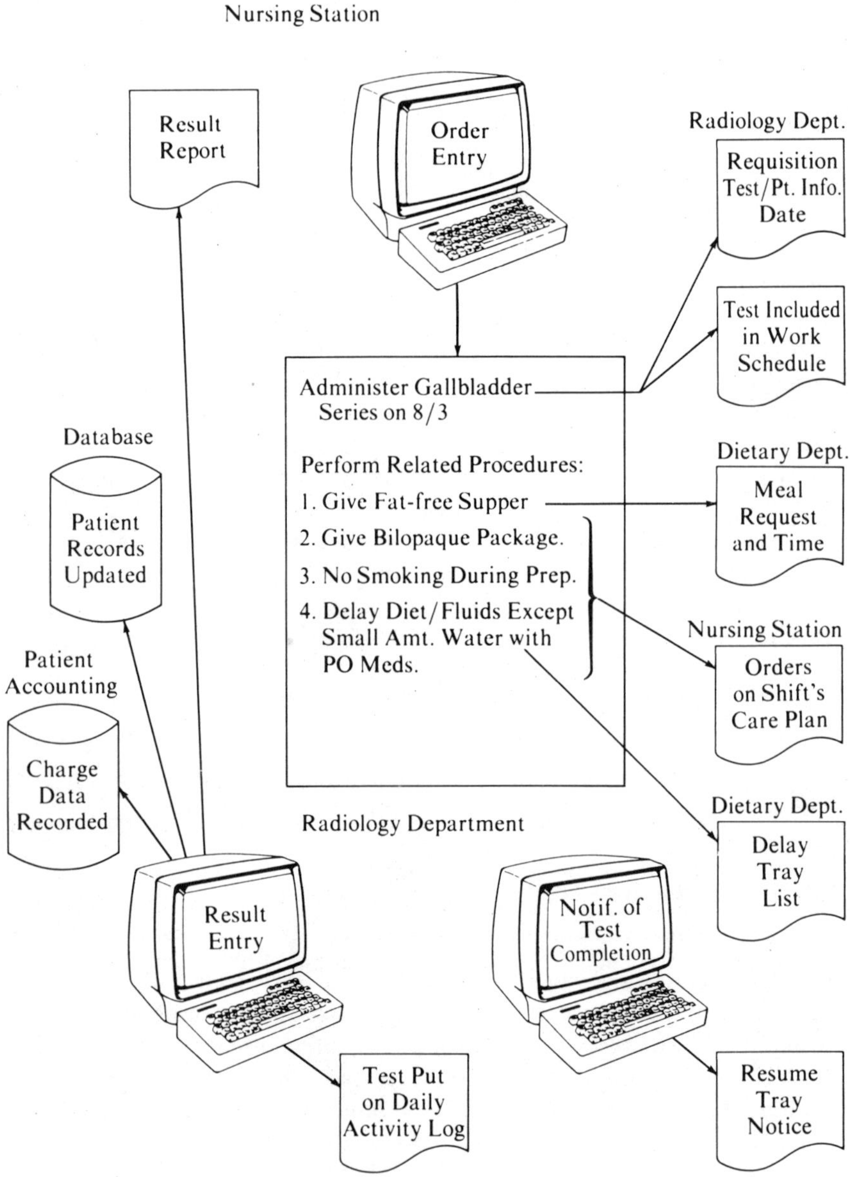

From *Burroughs Hospital Information System (BHIS) Overview Capabilities Manual*. Reprinted with permission of Burroughs Corporation.

nected electronically to make possible significant interaction among the units. A distributed system thus consists of *nodes*, which can be computers or peripherals, and *links*, which provide communication paths between the nodes. The user of a distributed system has access to independent, *local* processing from one of the units in the system and to facilities that are provided by the umbrella of the distributed system. There is "some level of single system image."[1] The mere interconnection of two processing units does not constitute a distributed processing system. Each subsystem unit should be complete and capable of a degree of independent processing, even though a single-system image is presented to users of any part of the entire system. Subsystem units can be interconnected by a bus of parallel circuits for machines in the same room, by in-house wiring between machines in the same building, by permanent common-carrier access in the form of a leased telephone line, or by intermittent common-carrier access provided through automatic-dial modems and a telephone line.

Distributed processing design can contribute added reliability and security. The presence of multiple processing units provides redundancy of hardware and software. Failure of the main processor in a distributed system that is organized hierarchically (that is, where there are higher-level and lower-level processors) will leave the lower-level units capable of performing many routine functions. In a *peer-coupled* system (where all units are the same or similar) the failure of a single unit will not disable the other units, but it may inhibit certain information requests from the units still functioning.

Certain usage and cost factors have accelerated the design and implementation of distributed processing:

1. Growth in demands for increased volume of computing services,
2. Growth in demands for increased versatility of computing services,
3. Reduced costs of processing hardware, and
4. Increased costs of data transmission.

The simultaneous increase in volume of services demanded and in demand for on-line services has stimulated development of distributed processing strategies. Relatively independent handling of data entry at the various nodes of a hospital system relieves the central system's processing facilities of a significant portion of the volume of processing associated with terminal operation and helps assure that response time for communication with the central computer remains acceptable. Where the same function can be provided by a small computer serving as a node of a distributed system or by a large mainframe computer, the *software path length* for handling the transaction on the smaller system can be shorter. This means that fewer software instructions may be required to perform a transaction in a smaller, simpler system. [2]

There are many possible logical and physical configurations for distributed processing systems. The nodes of a distributed system may be located close to one another in a single building, or they may be dispersed and connected only by microwave transmissions. Processing units of vastly different sizes and capabilities may be involved, although some distributed systems utilize a collection of identical subsystem units. There are a great many design options in establishing distributed processing, including assignment of unique, specialized tasks to individual subsystem units.

The handling of data in a distributed system can proceed according to one of several strategies. Files may be physically and logically distributed. Data may be replicated at the nodes of a distributed system. The implementations of such strategies carry with them challenges for maintaining the integrity and accuracy of data. Some fundamental patterns used in distributing data in hierarchical systems are as follows:

1. Certain data at lower-level sites are replicated subsets of data at higher-level sites in the system;
2. Certain voluminous data needed only at the local level are not replicated at the higher level; and
3. Certain data at the lower level are stored independently of the higher level but are available to the higher-level processor when needed.

In many cases, each lower-level processing site will maintain the same types of data for the department in which it is located.

In any distributed processing system, decisions must be made as to the degree of centralization of the system. The following topics are among those reviewed in planning the level of centralization:

1. Practical control by data-processing management: accountability for the entire organization versus accountability for individual departments;
2. Staffing size and quality;
3. Integrity of the entire system performance;
4. Autonomy of departments with specialized functions; and
5. Costs of processing hardware and communications facilities.

Additional specific advantages offered by distributed processing systems include:

1. Data transmission costs are reduced because independent processing at the nodes reduces the quantity and volume of transmissions and permits transmissions to be concentrated into brief bursts of data; and
2. Problems associated with peak load periods can be managed by storing data temporarily at some nodes of a system and forwarding them later to other nodes or the central node.

Whiting-O'Keefe et al. outline the respective advantages and disadvantages of the various configuration options available to hospitals: maxicomputer centralized commercial systems, maxicomputer centralized in-house systems, decentralized minicomputer systems, and distributed minicomputer systems with local networking.[3]

SYSTEM FLOWCHARTS

System flowcharts are used in the design and analysis of computer system functions. Text legends can be entered inside most of the symbol enclosures to specify the nature of the decision, file, type of processing, and so on. The components of a system flowchart fall into the following categories (see Appendix B, Key to Flowcharting Symbols):

- Flow symbols: flowlines, connectors, communication links
- Decision symbols
- Processing symbols
- File media and input-output symbols

Normally the diagrams are read from top to bottom, with *flowlines* showing the logical flow of data in a system. An entire system or a single component, or module, can be displayed by a system flowchart. Connectors are used to identify flowline logic from one module to another or to reduce the number of flowlines on a page and make flowcharts more readable. Communication link symbols are used to indicate connection of physically remote sites that could be connected by common carrier or even by long-distance or satellite microwave transmissions.

Decision symbols mark points in the process where a condition must be evaluated before the data are routed in one direction or another. If the condition statement, which always can be evaluated as true or false, is evaluated as true, the data flow along one flowline. If the condition statement is evaluated as false, then the data flow along another flowline.

The process symbol is used to indicate where in the system computer processing of data is taking place. A legend entered in the process symbol box identifies the particular type of processing in a concise fashion.

The two commonly used file media symbols are intended to resemble magnetic disk packs and magnetic tape reels. These symbols represent storage of a data file on the particular medium. According to placement in the system flowchart, a tape or disk symbol may either mark mass, secondary storage as the source of data for processing, or the destination of data to be stored. These symbols may be used to refer to permanent master files maintained indefinitely, to transaction files accumulated periodically for processing, or to temporary work files used only while data are being processed.

Input and output files are also designed to represent the visual images of the various media. Such symbols make it easier to identify the sources and destinations of characteristic data files. Input files may come from such external off-line sources as printed or handwritten documents, microfilmed documents, punched cards, punched paper tape, and, of course, from direct keyboard entry at a CRT or printer terminal. Output may occur as printed paper, microfilm, microfiche, punched cards, paper tape, and CRT or other display. Examples of system flowcharts are shown in Figures 6-1, 6-2, 7-7, and 8-3.

FILE ORGANIZATION AND DATABASE CONCEPTS

Data reside in programs only as long as the programs are executing. As soon as a program stops execution and delivers its output, the memory locations the program used are reclaimed by the operating system and allocated to other uses. Data files make it possible to retain data between the execution of programs.

Two concepts are common to file structures: *record* and *field*. The logical entities that a file contains are called records. Each separate component within a record is referred to as a field. Any element in a logical file can be identified in terms of the hierarchy of file, record, and field. If one imagines a simple file containing information on three hospitals, it could appear as follows:

File Number	*Record Number*	*Field A (Name)*	*Field B (City)*	*Field C (Telephone)*	*Field D (Beds)*
1	1	County	Roxton	342-5574	142
	2	Memorial	Lakeview	237-4900	205
	3	Bradbury	Bradbury	522-6100	120

In this particular file, each record has four fields. For any file stored and used by a computer, the structure of the file must be predictable. The computer program used to create or to access the file must be able to locate the records and, within the records, to locate the individual fields.

FIGURE 6-4
File Structure: Fixed-Length and Variable-Length Records

Method I — Fixed-length records, 25 characters long, separated by pairs of slashes as delimiters:

/Good Samaritan //St. Luke's /
/County Memorial //Municipal General /
/Tri-County Authority Comm //

Method II — Variable-length records, length in characters given in parantheses at the beginning of each record, records separated by two slashes as delimiters:

/(14)Good Samaritan//(10)St. Luke's//(15)County Memori
al//(17)Municipal General//(30)Tri-County Authority Co
mmunity/

Treatment of fields affects control of record length. Record 1, as compared with Record 2, has multiple repeating fields. Record 2 has an embedded, vacant (empty) field.

Field	Record 1	Record 2
Name	John Smith	Susan Jensen
Address	342 Main St.	1156 Elm St., Apt. 5
City	Boulder	Carpenter
(Phone)	441-6272	(none)
(Spouse)	Diane	George
(Child 1)	Jim	Mark
(Child 2)	Sarah	
(Child 3)	Fred	

Records may have a fixed number of fields, and fields may have fixed lengths. Where the number of fields in a record or the length of text data in a field must vary, information must be stored with the record or field to describe the variation. For example, names have different lengths. There are two ways of storing names so that their precise extent can be determined in the process of retrieval: make all the name fields automatically the same length, or store the length of the name as well as the name. Imagine the same names (Good Samaritan, St. Luke's, County Memorial, Municipal General, Tri-County Authority Community) stored according to each method (see Figure 6-4). As the figure shows, fixed-length records or record fields have the advantage of simple structure. However, the preestablished field will usually be too long or sometimes too short for the data stored, causing wasted space or truncated text. Variable-length records or fields have the advantage of using only as much space as the actual length of the name requires, but the possible disadvantage of a more complex structure and of the need to consume storage space for the lengths.

If a consistent structure is designed for a mailing list, for example, records may have unused fields, which must be accounted for, or repeated field entries of the same type. Compare the two mailing list records in Figure 6-4. In creating files of records such as these, variations in the number of fields can be encountered: the mailing address may require four lines; there may be no spouse; there may be no telephone number; in some cases another telephone number may need to be listed; the number of children may vary; or there may be no children to list. Either a field must be allowed for every possibility, or there must be a method for determining which fields are present for a given record. If fields are not used, the omission must be signified in some way: by the presence of two adjacent delimiters, by a record code, or by storing an appropriate message in the field as a sort of place holder.

When there are limited possibilities for the information to be stored, as with sex, status as a resident of a district, status as insured or not insured, or status as previously admitted, a code provides a compact method of storage. Thus information fields in a record can be as short as a single character (letter or digit).

Records, which are structured to store information, are often referred to as *logical records*. For technical reasons having to do with the characteristics of magnetic tape and magnetic disk storage systems, performance is enhanced by accumulating logical records into groups called *blocks* or *physical records*. Logical records are designed to store individual units of information and may be too short for efficient access. Physical records are larger and more practical for processing. The blocking of logical records into groups reduces the amount of wasted tape consumed by interrecord gaps on tape systems and provides for more efficient use of the access mechanism on disk systems. The number of logical records contained in a block is called the *blocking factor*. Where it is practical to group blocks into larger physical units, such units are called *buckets*.

Commonly used file structures are *sequential, direct*, and *indexed sequential*. Sequentially organized files are well suited to the storage conditions of magnetic tape. All records in the file must be read in sequence until all the desired records have been located. Sequential files are normally organized in the order of a selected field in each record, called the *key*. To implement a direct file structure on disk storage, an index system is created. The index is itself a file containing records with at least two fields: the key of a record stored in the main file and the physical address of the record referred to by the key. Direct file systems use various methods to disperse stored records in such a way as to have efficient storage and retrieval.

With indexed sequential files, it is not necessary to store a key and address for every record. Partial, rather than full, indexing is used. The indexes may refer to a track or bucket by giving the address of one logical record in a large physical record. Where there are large numbers of relatively small records, the size of the index that must be searched can be relatively small.[4]

In some files, each record may contain a *pointer* field. The pointer field contains the address of another record. Pointer fields are used to create compact files which can serve as directories for other files. For example, if records in a file were added (and therefore arranged) in order of arrival, a directory according to some key order could serve as an efficient reference file for searches by that key. Records in the directory could consist only of a key field and a pointer field. Pointer fields are also used to create chained or linked lists. In such lists, each record has a field containing the address of the next record in sequence. One of the uses of such chains of records is to add overflow records to a file. (See Figure 6-5.)

Files that are used in database systems are in *normal form*. Normal form files or tables have a fixed number of fields per record; variable numbers of fields are not permitted in records used in database systems. Beyond this fundamental requirement, additional levels of normal forms are defined by restrictions on *dependencies* of files. All fields in a record contain either (1) information as to what the *key* is or (2) other information. Any field within a record that determines, or helps to determine, the key of the record is called a *key field*. The other fields of the record are referred to as *nonkey* fields. When the design of a record has satisfied normal form requirements, the nonkey fields of the record may not contain information relevant to a portion of the key or to other nonkey fields. In general, such restrictions on the design of table-form data stored in files make it possible to (1) have better control over updating records, (2) avoid redundant storage of data, and (3) design consistent ways of extracting information from the entire database when needed.[5] In practice, the final decision as to data file structure must take into consideration the volumes of respective files and the number of disk accesses that would be generated by operations that occur frequently in the local system applications programs. Database structure and processing flow are shown in Figure 6-6.

File Processing

A file-processing program serves as intermediary between the user of a data file and the logical file stored in a computer system. Operations fundamental to file processing are the establishment of a new file and the operations necessary to maintain the file as conditions change.

In order to establish a new file, space must be reserved in the mass

FIGURE 6-5
File Structure: Use of Pointers

Use of Pointers to Create Linked List

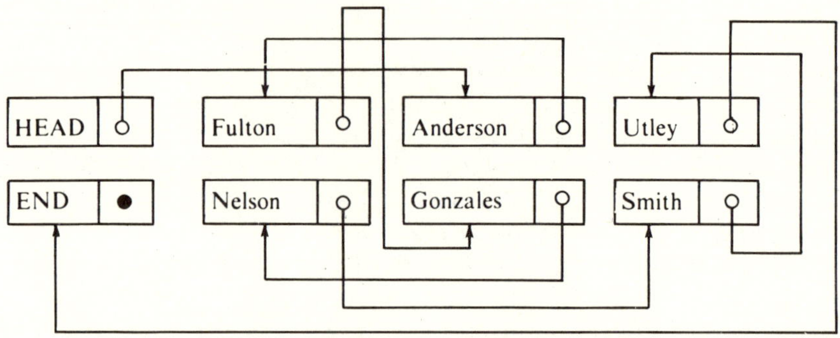

Use of File of Pointers to Index Data File

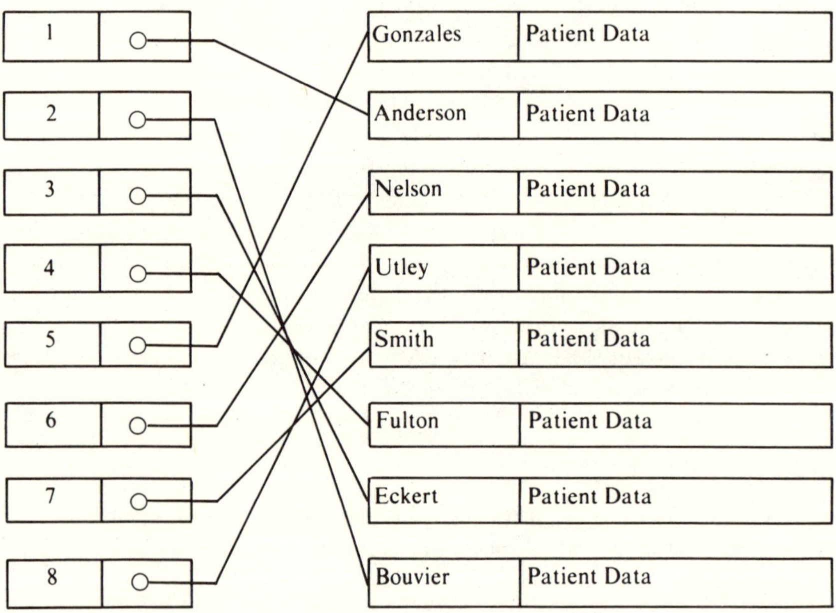

FIGURE 6-6
Database Structure

ACCESS FILE — ACCESS FILE DEFINITIONS

```
PTID   SET OF PAT    KEY IS (PAT—HOSPNO. PAT—PTID)
       INDEX SEQUENTIAL DATA (PAT—PTTYP, PAT—STATUS, PAT—STAMFLAG,
       PAT-PTFCCNGFLG, PAT—REVIEWDT, PAT—BILLFLAG, PAT—TOBEBILLDT,
       PAT—PSTOTHACCT)
       POPULATION=200000 TABLESIZE=52
       LOADFACTOR=90   PACK=BHISDB
COMMENT    START OF PAT DATA FIELDS:
```

DATA NAMES:

BASE NAMES	TYPE	SIZE	INITIAL CONTENTS
PAT—HOSPNO	NUMBER	(2)	REQUIRED:
PAT—SCHCNT	COUNT	(100)	
PAT—PTID	NUMBER	(10)	INITIAL VALUE 0;
PAT—STATUS	NUMBER	(1)	INITIAL VALUE 0;
PAT—PTTYP	NUMBER	(1)	INITIAL VALUE 0;
PAT—PSTOTHACCT	NUMBER	(1)	INITIAL VALUE 0;
PAT—PTTYPPOST	NUMBER	(1)	INITIAL VALUE 0;
PAT—OPPATCL	NUMBER	(2)	INITIAL VALUE 0;
PAT—NAMEPT	ALPHA	(24)	INITIAL VALUE BLANKS;
PAT—PTCARECL	NUMBER	(2)	INITIAL VALUE 0;
PAT—TITLE	ALPHA	(4)	INITIAL VALUE BLANKS;
PAT—SEX	ALPHA	(1)	INITIAL VALUE BLANKS;
PAT—PTTRAVEL	ALPHA	(2)	INITIAL VALUE BLANKS;
PAT—AGE	ALPHA	(3)	INITIAL VALUE BLANKS;
PAT—BRTHDT	NUMBER	(5)	INITIAL VALUE 0;
PAT—SSNPT	ALPHA	(10)	INITIAL VALUE BLANKS;
PAT—PTCATEGORY	NUMBER	(1)	INITIAL VALUE 0;
PAT—FINCLAS	ALPHA	(2)	INITIAL VALUE BLANKS;
PAT—FINCLASPOST	ALPHA	(2)	INITIAL VALUE BLANKS;
PAT—CREDIT	NUMBER	(2)	INITIAL VALUE 0;
PAT—MEDHISTID	ALPHA	(10)	INITIAL VALUE BLANKS;
PAT—DSGDT	NUMBER	(5)	INITIAL VALUE 0;
PAT—DSGTM	NUMBER	(4)	INITIAL VALUE 0;

DASDL Data Dictionary

BASE NAME	FIELD SIZE	FILES IN WHICH FIELD APPEARS
BEDCLEAN	9(1)	HSP
BEEPERNO	A(5)	CNX, PRF
BEEPERNOAD	A(5)	CNX
FNOTBILLD	S9(8)V99	HSP

DATA ELEMENT DESCRIPTION:

BEDCLEAN 9(1) HSP
FLAG INDICATING WHETHER HOSPITAL HAS COMPUTER FUNCTION FOR MAKE BED CLEAN; IF SO, MAY NOT ADMIT OR TRANSFER PATIENT TO BED THAT IS EMPTY DIRTY;
YES=1, NO=0.

BEEPERNO A(5) CNX, PRF
NUMBER OF THE BEEPER ASSIGNED TO THIS PHYSICIAN. USER DEFINED CODE RANGE.

BEEPERNOAD A(5) CNX
NUMBER OF THE BEEPER ASSIGNED TO THIS ADMINISTRATOR. USER DEFINED CODE RANGE.

FNOTBILLD S9(8)V99 HSP
TOTAL BALANCE FORWARD NOT BILLED AT START OF RUN, PART OF BALANCES GROUP.

From *Burroughs Hospital Information System (BHIS) Overview Capabilities Manual*. Reprinted with permission of the Burroughs Corporation. © 1978 Burroughs Corporation.

storage of the computer system. The file must be named so it can be identified in further transactions. Maintaining or updating the file involves three typical transactions: adding a new record, revising an existing record, and deleting an existing record.

Files are often categorized according to their function in the system. The *master file* contains information regarded as permanent. The master file maintains records for processing. Periodically, individual transactions will be collected into a batch for processing in order to update the master file. Such a periodically accumulated file is referred to as a *transaction file*. Commonly used tables of information used in processing may form a separate *table file*. A *history file*, which can consist of a collection of previously used transaction files, is preserved in case it is necessary to reconstruct files. A *log file*, or *journal file*, is normally kept to document all computer activity. Carren describes the way in which up to 24 hours of data can be recovered by using the current job log file in conjunction with the previous night's backup files.[6]

Most file processing is (1) batch preparation of reports and file maintenance, (2) on-line entry of a new file or of additions to an existing file and file interrogation, and (3) database system operation. Batch processing typically deals with the master file and a transaction file. Both files are sorted into sequence according to the same key field or fields. As processing occurs, key fields in the respective files are matched. The file-processing program is designed to respond to the pattern of results of matching the key fields of records from the two files. In updating a file, the master file record is updated when a match is detected. If a key field that is not present in the master file is detected, either an error has occurred or a new record needs to be added to the file. In on-line systems, single requests for file processing are handled as they arise. Database management systems make it possible for new combinations of information to be produced automatically in response to properly formatted inquiries.

Evaluating and Selecting a Computer System

When acquisition of a computer system or of computing services becomes necessary in order to automate existing activities, to increase computing capacity, or to replace outmoded facilities, thorough documentation of functions to be performed is the first step. The principal options are as follows:

1. Purchase or lease of a computer system, assuming in-house management and maintenance of software;
2. Contract for shared computer services, interactive or batch or both; or

3. Contract for facilities management.

Some hospitals acquire systems and manage in-house services for certain functions, while contracting for shared services for other requirements. When the needs to be met through acquisition of a computer system have been adequately described by management and by health care specialists in the departments affected, there is a foundation for evaluation and selection. Recommendations for documentation of function at the departmental level have been described in Chapter 5 under "Guidelines for Acquiring Software."

In order to implement the selection and evaluation process, a Request for Proposal (RFP) is prepared. The RFP announces the acquisition plan and states guidelines for the responses. The design of the RFP is important in the process of acquiring a computer system. The RFP should (1) introduce the vendor to the environment for which the system is intended, (2) state general requirements for information to be supplied, (3) describe any performance bond or equivalent requirement, (4) state conditions of an equipment demonstration, (5) outline the method of financing, (6) specify training and orientation expected, (7) specify warranty and maintenance expected, (8) cite evaluation criteria to be used in evaluating proposals, (9) state the standards of performance that will be used in deciding whether the system is acceptable, and (10) state specifications for particular hardware and software components.[7]

In the introduction to the RFP, the vendor should find information on how the system is to be used and who will use it. The proposed location should be briefly described. Vendors may be invited to inspect the installation site so that they can include necessary changes or additional specifications in their proposals. The vendor should understand all functions expected of the system. Thus the introduction should contain a thorough outline of all computer-based transactions, organized by department or other units of the hospital. Statistics on normal and anticipated levels of activity (bed capacity, occupancy rate, admissions-discharges, outpatient service levels, numbers of records on file, number of personnel, levels of activity by category in departments) are necessary to "size" the system needed; they will be required by the vendor to determine the adequacy of the system proposed and to project the proper configuration.[8] A description of the current computer configuration will help in orienting vendors to the operation and will provide detailed information on interface and conversion problems. The implementation schedule should be outlined. If collaborative proposals (in which more than one vendor is responsible for the system) will not be accepted, a statement should be included stating that all hardware, software, and maintenance is to be supplied by a single vendor. On the other hand, if facilities management can be bid either by the system vendor or separately, a statement to this effect should be included.

It is prudent to stipulate that the successful vendor will be responsible for any interface problems between the system acquired and any existing installations. Where modems and communications lines are involved, there is a tendency for each party involved (installations at both ends and the communication facility, such as a telephone company) to assume that the problem is in someone else's territory. To avoid unexpected charges in conjunction with the proposal and bid process, a clear statement should be included disclaiming responsibility for expenses of the vendors for demonstrations or delivery of information. The name, address, and telephone number of the contact for proposals should appear in the introduction, together with rules designed to prevent problems with clarifications and exceptions. In the case of public-supported and nonprofit institutions, it may be necessary to state that no amounts identified as taxes can be paid as part of the purchase. The key elements of the proposal evaluation process may be summarized, with a reference to the details of evaluation.

General requirements for proposals should specify the format for the reply to the RFP. If all the vendors adhere to the reply format, it will be easier for the buyer to compare proposals. Among the items required should be a vendor profile, an outline of the response, explanation of maintenance coverage, recommended training, a list of users, environmental and physical specifications, the vendor's cost schedule for the hardware and software bid, and assurances of quality. The description of the format for the reply should encourage vendors to supply all relevant information, but it should request that stated section headings, such as those given above, be used in the order listed. A table of contents and divider tabs may be requested. If multiple copies are required, then the number needed should be stated. Complete sets of brochures, description information, operation manuals, and technical reports will aid evaluation of competing proposals. An offer to return materials, except in the case of the successful bidder, may be included.

The vendor profile is intended to assure that the company is stable financially and is capable of providing the kind of long-term support needed for computer products. Examples of pertinent information are the most recent annual report and the company's Dun and Bradstreet rating. A copy of a maintenance contract will aid in assessing a company's policies on maintenance coverage. It is necessary to understand a vendor's capability for providing maintenance at the proposed site. Information on where spare parts are available and on the time necessary to obtain replacement parts should be supplied in the proposal. The vendor's practices with regard to on-site repair and the average response time should be included in the information furnished. The request for a user list or client history should specify any desired limitations to the type of system to be installed or to hospitals with a certain minimum size (in number of beds). The vendor should state what types of training will be necessary for the system, what training materials will be needed, and the minimal skill levels of the persons to be trained. It should be clear where training is to be conducted, how long it will last, and what it will cost. The vendor's quality control program should be adequately described to satisfy the purchaser. Information about the *life-cycle*, or history of availability, of the model offered can be useful. Within the context of the vendor's established practices regarding systems marketed, this information may assist the buyer in evaluating the level of maintenance support that will be sustained for a particular model over the period of use intended by the hospital. If the system proposed has appeared on the market recently, attention will be focussed on assurance of reliability of hardware and software and availability of software.

A performance bond for an amount equal to a substantial fraction of the total purchase price was formerly considered vital to purchasers in those cases where there is a serious performance need with regard to quality, capacity promised, delivery schedule, or maintenance obligations. Under today's financial conditions, vendors will not normally agree to a sizable performance bond. To provide equivalent protection to the purchaser, a carefully prepared contract dealing with acceptance will be needed. For a large system, this may require the services of a specialist, such as an attorney who specializes in computer contracts. According to Vogel, the "establishment of realistic milestones for periodic measures of performance is essential to a successful computer system installation."[9] The standards of performance that will be used to determine whether the system purchased is acceptable should be outlined. The purchaser may specify a performance period during which the level of performance will be measured against the agreed-upon standard.

The method of financing the purchase of the system and of paying recurring costs, such as maintenance, should be stated. Purchase, lease-purchase, and lease are options to be considered. Systems may be leased from the manufacturer or from a third party. Normally the vendor retains title to the computer hardware until the full purchase price has been paid. According to Frankenhuis, the purchaser retains more leverage when a balance is due after the date of delivery.[10] The RFP should include a request for an outline of estimated economic benefits to be gained through installation of the proposed system. Among the estimate categories which may be desired are recovery of lost or late charges, improvement of cash flow, projected labor savings, projected savings in purchase of consumables or in charges for services, and cost containment.

The purchaser may wish to have the option of a system demonstration. Any demonstration should be on a system identical to the one proposed for purchase. The purchaser will want the demonstration to utilize software and source code programs that will assure useful function under normal conditions. The conditions of transfer to backup systems in emergencies should be determined.

In the discussion of training and orientation, the purchaser can elaborate on the number and categories of personnel to receive training. All procedures and categories of personnel should be included in order to obtain accurate training costs.

The more obvious topics to deal with under maintenance are specific provisions desired for warranty and maintenance and responsibility for costs. It may also be prudent to request that all documentation necessary for maintenance be supplied to the purchaser when the maintenance contract period ends, stipulate an agreement on availability of maintenance parts for a set period after the maintenance contract period ends or manufacture of the hardware is halted, and assure access to engineering improvements to the system purchased during the maintenance contract period.

The buyer's task is to determine which proposal offers the lowest cost and the best system to meet the needs of the hospital. The evaluation criteria sections of the RFP should clearly state how costs are to be determined from the information supplied or obtained. A computation of energy consumption costs for each system considered may be included in determining overall costs. The purchaser may wish to determine and add on the costs of any services specified in the RFP but not included in the proposal received. In order not to be held to cost alone, the buyer should outline additional factors that will be considered, such as quality of services, conditions attached to the proposal, promptness of service provided for similar installations, economic benefits, and reputation and resources of the vendor. An evaluation matrix based on cost analysis is described by Reps.[11] Benson proposes an evaluation method using a weighted key factor list.[12]

Specifications and requirements for the system as a whole and particular components should be listed, so that the vendor will know what requirements must be met or exceeded. If examples are given to aid the vendor in understanding what performance is expected, these examples should be carefully chosen to conform to the specifications given. Specifications may be presented in the form of a checklist, so that the vendor using the format affirms by checking off each item that it meets or exceeds the requirements. Space can be included for references documenting the adequacy of vendor information. Forms for supplying a list of user hospitals and for detailing costs can be supplied to vendors with the RFP.

SUMMARY

An understanding of information processing systems is essential for the contemporary hospital manager. Computer systems employ five types of hardware components: one or more computers, input devices such as CRT terminals and remote sensors, output devices such as printers and COM, external memories, and communication links. A computer system consists of the hardware components and the software necessary for operation.

A computer transaction that processes data as soon as they are entered and then sends an acknowledgement or results back to the user is called an interactive transaction. Batch transactions, on the other hand, are processed at fixed intervals. Modern computer systems offer both modes of operation. Through management of an integrated database, the same file structure may serve both interactive and batch operations. Which approach is adopted for a particular application depends on the nature of that application. Financial activities, for example, are handled in batch mode to produce periodic reports and in interactive mode to respond to immediate management needs. The tendency in general is to replace batch reports with interactive access to information.

Computer systems based on multiple processing units are called distributed systems. Distributed information processing makes possible a sharing of load or of computer resources among the computers involved in the system. Increased demand for computer services, increased reliance on interactive transactions for routine health care and management needs, and improvements in technology and software have led to growth in use of distributed processing in hospitals.

File systems enable a program to retrieve data stored previously by nother program. Consistent file structure is required so that the location of elements of a file can be predicted automatically by software in response to user inquiries. Database systems make it possible to reduce redundant storage, avoid problems associated with updating the same information in several locations, and facilitate responses to new requests for information. Files used by a database system must have a normalized table structure so that ambiguities of interpretation are prevented and relationships between data objects stored can be assessed through software.

Thorough, well-organized descriptions of functions to be performed are vital to the acquisition of computer facilities or services. A clearly stated format for proposals from vendors can reduce the labor of evaluating competing proposals and help assure a sound basis for acceptance and rejection of proposals.

DISCUSSION QUESTIONS

6-1 What is the significance of such terms as "8-bit", "16-bit", or "32-bit" in classifying computer systems?

6-2 What are the principal advantages of distributed processing systems? What are some limitations or disadvantages of distributed processing systems?

6-3 Discuss the role of *software path length* in system performance.

6-4 What are some strategies for handling data in a distributed processing system?

6-5 What is the fundamental purpose of data files in a computer system?

6-6 What must be taken into account in designing a file? What options are there with regard to record structure?

6-7 What restrictions are there on the design of files to be used in database management systems?

6-8 What are the major categories of file in a computer system, and what are the functions of each category?

6-9 Distinguish between file structure and file access method. Give examples of each.

6-10 Discuss the pros and cons of disclosing the acquisition budget figure in the RFP.

6-11 How are the performance requirements of a desired computer system described in the RFP?

6-12 What can be gained in the proposal evaluation process by reviewing information on the life cycle of the model proposed by a vendor (that is, the history of availability of the model)?

6-13 What can be gained in the proposal evaluation process by reviewing vendor profile information?

6-14 What are the practical problems of evaluating proposals after they have been received? How can the specification section of the RFP be designed to facilitate evaluation of competing proposals? In what other ways can the design of the RFP help in obtaining proposals that are easier to evaluate?

6-15 Cite the respective merits of these options in obtaining computer services: purchase or lease of a system to be used in conjunction with in-house software management, shared services contract, and facilities management contract.

6-16 Why might it make sense to announce in the RFP that collaborative proposals (those involving more than one vendor) will not be accepted? Under what circumstances would it make sense to omit such a stipulation in drafting the RFP?

PROBLEMS

For problems 6-1 to 6-6, refer to Figure 6-1. Models other than those given in Figure 6-1, if relevant to hospital information systems, may be used as examples. Recommended sources of information are management aids, such as those provided by Auerbach, Data Decisions, Data Sources, Datapro Research, and others; vendor brochures or publications; directories of corporations; articles in journals; telephone directories; and other current materials.

6-1 For any three large mainframe models, determine:
(a) Typical or entry-level configurations
(b) Specialized architecture features
(c) Computer languages (compilers, interpreters) available for each system
(d) Type of main storage
(e) Capacity of main storage
(f) Cycle time
(g) Error checking or protection
(h) Communications or message control software
(i) Editing facilities

6-2 For any three minicomputer models, determine:
(a) Typical or entry-level configurations
(b) Number installed (as of the date of the reference used)
(c) Date the model became available
(d) Type of internal code (ASCII or EBCDIC)
(e) Type of main storage
(f) Capacity of main storage
(g) Cycle time
(h) Availability of virtual memory
(i) Rate of transfer of data for input and output

6-3 As best you can, design a configuration for a given model. Determine the following for the equipment configuration you select:
(a) Purchase price
(b) Monthly lease on a 1-year lease basis
(c) Monthly lease on a 5-year lease basis
(d) Monthly maintenance charge

6-4 For the configuration described in Problem 6-3, compare lease and purchase costs and formulate a recommendation as to which acquisition method to use.

6-5 Select software acquisitions for a particular system.
Determine all fees involved for the first year of operation.
Specify for each software item whether any particular type of license is required. Include initial fees and monthly charges, as appropriate.

6-6 For any three vendors, determine:
(a) Headquarters address
(b) Headquarters telephone number

(c) Name of the executive(s) in charge of marketing data-processing hardware and software
(d) Ownership status of the firm
(e) Percent of gross sales due to marketing of data-processing products and services
(f) Number of employees the firm has
(g) Date the firm was established
(h) Lines of data-processing products or type of data-processing services of the firm
(i) Countries outside the United States where the firm has operations
(j) Closest office address (headquarters or branch office)

6-7 Identify six firms offering time-sharing and remote computing services for hospitals. For each firm, determine:
(a) Name of the service
(b) Geographical areas served by the service
(c) Type(s) of terminal(s) supported
(d) Year the service became operational
(e) Charges for the various applicable charge categories
(f) Number of simultaneous users

6-8 Select three software products that perform the same or comparable tasks. Compare these products with regard to user ratings of reliability, ease of use, documentation, and maintenance of the product by the vendor. On the basis of this information, specify which of the three you would recommend for acquisition.

6-9 Identify three models of computer output microfilm (COM) units. For each model, determine:
(a) Whether the model can be used on-line or off-line or both
(b) Input data transfer rate for on-line and off-line uses
(c) Character generation technique used
(d) Width, form and frame orientation of film
(e) Text (alphanumeric) capabilities with respect to number, types and sizes of character fonts
(f) Graphics and forms overlay capabilities
(g) Performance characteristics
(h) Purchase price
(i) Number of installations as of the date of the reference used

6-10 Decide whether it is to the advantage of a hospital to use commercial COM services for microfiche record production or to acquire in-house equipment for on-line use for the following monthly levels of use:
500 masters, 8 copies of each master

2000 masters, 10 copies of each master
4000 masters, 12 copies of each master

Use the equipment acquisition prices obtained in problem 6-9 and area COM service bureau charges. Consider the following criteria:

(a) Prime-time and off-shift maintenance costs

(b) Salaries (regular and other shifts, including fringe benefits) for operating personnel and systems or data processing personnel involved in setting up production

(c) Management and accounting overhead

(d) Floor space

(e) Utilities

(f) Special facilities, such as air conditioning, required venting, sinks, and storage

(g) Insurance and taxes, if applicable

(h) Consumables (chemicals and other supplies)

6-11 Select one model for each of the following: (1) train impact line printer; (2) electrostatic page printer; and (3) laser printer. Discuss the advantages and disadvantages of each. State under what operating conditions you would recommend one over the others. Consider the performance characteristics, type of paper used, price, and volume of output per day of the installation for which the printer is intended.

NOTES

1. Harold Lorin, *Aspects of Distributed Computers* (New York: Wiley-Interscience, 1980), p. 4.
2. James Martin, *Computer Networks and Distributed Processing* (Englewood Cliffs, New Jersey: Prentice-Hall, 1981), p. 24.
3. Quinn E. Whiting-O'Keefe et al., "The Argument for Modular Distributed Hospital Information Systems (HIS)," in *Proceedings of the Fifth Annual Symposium of Computer Applications in Medical Care* (New York: Institute of Electrical and Electronics Engineers, 1981), pp. 913-916.
4. Owen Hanson, *Design of Computer Data Files* (Rockville, Maryland: Computer Science Books, 1982), pp. 206-207.
5. William Kent, "A Simple Guide to Five Normal Forms in Relational Database Theory," *Communications of the ACM* 26, February 1983, pp. 120-125.
6. Donald M. Carren, "Multiple Minis for Information Management," *Datamation*, September 1975, pp. 54-57.
7. Lowell N. Ballew, "Outline of a Request for Quotation," unpublished study guide for Computer Science 542, Data Processing Management, East Texas State University, Commerce, Tex., 1980.
8. "Burroughs Hospital Information System: Executive Questionnaire," information-gathering form used by Burroughs Corporation.

9. Peter S. Vogel, "Computer Wars: Vendor vs. Lawyer," *The National Law Journal*, November 2, 1981, p. 22.
10. Jean-Pierre Frankenhuis, "How To Get a Good Mini," *Harvard Business Review*, May-June 1982, p. 147.
11. David Reps, "Sort DP Proposals with this Input/Output Cost Matrix," *HFM*, January 1977, p. 39.
12. Donald Benson, "Hospital Computer Evaluation and Selection," *CRC Critical Reviews in Bioengineering*, June 1975, pp. 256-257.

ADDITIONAL READINGS

Auer, Joseph and Harris, Charles E. *Major Equipment Procurement*. New York: Van Nostrand Reinhold, 1983.

Bradley, James. *File and Data Base Techniques*. New York: Holt, 1982.

Brickman, Bruce K. *Solving the Computer Contract Dilemma*. Rochelle Park, New Jersey: Hayden, 1983.

Finkel, LeRoy and Brown, Jerald R. *Data File Programming in BASIC: A Self-Teaching Guide*. New York: Wiley, 1981.

Jacobs, Stanley E. "Facilities Management of Hospital Data Processing." In *Proceedings of the Fifth Annual Symposium on Computer Applications in Medical Care*, Henry G. Heffernan, ed. Los Angeles: IEEE Computer Society, 1981, pp. 907-911. This article contains a listing of vendors who provide facilities management for hospital data processing, p. 911.

Ullman, Jeffrey D. *Principles of Database Systems*, 2nd. ed. Rockville, Maryland: Computer Science Press, 1982.

Welburn, Tyler. *Advanced Structured COBOL: Batch, On-line, and Data-base Concepts*. Palo Alto, California: Mayfield, 1983.

Wiederhold, Gio. "Database Technology in Health Care." *Journal of Medical Systems*, 1981, pp. 175-196.

III

Information Systems Analysis, Design, and Implementation

7

Information Systems Analysis

Systems analysis is a necessary first step in the design and implementation of any hospital information system.* Guided by the principles and priorities set forth in the hospital's master plan for information system development, systems planners should conduct a careful study of functional system requirements in advance of the design stage of a project. Technically trained staff (systems analysts and management engineers) and hospital operating personnel who will be using the information system must join in this effort. Systems analysis will pay dividends whether or not any automated information system is the result.

System development projects in the hospital should be pursued by a project team. The team should include a balanced combination of people who know the hospital well and people who have technical knowledge of systems analysis and design techniques. The team should study the functional requirements of the system before the system characteristics are specified, just as an architect would join with hospital personnel to determine the specific functional requirements for a new building (taking a complete inventory of activities that will be carried out in the new facility and examining them in detail) before the specific design characteristics of the building are drawn up.

Organizing a Project Team

A senior systems analyst should serve as project leader (if the project is to be carried out using in-house staff). The person chosen for this task should not be a narrow specialist in computer technology, but rather should combine systems knowledge with experience and understanding of hospital operations and the idiosyncracies of the complex hospital environment.

---

* See Chapter 3 for a review of the five steps in the cycle of information systems development.

At least one representative of each department to be using information or generating data in the new system should be assigned to serve on the project team. Departmental representatives should be key staff members who understand departmental procedures and policies in their totality rather than individuals who are specialists in only a small phase of departmental activity. It may be important that the department manager serve on the project team. Alternatively, a top assistant might serve in this role well and might not be burdened with day-to-day operational problems, as would the department manager. An important responsibility of each departmental representative is to provide a liaison between the project team and the department.

Finally, every project team should include a representative of the hospital administration who can interpret hospital-wide policy and serve as a liaison with the administrator as the new system develops. This could be the administrator, but in larger hospitals it often would be an assistant or associate administrator or a major staff aide.

If a systems project is to be carried out under contract, the contract specifications should call for a similar form of project organization. The contractor should provide the project leader and technical staff, but hospital operating personnel should be involved in the same way as they are for an in-house effort. If this is not done, the result often will be a system which is elegant in its technical design but out of touch with the realities of a particular hospital and its environment. Early involvement of hospital personnel in a contractor-developed system also will aid immeasurably in system maintenance after the new system is working and contractor personnel have departed.

Once the project team has been organized, agreement should be reached on a regular schedule of periodic meetings to assess progress and to report on various phases of the project. Also, estimates should be made of their time requirements for each member of the team and these should be formalized in writing and agreed to by the appropriate department manager as well as the hospital administrator. Formalizing a time commitment for each member of the team will help to insure availability of key personnel when they are needed, particularly when other demands for their time compete with the system project, as inevitably they will. The best insurance a hospital can have against a poorly designed system is the active and enthusiastic involvement of its own personnel, particularly in the early stages of analysis and development of system requirements.

THE SYSTEMS ANALYSIS PROCESS

Systems analysis should provide answers to a series of questions regarding the proposed new system. What are the weaknesses of the present system? What are its strengths? Why is a new system needed? What specific kinds of information should the system generate? When does this information need to be available? Who will use it? In what ways will it be used? Where does the needed data originate? Answering questions such as these is the basic task of systems analysis.

Note that the question, "How will the new system provide the requisite information?" is not included here. This is the basic task of the design phase of the project. The details of how information requirements are to be met should not constrain a systems project too early. Rather, requirements should be stated and ways should be found to meet these requirements. More problems in hospital information systems have resulted from inadequate analysis and lack of specification of system requirements than from shortage of available information systems technology.

Systems analysis is the process of *collecting, organizing*, and *evaluating* facts about information system requirements and the environment in which the system will operate.[1] If the proposed information system is to replace an existing one, regardless of whether information is obtained manually or through machine processing, then the first step of systems analysis should be a complete study of existing procedures, their strengths and weaknesses.

Collecting the data. Data on system requirements are collected through a variety of mechanisms. Key personnel in the hospital departments involved in the information system should be interviewed as one means of documenting present procedures and obtaining input on new system characteristics that are desirable. Interviews should be carefully planned, and a structured interview guide should be prepared in advance to facilitate the interview and to be sure that key points are covered. An example of an interview guide to be used in obtaining information from the director of a hospital's clinical laboratory is shown in Figure 7-1. Following a structured format, data are obtained on departmental organization, staffing, workload, facilities, current procedures, information flows, problems, and unmet information requirements.

Data can also be obtained through the use of questionnaires. Time and resources permitting, however, a face-to-face interview is preferable, since it permits elaboration and dialogue not possible with a questionnaire. Questionnaires can be particularly useful in obtaining a representative sample of data from a larger group—for example, patient opinions on an existing service or proposed new procedure.

In addition to using interviews and questionnaires, those involved on the project team, particularly the project leader and other members of the technical staff, should observe operations in the departments to be involved

FIGURE 7-1
Interview Guide—Director of Hospital Clinical Laboratory

Background Information

1. How is the laboratory organized? Chart available?
2. What are current staffing levels (numbers of personnel by job category and levels of training)? Position descriptions available?
3. What are current lab workloads? Volume of work by type of test? Percentage of stat orders? Statistical summary available? Frequency distribution over the workday.
4. What kinds of equipment and other specialized facilities are used? Any urgent needs for new equipment at present?
5. Describe relationships with other units of hospital: (a) frequent interaction (e.g., daily); (b) less frequent interaction.
6. Describe goals and objectives of laboratory. Copy of goals statement available?

Departmental Procedures

1. How are specimens obtained from patients?
2. How are stat orders handled?
3. What degree of automation is used in testing?
4. How are test results transmitted back to the patient's chart?
5. How are charges transmitted to the business office?
6. What kinds of quality control procedures are used?
7. Procedures manual available?

Information Flows

1. What reports are generated in the lab?
2. What other kinds of information are produced? Telephone communications? Verbal reports?
3. What kind of input information do you receive from other departments? Sample forms available?
4. What kind of data coding systems are used? Code lists available?
5. What master files do you maintain in the lab?

Assessment and Problems

1. What are your major problems in lab operations? What are some of your less serious problems?
2. Any specific problems in information flow?
3. What are the major gaps and inefficiencies in your lab information system? Are error rates too high? Are input forms or reports consistently late?
4. How could a new or revised information system serve you better? What would you like to see in such a system?
5. Other comments or suggestions?

---

in the information system. Observation will supplement information obtained through interviews and often will point up the need for system characteristics which did not surface during conversations with hospital personnel. Of particular importance, systems analysts should pay close attention to environmental factors while observing departmental operations. Physical facilities, leadership styles of supervisors, degree of formality or informality in departmental procedures, and other elements of the day-to-day working environment can have a tremendous impact on how a system will function in a given organization.

Notes should be taken throughout the data collection process, and other written documentation should be obtained, including sample reports, completed forms, procedural manuals, and organizational charts.

Organizing the Data. The collected data should be analyzed according to standard formats, and summary tables should be prepared for these. Figures 7-2, 7-3, and 7-4 are examples of standard forms for summarizing data obtained from reports, input documents, and master files. Figure 7-5 is a possible format for a table summarizing data on current reports. Figure 7-6 is a graphic analysis of fluctuations in workload in a hospital clinical laboratory. Workload summaries such as these are important for obtaining estimates of the volume of activity to be included in an information system. In addition to tabular and graphic organization of data, interview reports and observations of department operations should be written up in concise narrative format.

One of the most useful tools in systems analysis is the flowchart. Flowcharts provide a concise, logical, and standardized mechanism for depicting and analyzing current information flows. They help to pinpoint errors, inconsistencies, and inefficiencies in information flows and are very helpful in estimating the effects of changes on current departmental operations. Flowcharts illustrate relationships among various hospital functions as far as information interchange is concerned. This is a critical element of information system analysis, since the identification of interfaces among functions is most important when attempting to achieve modular or total systems integration.

Figure 7-7 is an example of an actual system flowchart produced by graduate students in hospital administration as part of the requirements for a class in hospital systems analysis. A project team of four students conducted an in-depth study of the procedures and information flow in the clinical laboratory of a 273-bed general medical and surgical facility. The flowchart indicates the process followed in ordering lab tests, obtaining specimens, conducting the tests, and reporting results. The flow of information throughout this process is shown in a concise and logical format through the flowchart.

FIGURE 7–2
Report Analysis Form

<table>
<tr><td>Report No.</td><td>Name:</td></tr>
<tr><td colspan="2">Generated by (department):</td></tr>
<tr><td colspan="2">Purpose:</td></tr>
<tr><td>General Content:</td><td>Source of Data Contained in the Report:</td></tr>
<tr><td>Distribution to:</td><td>Schedule:
—Daily ___
—Weekly ___
—Monthly ___
—Quarterly ___
—Annual ___
—Other (specify)
______________</td></tr>
<tr><td>Volume (average number of pages)</td><td>Processing:
—Manual ______
—Computer ______
—Other (specify) ______________
______________</td></tr>
<tr><td>Problems:</td><td>Other comments:</td></tr>
</table>

FIGURE 7–3
Input Document Analysis Form

<table>
<tr><td>Form No.</td><td colspan="2">Name:</td></tr>
<tr><td colspan="3">Prepared by (department):</td></tr>
<tr><td colspan="3">Purpose:</td></tr>
<tr><td colspan="3">How is data obtained?</td></tr>
<tr><td colspan="2">Distribution—copies to:</td><td>Volume:
_____ forms per ____________
(time period)

____
Schedule for completing form:</td></tr>
<tr><td colspan="2">Problems:</td><td>Other comments:</td></tr>
</table>

Several problems were identified as a result of the analysis. These included breakdowns in communication between ward and lab personnel, lost charges for tests performed, problems with the pneumatic tube system used to transmit information, and the need for more preadmission testing. With the aid of the flowchart and other tools of systems analysis, immediate solutions to each of these problems could be recommended to hospital management. In addition, the flowcharts and other analyses can serve as the basis for an automated information-processing system in the laboratory

FIGURE 7–4
Master File Analysis Form

Master File No.	Name:
File maintained by (department):	
Purpose:	
Content:	
Form: Computer (disk) ___ 3 x 5 cards ___ Computer (tape) ___ File folders ___ Kardex ___ Other (specify) ______	
Volume:	Frequency of updating:
Data in file accessible to:	
Problems:	Other comments:

should a decision be reached in the future to design and implement such a system.

Evaluating the Data. After data have been collected and organized into tables, graphs, flowcharts, and narrative summaries, analysis and eval-

FIGURE 7–5
Reports Inventory

INFORMATION SYSTEMS ANALYSIS OF ________________
(Functional Area)

Report No.	Name	Purpose	Generated by (Department)	Volume	Processing Mode			Comments*
					Manual	Computer	Other	

*Include estimates of time and manpower required to prepare the report, if available.

uation can begin. The analysis should include a complete examination of all aspects of the present system and documentation of new system requirements. The following elements should be included.

1. Analysis of workloads: Are loads evenly distributed across work stations, or are there bottlenecks at critical points in the process? How are workloads distributed over time and why are they so distributed? Are there peak load periods and slack periods? How does information aid or impede the work of the departments involved in the system? How could a revised information system facilitate workload?
2. Report utilization: How are current reports actually used? Are there some which really are not used at all? Are the costs of generating a particular report worth the benefits received from having it? What are the deficiencies in current reports? What new reports or revisions to existing reports should be included in the new system?
3. Input and data collection analysis: What are the current problems in data collection? Are forms efficiently designed? Are data transcribed from document to document more than is necessary? What are the error rates on data entry? Are the same data captured

FIGURE 7–6
Workload Summary—Clinical Laboratory

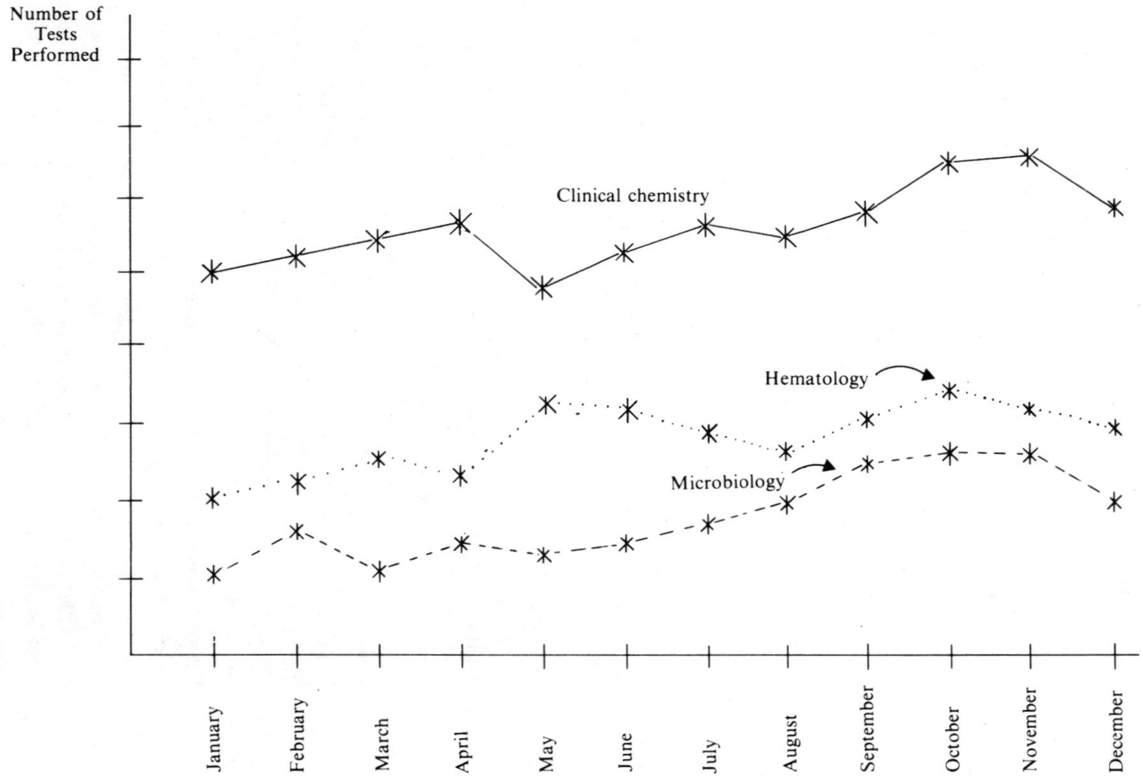

FIGURE 7–7
System Flowchart—Ordering Tests and Obtaining Specimens

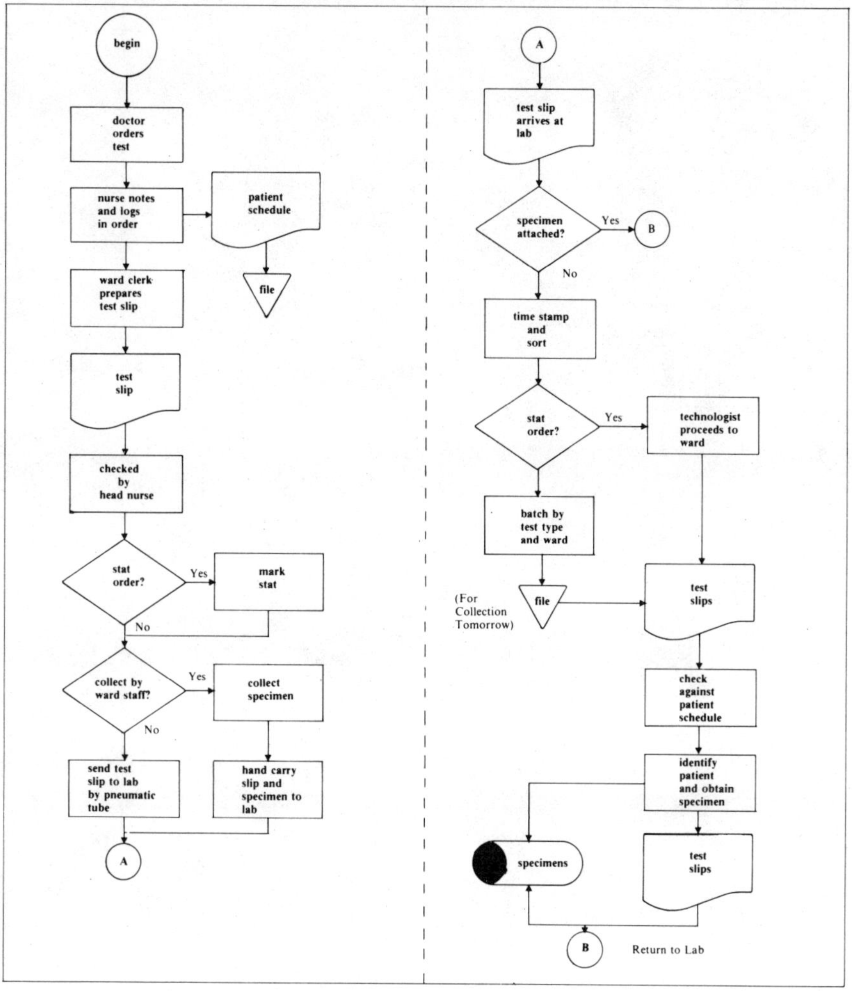

repetitively by various organizational units? How can data collection be improved? What new kinds of data are needed to meet system requirements? What data elements currently collected can be eliminated?

4. Code analysis: What codes and coding systems are presently used? Are they consistent throughout the hospital? Are codes designed

FIGURE 7–7 (continued)
System Flowchart—Testing and Reporting

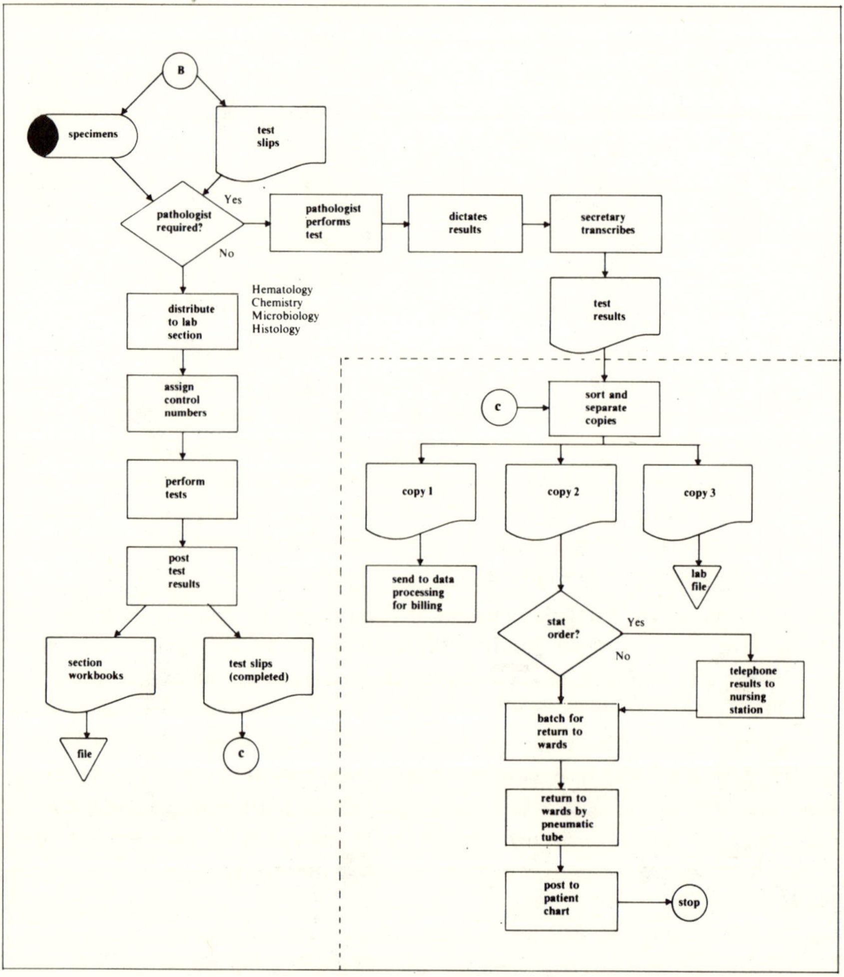

simply to identify data elements or do they also categorize? Are checking systems built into coding structures? Are codes flexibly designed and expandable to handle an increased volume of transactions? Are codes consistent with other hospitals' for comparative purposes? Are the codes consistent with external reporting needs? What kinds of coding systems are needed in order that the new information system may be designed?

5. Master file analysis: Are data elements duplicated in master files throughout the hospital? Is such duplication necessary? Are files updated according to a periodic schedule? Have files become cluttered with out-of-date material? Are the files properly indexed and accessible for retrieval of needed information? What data are being retained in master files needlessly? How can files be improved? What new files are needed for the new system?
6. Procedures and information flow analysis: How efficient are current operating procedures? What improvements are needed? Does information flow smoothly and on a timely basis? How can information flow be handled more expeditiously so that information truly supports operations and management decisions?
7. Cost analysis: What are the current costs to the hospital of processing information in the area under study? Are these costs reasonable? Higher than expected? The cost analysis should be a complete study of all costs incurred in collecting, storing, processing, retrieving, and utilizing information under procedures presently employed by the hospital. Cost data gathered at this phase of a system project provide important benchmark information for later comparison with costs of the proposed new system.

This is only a brief description of the process of systems analysis. The reader interested in more detail is directed to one of the several references on this subject included in the Additional Readings at the end of the chapter. The system analysis process itself has been subjected to automation. There are computer programs available to aid in the organization and analysis of data obtained in a systems study. Not only do these systems facilitate the analysis of data, they also provide a standardized protocol for collecting the data. Their use should be investigated by any project team about to undertake a systems analysis of a major functional area of the hospital.

Benefits of Systems Analysis

There are many benefits which accrue from systems analysis, whether or not the system is adopted. Systems analysis requires careful self-examination of current hospital procedures. Any such analysis, properly performed, will result in procedural changes and methods improvement which in themselves should be worth the cost of the analysis. Systems analysis will also result in the development of standards for the hospital, for both procedure and performance. In most hospitals, such standards are needed badly in order to improve management control and accountability of operations.

The analysis also provides documentation of existing procedures and information flow which many hospitals do not compile in a systematic manner. Finally, systems analysis permits decisions about information systems to be based upon objective data and careful examination of requirements rather than intuition. As such, it provides a strong foundation upon which a new information system can rest.

SUMMARY

Systems analysis is the process of collecting, organizing, and evaluating facts about information system requirements and should provide answers to fundamental questions. Systems development projects should be carried out by a project team, headed by a senior systems analyst and including representatives of relevant hospital departments and a representative of hospital administration. If an outside contractor is to be employed for systems development work, the same form of project organization should be a requirement of the contract.

Data about system requirements are obtained through interviews, questionnaires, observation of hospital operations, and review of written documentation. Once data from a systems analysis have been collected and organized, a variety of analyses are carried out. These include analysis of workloads, report utilization, input and data collection analysis, code analysis, master file analysis, procedures and information flow analysis, and analysis of present system costs.

Systems analysis provides the benefits of self-examination, improvement of operations, and development of standards. Of greater importance, systems analysis provides a strong foundation upon which to build automated information systems for the hospital.

DISCUSSION QUESTIONS

7-1 What is the purpose of systems analysis in hospitals?

7-2 Give examples of the kinds of questions which systems analysis should address.

7-3 Why is a project team organization important in the conduct of a systems analysis in the hospital? How should a team be organized? Why should a systems analyst be assigned as team leader?

7-4 What kinds of data are collected in hospital systems analysis?

7-5 How are these data organized for subsequent analysis?

7-6 What are some of the specific analytical tools and techniques that can be employed once data are collected and organized?

7-7 Why is documentation of present system costs important?

7-8 What are some of the benefits to the hospital from a well-conducted systems analysis? Should the analysis always lead to development of an automated information system?

PROBLEMS

7-1 Draw up an organization chart and work plan for a systems analysis of the billing and accounts receivable functions in a community general hospital of 350 beds.

7-2 Design a set of standardized forms for gathering data in a systems analysis of the admitting process of a general hospital.

7-3 Conduct a study of information flow in a functional area of a hospital. Develop a systems flowchart with accompanying narrative notes. Describe improvements which could be made in the present system as a result of your study.

NOTE

1. See Robert H. Gregory and Richard L. Van Horn, *Automatic Data Processing Systems: Principles and Procedures* (Belmont, California: Wadsworth Publishing Co., 1965), p. 175.

ADDITIONAL READINGS

Adler, David A. and Edwards, Carl N. "Issues Encountered in an Attempt to Implement a Second-Generation Management Information System." *Public Health Reports*, July-August, 1981, pp. 369-375.

Bennett, Addison C. "Systems Approach is Needed for Data Processing Function." *Hospitals*, February 1, 1979, pp. 48-51.

Bingham, J.E. and Davies, G.W.P. *A Handbook of Systems Analysis.* New York: John Wiley & Sons, 1972.

Carlsen, Robert D. and Lewis, James A. *The Systems Analysis Workbook.* Englewood Cliffs, New Jersey: Prentice-Hall, 1973.

Davis, G.B. "Strategies for Information Requirements Determination." *IBM Systems Journal*, Vol. 21, No. 1, 1982, pp. 4-30.

Donaldson, Hamish. *A Guide to the Successful Management of Computer Projects.* New York: John Wiley & Sons, 1978. Note particularly Chapter 5, "Survey Stage of Project Development."

Fitzgerald, John M. and Fitzgerald, Adra F. *Fundamentals of Systems Analysis.* New York: John Wiley & Sons, 1973.

Garrett, Raymon D. *Hospitals—A Systems Approach.* Philadelphia: Auerbach Publishers, 1973. Note particularly Chapter 8, "System Analysis, Design and Implementation."

Gildersleeve, Thomas R. *Successful Data Processing Systems Analysis.* Englewood Cliffs, New Jersey: Prentice-Hall, 1978.

Gore, Marvin and Stubbe, John. *Elements of Systems Analysis for Business Data Processing* (Second Edition). Dubuque, Iowa: Wm. C. Brown Co., 1979. Note particularly Unit Three, "The Study Phase."

Lott, Richard W. *Basic Systems Analysis*. San Francisco: Canfield Press, 1971.

Lucas, Henry C. *The Analysis, Design, and Implementation of Information Systems*. New York: McGraw-Hill, 1981. Note particularly Chapters 6-8.

Thomas, J. William and Lowery, Julie. "Determining Information Needs of Hospital Managers: The Critical-Success Factor Approach." *Inquiry*, Winter 1981, pp. 300-310.

Thierauf, Robert W. and Reynolds, George W. *Systems Analysis & Design: A Case Study Approach*. Columbus, Ohio: Charles E. Merrill Publishing Co., 1980.

Webb, Robert E. "Cost Justification for a Hospital Information System." *Hospital Topics*, January-February 1982, pp. 22-26.

Wetherbe, James C. *Systems Analysis for Computer-Based Information Systems*. St. Paul, Minnesota: West Publishing Co., 1979.

8

Information Systems Design

Design of a hospital information system should flow readily from a carefully executed analysis of information system requirements. Following guidelines provided by the hospital's master plan for information systems development, the next step of the five outlined in Chapter 3 should be selection of a design approach.

SELECTION OF A DESIGN APPROACH

The alternatives available in selection of a design approach cover a spectrum ranging from minor improvements upon an existing manual system to complete redesign of a new, automated information system unconstrained by current policies and procedures. If the systems analysis shows that the existing system is working well or if the analysis indicates that the cost of a new information system would be prohibitive, then the project team should recommend that specific changes and improvements be made to the existing system. After these changes are in place, the project team should be disbanded and no further efforts put forth on development of a new system. Assuming that the systems analysis indicates that the project of designing a new information system should proceed, then several alternative design strategies can be considered. One such strategy would be full or partial *mechanization* of the existing information-processing system. That is, computer processing would be substituted in part or in full for work now carried out manually. Under this alternative, current policies and procedures would not be changed. The only change would be introduction of machine processing into existing procedures. Although there are situations in which this alternative may be the best one for a hospital to follow, it should be carefully scrutinized before it is adopted.

If a systems analysis has been executed properly, it is quite likely that the analysis will uncover needed changes in existing procedures and practices, such as reports which are no longer useful, bottlenecks in current work flow, new reports which are needed, rescheduling of information flow in order to generate data on a more timely basis, and inefficiencies in existing organizational arrangements. If the choice is simply to introduce machine processing of data and not to attack these other problems, then the hospital will not have taken full advantage of the systems analysis.

However, in certain cases (particularly in well-defined, self-contained systems), the simple mechanization approach may be the chosen alternative. For example, a hospital might presently operate a well-defined timekeeping and payroll system. A systems analysis indicates that machine processing of data would reduce clerical labor requirements and speed the availability of information, but no basic changes in reports or information flow are needed. In this case, the mechanization alternative might be selected, particularly if there are no plans to integrate the payroll system with other applications to be developed later.

In most situations, however, hospitals are well advised to go beyond the simple mechanization approach and look to broader improvements, which are available through reexamination of current policies and procedures. In these cases, the choices are *partial redesign* or *complete redesign* of the existing manual system into a new, automated information system. In the latter case, the project team members are not constrained by current policies, methods, or organizational arrangements and are free to consider completely new approaches in the system design. Obviously, changes in policy would have to be justified through careful cost-benefit analysis, as discussed later in this chapter. However, constraints would not be imposed initially on the creative work to be carried out by the design team. Thus major improvements in patient care or administrative operations might be effected through new procedures and organizational arrangements made possible by new approaches to information reporting and availability.

The selection of an approach to systems design should, of course, be guided by the principles set forth in the master plan for systems development. If the plan calls for development of individual applications with no attempt to interchange information across systems, obvious limits are placed on the design choices available. If, on the other hand, the hospital has chosen to follow the modular design approach, then specific design work on this system must be carried out in the broader framework of the impact of this system on others to which it relates. For example, under the modular design approach, the design of a laboratory information system would be planned in reference to related systems (existing or planned) for ordering services for patients and for capturing information for charging and billing purposes.

THE PROCESS OF SYSTEM DESIGN

System design is the creative, technical process of converting information system requirements into a detailed set of specifications for a system. It is analogous to the preparation of architectural drawings and mechanical specifications for a new building in a hospital construction program. The project team organization should be continued during the design phase of a project. However, emphasis will shift to the more technical tasks requiring the skills of trained systems analysts or management engineers. Additional technical personnel may be needed at this point in the project. Hospital operating and administrative personnel should continue to serve as a sounding board for the specific design characteristics developed by the systems analysts working on the project. The final result of the design phase should be a formal, detailed set of system specifications. The content of the specifications is summarized below:

1. Statement of System Objectives
2. Output Specifications
    a. Purpose
    b. Content
    c. Format
    d. Distribution and reporting schedule
    e. Estimated volume
3. Input Specifications
    a. Sources of data
    b. Forms
    c. Procedures for converting to machine readable form
    d. Coding systems
    e. Schedule and estimated volumes
4. Master File Specifications
    a. Content and format
    b. Access requirements (including data privacy protection)
    c. Estimated volumes and file size
    d. Updating and purging schedules
    e. File security procedures
5. Procedures and Data Flow
    a. Flowcharts

   b. Narrative description
   c. Computer program specifications
6. Cost-Benefit Analysis
   a. System development costs
   b. System operating costs
   c. Maintenance costs
   d. Anticipated benefits
7. Management Approvals (Signatures)
   a. Operating departments involved
   b. Hospital administration

The first step in the process must be the definition of system objectives. What are the specific goals the hospital expects to achieve through the design of the new information system? Objectives should be as specific as possible and should be measurable later, when the system is operational. System objectives may relate to effectiveness of operations, to increased efficiency, or both. If savings in personnel time are anticipated, then these should be specifically stated: How many man-hours of labor, by job category, are to be eliminated by the new system and what will be the savings in payroll costs? If new benefits are to be realized by the availability of timely information, these should be stated as specific objectives of the new system. A well-stated objective should meet the criterion of measurability. If a specific evaluation criterion can be stated, then the objective is adequate to guide the design process. Otherwise, system objectives are nothing more than nonoperational platitudes which are of little help to those designing the new system.

Output specifications should flow readily from a specific statement of system objectives and a completed systems analysis. Reporting requirements will be specified by departmental representatives on the project team working with the systems analyst.

Each report or other form of output to be produced by the system should be specified in detail. The purpose of each report should be stated. Who in the hospital will receive copies of the report and to what use will it be put? The specific content and format should be specified, and sample copies of completed reports should be drawn up by the systems analysts. These sample reports should look exactly as they will when generated by a computer printer, data communications display, or other computer output device. Report formats should be designed with the user in mind. They should be easy to read and self-explanatory whenever possible. Meaningless code numbers should be avoided, and descriptive headings should be printed at the top of each column of the report.

The systems analyst should consider the alternatives of preprinted versus computer-printed report forms. Computer-printed forms are generally less expensive than preprinted forms and are easier to change. However, preprinted forms are more compact and easier to read, and these kinds of trade-offs must be considered in report design. Output specifications also should include the distribution, schedule, and estimated volume of each report to be generated by the system. The same principles should be followed in specifying computer output to be displayed on video screens if online retrieval is part of the system design. The exact format of each video display should be spelled out in the system specifications.

Input specifications are derived from system objectives and output formats. Specific input data requirements are derived from the content of output reports and from data retrieval specifications. For each set of input data to be processed by the system, the source of the data must be specified and forms or other means of capturing the data must be designed. As a general rule, it is desirable to capture data as close to the original source as possible, and it is also wise to minimize transcription of data before entering it into the computer for processing. Direct input of data through terminals or capture of data in a machine readable format, if possible, is highly desirable. Good forms design also is an important step in the capture and entry of data into the system.

Input specification also includes development of codes and coding systems. Codes should be simple and easy to use. They should be flexible and easy to expand as the volume of transactions increases. Consideration should be given to the use of self-checking codes for critical data items such as patient identification numbers or hospital service codes. In such systems, a check digit is added to the code number. This digit can then be checked when data are entered into the computer to be sure that an error has not occurred in data recording or transcription. Input specifications should also include the schedule for data entry and estimated volume for each input element.

The design team must also specify how each set of data will be converted to machine readable form. Choices range from manually recording data on forms for later keypunching to various methods of source data automation (techniques for simultaneous capture of information and conversion to a form for direct entry into the computer). Examples of source data automation include mark sense cards or forms, precoded plastic cards to record data with embossers, and optical recognition of bar code labels and printed or typewritten characters.

The fourth major element of system specifications is the design of master files. Each master file must be specified in detail, including content and format of the file structure, estimated volume of transactions, and average file size. Consideration must be given to access requirements as well. If files are to be accessible for on-line updating and retrieval of information, then direct access computer storage devices must be used.* Alternatively, if access to files will occur only through batch processing, then other forms of electronic storage, such as magnetic tape, can be utilized.

The system design should also include a procedure and schedule for periodic updating and purging of files. The latter is often neglected, and the resultant system must cope with cluttered files of outdated information. File security procedures are another essential element of master file specification. Protection of the patient's right to privacy must be paramount in the construction of computer files, and safeguards should be built into the initial design to insure that files are accessible only to authorized hospital employees.

Inputs, outputs, and master files are system elements which must be related to one another through the specification of procedures and data flow. Flowcharts, similar to those used in systems analysis, are the basic tools employed in specifying information flow in the new system. In addition, narrative descriptions and elaboration of procedures, revised policies, and new organizational structures should be detailed in this section of the specifications. Also included should be written specifications for computer programs which will be required for processing data. These usually take the form of *computer run diagrams* with accompanying narrative notes which detail the function of each computer program required.

It is essential that the project team be realistic in specifying procedures for the new system. The importance of environmental analysis has been emphasized in the discussion of systems analysis. Data obtained from that analysis should be utilized in developing procedures that are realistic and workable in a given organizational setting. Consideration must be given to physical space limitations, management philosophy, training and attitudes of personnel involved in the system, and other formal and informal elements of the work place which will affect new policies and procedures. Hospital information systems are man-machine systems, as previously defined, and the importance of good "human engineering" in the construction of such systems cannot be overemphasized.

The final step in the development of system specifications should be a thorough cost-benefit analysis of the system which has been designed.[1] Three kinds of costs should be estimated: system development costs, operating costs, and maintenance costs. Development costs include the remaining costs of design and implementation, including computer programming,

---

* See Appendix A: Glossary of Technical Terms for definition of technical terms, such as *direct access computer storage*.

training of personnel, procedures writing, system testing, conversion of data files, and other similar tasks. Operational costs include labor, materials, and a prorated share of computer time used for the new system. Maintenance costs are often overlooked. These are the personnel costs incurred in keeping qualified systems analysts and programmers available to make necessary changes in the system after it goes into operation and to evaluate it periodically for improvements.

These costs must be matched against the anticipated benefits of the system, both tangible benefits which can be translated into dollar savings for the hospital and also intangible benefits which cannot be measured directly in financial terms but which are expected to improve the effectiveness of service delivery. At this point planners should again critically evaluate whether or not to proceed with implementation of the system. It is quite possible that a system which looked attractive after an initial systems analysis could be found to be prohibitively expensive or not feasible after a detailed design is completed. In such a situation, the project team and hospital administration must be bold enough not to proceed with implementation. A decision to proceed because a major investment has been made in the design phase is foolish; unfortunately many hospitals have implemented computer systems when the results of a design effort dictated against such action.

The final element of the specifications should be a formal section for management approvals. The specifications should be submitted for formal review to the manager of each department and hospital service involved and also to administration. Meetings should be scheduled to elaborate on the specifications, answer questions about them, and discuss possible problems with the system design. Once necessary changes have been made, signatures of approval should be required before the implementation phase begins. If busy department heads and administrators know that they must formally indicate their concurrence with the design of the new system, they are much more likely to take the time to review the specifications carefully. This will help to insure that the system can meet the objectives laid down for it and will be workable within the operating environment of the hospital.

Use of Contractual Services

As discussed in Chapter 3, some hospitals may choose to carry out detailed design and improvement of information systems through contractual services. This often involves the development of formal specifications in the form of a Request for Proposals or RFP. There is considerable debate about the degree of specification that is desirable in an RFP. Some argue for minute specification of every detail for the proposed system in order to insure that the hospital knows in advance exactly what it is getting. The counter argument calls for great flexibility and latitude in the specifications so that vendors are free to propose a variety of approaches in meeting the functional requirements included in the RFP. Although no general rule can be stated, since each situation must be evaluated on its own merits, the answer usually lies somewhere between these two extremes. Specifications should be reasonably tight to insure that hospital objectives are met and to provide a common base for evaluating proposals. Some flexibility should be included, however, to permit creative approaches on the part of prospective bidders.

Criteria for evaluating responses to an RFP should be drawn up in advance of its issuance. Consideration should be given to use of a weighted value system whereby each major criterion is assigned a percentage weight in relation to the overall evaluation. For example, in the selection of a system, percentage weights might be assigned to such factors as (1) demonstrated understanding of system requirements and overall system design, (2) hardware proposed as part of the system, (3) the general reputation of the company, (4) qualifications and experience of staff members who would be assigned to the project, (5) installation requirements, (6) support services available after the system is operational, (7) the number of similar systems installed in other hospitals, and (8) the costs to install, operate, and maintain the system. Each of these criteria would then be subdivided into more specific items, and specific measurement factors would be drawn up with a point value system established to rate how well each proposal responds to that factor.

General guidelines for hospitals to follow in evaluating responses to RFPs for contract services were discussed in Chapter 3. These include examination of the previous experience of the contractor, review of the experience and training of specific individuals to be assigned to the project, and a check to see whether the contractor plans to follow well-established principles of systems analysis and design. If necessary, the hospital should utilize a neutral consultant to assist in the technical evaluation of proposals.

One major health care provider, Kaiser-Permanente Medical Care Program, reports increasing use of outside contractors for software development to be shared by its seven regional prepaid health care plans. According to the vice president for information services, " . . . Kaiser-Permanente is switching to outside software developers . . . because its studies show they can do the work for considerably less than the in-house staff that traditionally has been used."[2]

Implementation of a system may also involve serious consideration of predesigned or packaged information systems available for a variety of hospital functions. Of particular importance, the following questions must be asked: Does the proposed packaged system meet our hospital's specific requirements? If not, are we willing and able to adjust to the general requirements of the packaged system? By their very nature packaged systems must be generalized so that they can be applied in a variety of hospital settings. While hospitals are not dissimilar in their overall functions, specific policies and operating procedures may vary widely. Thus the question of adaptation becomes a critical one in considering the use of generalized systems. While such adaptation is often possible, recognition by hospitals of the need to make adjustments to current policies and practices is very important before purchasing a packaged system. It may be possible also to have the contractor tailor the packaged system to the needs of an individual hospital; however, additional costs would be incurred in the process.

Other important factors in evaluating packaged systems include consideration of how the system will be maintained and whether documentation is adequate. Will hospital staff be able to make changes in the system, or will an additional contract with the supplier be necessary? What guarantees are there that these changes will be made by the supplier of the package? As a general rule, provision for in-house maintenance by hospital staff is a wise course to follow.

Whenever outside services are used, hospitals should protect themselves by (1) developing clearly stated and detailed specifications for the work; and (2) developing a written contract with performance requirement detailed so that both parties have identical expectations for the results of the systems work or software package to be developed.[3]

CASE STUDY—SYSTEMS DESIGN SPECIFICATIONS

We will now turn to a case study constructed to illustrate the principles of systems design. The example represents a completed set of system specifications for a Management Reporting System of Aged Accounts Receivable in a community general hospital. The example is completely fictitious and presented for illustrative purposes only. Simplifications are made in order to keep the size of the problem manageable.

The following assumptions are made about the hospital in which this system is being developed:

1. The hospital is a nonprofit community general hospital offering acute medical and surgical services.
2. The hospital already has installed a general purpose electronic computer system and has developed an in-house staff capability for systems analysis and computer programming.

3. The hospital has an operational computer system for collecting patient charges and preparing bills for patients and third parties.
4. A systems analysis has already been completed. The hospital has a master plan for information systems development and is following the modular approach to systems design and integration of information.

System Specifications,
Management Reporting System—Aged Accounts Receivable

I. System Objectives

A. To provide hospital administrators, financial managers, and Board of Trustees Finance Committee members with periodic summary information on the status of accounts receivable in the hospital through preparation of a monthly statistical report.

B. To provide the Administrator and Controller's office the capability of retrieving information on the current status of any payment category through on-line display at a computer terminal.

II. Output Specifications

A. Monthly Summary Report (see Figure 8-1)

1. Purpose: to provide a summary statistical report for periodic review of the current status of accounts receivable in order to provide early warning of cash flow problems.
2. Content: total dollar value of accounts receivable by payment category, distributed according to five time intervals measured from the date of first billing.
3. Format: computer printed form (no preprinted form to be used); matrix columnar format.
4. Distribution: Administrator, Controller, and Board Finance Committee members.
5. Schedule: printed on the third working day of each month; sent out in advance of the Board Finance Committee meeting held on the second Tuesday of each month.
6. Volume: one page per month.

B. On-line Displays (see Figure 8-2)

1. Purpose: to provide current status information (by payment category) on a demand basis to the Administrator and Controller.
2. Content: for a single payment category and specified time

FIGURE 8–1
Sample Monthly Report

MONTHLY REPORT—AGED ACCOUNTS RECEIVABLE

PAYMENT CATEGORY	DAYS FROM DATE OF FIRST BILLING				
	0–30	31–60	61–90	91–120	OVER 120
PATIENT PAY	$XXXXXX	$XXXXXX	$XXXXXX	$XXXXXX	$XXXXXX
MEDICARE—TITLE 18					
MEDICAID—TITLE 19					
BLUE CROSS—PLAN A					
BLUE CROSS—PLAN B					
BLUE CROSS—PLAN C					
COMMERCIAL INSURANCE					
OTHER					
TOTAL					

FIGURE 8–2
Computer CRT Display

CURRENT STATUS—ACCOUNTS RECEIVABLE

PAYMENT CATEGORY: ______________________

TIME INTERVAL SPECIFIED: ______ TO __________ DAYS ________
TOTAL NUMBER OF ACCOUNTS: ______________________

DISTRIBUTION BY ACCOUNT SIZE:

	(NUMBER OF ACCOUNTS)
$ 0–$ 500	__________
$ 501–$ 1,000	__________
$1,001–$ 2,000	__________
$2,001–$ 3,000	__________
$3,001–$ 4,000	__________
$4,001–$ 5,000	__________
$5,001–$10,000	__________
Over $10,000	__________

interval, total dollar value of accounts receivable, total number of accounts categorized by dollar amount of the accounts.

3. Format: cathode-ray tube display.
4. Schedule: on demand at the computer terminal in the administrative suite.

III. Input Specifications

A. Sources of data: input data are derived from the patient accounting and billing system already in operation; the master patient account file, a direct access computer file organized by patient identification number, will provide the basic data required for on-line retrieval and preparation of the monthly report.

B. Forms: no new input forms required.

C. Procedures for converting to machine readable form: none required since input data are provided from an existing computer file.

D. Coding systems: no new codes required.

E. Estimated volume: on average, 8,000 to 10,000 unclosed patient accounts at any given time.

IV. Master File Specifications

A. Patient accounts master file: already created by the patient accounting and billing system.

B. Content and format: a direct access file organized by patient identification number; contains summary of patient charges, third-party and patient pay billing information, and current payment status.

C. Volume and file size: an estimated 50 to 75 new accounts are added to this file each working day; total file size averages 8,000 to 10,000 accounts at any given time.

D. File security procedures: terminal interlocks and inquirer identification systems are used to protect the privacy of information contained in this file.

V. Procedures and Data Flow (see Figure 8-3)

A. This system will be designed as a new module within the financial information system of the hospital.

B. The monthly report will be generated routinely by the hospital data-processing center using data from the patient accounting and billing system.

C. The retrieval of current status information from the computer terminal in the administrative suite will be triggered through entry of an inquiry message at the terminal; the request will specify the payment category and time interval since first billing to be displayed.

VI. Cost-Benefit Analysis

A. System development costs

1.	One man-month of detailed design work and computer programming	$2,000
2.	Computer time for testing system	200
3.	Supplies, materials, miscellaneous	150
		$2,350

B. System operating costs

1.	12 monthly reports @ $50 each	$ 600
2.	100 on-line inquiries @ $20 each	2,000
		$2,600

C. System maintenance costs (per year)
50 man-hours of maintenance @ $15/hour $ 750

FIGURE 8–3
System Flowchart

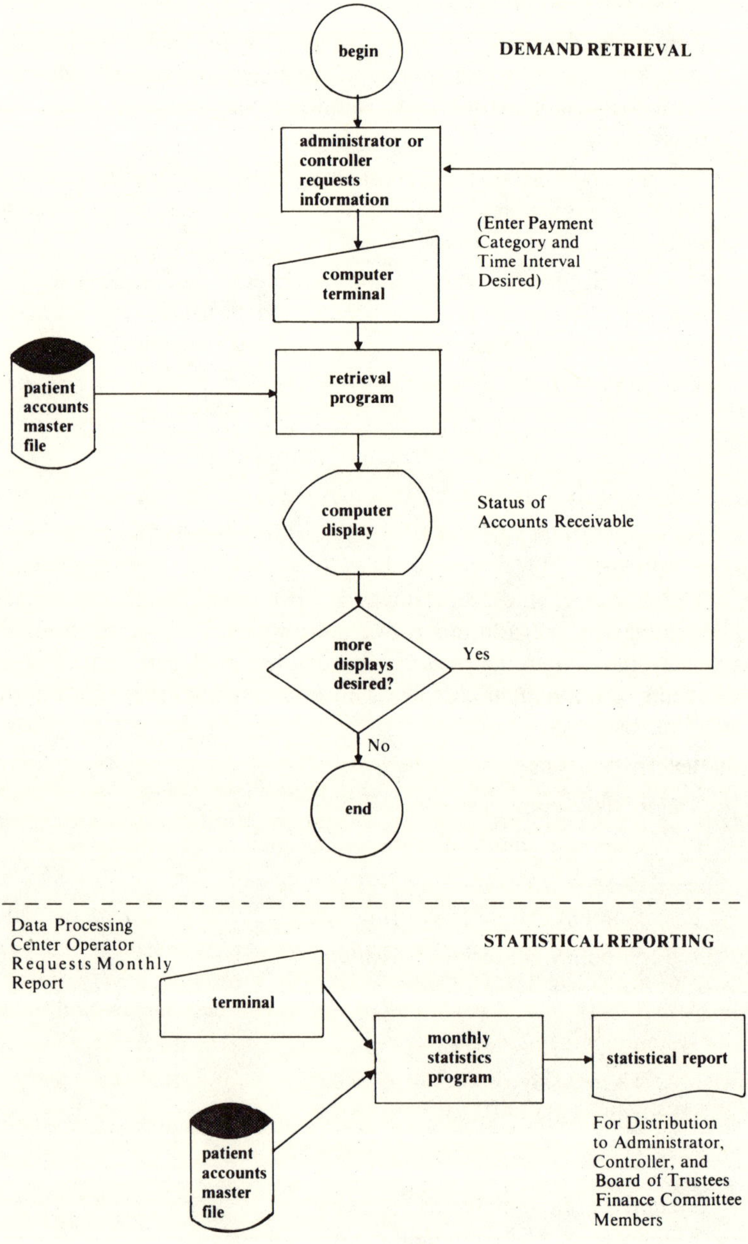

D. TOTAL ANNUAL COSTS (assumes development costs are prorated over five years) $3,820

E. Anticipated benefits

1. Tangible: none that can be directly measured.

2. Intangible: better control of cash flow; improved information to support financial planning.

VII. Approvals
These specifications have been reviewed and we concur with the decision to implement this system.

SUMMARY

Selection of a design approach for a hospital information system should be based upon completed systems analysis and should be carried out in accordance with the hospital's master plan for information systems development.

The alternatives available in selecting an approach to systems design range from minor improvements upon an existing manual system to complete redesign unconstrained by existing policies and procedures. In a limited number of cases, simple mechanization of existing work processes might be the approach followed, although, in most cases, benefits are realized through changes in policies and procedures as well.

Systems design is the technical process of converting information system requirements into a detailed set of specifications for the new system. A project team organization should be continued during the design phase, with hospital operating and management personnel used for "reality checking" of the design specifications. The final product of the system design effort should be a formally prepared set of system specifications. Decisions as to whether or not to proceed with implementation should be reached upon completion of the system design.

Some hospitals will choose to carry out detailed design and implementation work through the use of contractual services, often involving the development of a Request for Proposal (RFP). Hospitals also will frequently investigate the use of predesigned, packaged systems to minimize the costs of systems design and implementation. System documentation is very important, and consideration must be given to the method for maintaining the packaged system after it is installed.

DISCUSSION QUESTIONS

8-1 What are some of the alternatives in selecting an approach to information systems design?

8-2 Should the choice of a design approach be influenced by the hospital's master plan for information systems development? In what ways?

8-3 Why is simple mechanization of existing procedures often not the optimum course to follow in system design?

8-4 What kinds of activities are carried out in the system design phase of a project? What roles should various members of the project team play in these efforts?

8-5 What should be included in the specification of output reports for an information system?

8-6 What elements should be included in specification of system inputs?

8-7 What are the major elements of a cost-benefit analysis to be included in system specifications?

8-8 Why are formal review and sign-off procedures so important?

8-9 How much flexibility should be built into a Request for Proposals (RFPs) for contract services in order to permit creative approaches on the part of those submitting proposals?

8-10 How should the responses to an RFP be evaluated? What criteria should be used in the evaluation?

8-11 What are some of the things to look for when considering the use of predesigned (packaged) information systems in hospitals?

PROBLEMS

8-1 Develop a written work plan for the in-house design of an outpatient clinic scheduling and patient registration system. Include in the plan the project team composition and the major responsibilities of each team member.

8-2 Write an RFP for the design and implementation of a pharmacy information system in an acute care general hospital.

8-3 Develop a model set of system specifications for an information system to support one functional area of a hospital, either administrative or clinical. (You may wish to draw upon the systems analysis carried out for Problem 7-3.)

NOTES

1. For a discussion of specific techniques in cost-benefit analysis, see John R. Griffith, "Cost-Benefit Analysis," in *Quantitative Techniques for Hospital Planning and Control* (Lexington, Massachusetts: Lexington Books, 1972), pp. 225-238.
2. John Boeschen, "Kaiser Is Shifting to Outside Contractors," *Modern Healthcare*, November 1981, pp. 100-102.
3. Roy N. Freed, "Fully Detailed Contracts Limit Misunderstanding," *Modern Healthcare*, May 1981, pp. 122-124.

ADDITIONAL READINGS

Clifton, H.D. *Systems Analysis for Business Data Processing.* Princeton, New Jersey: Auerbach Publishers, 1969. Note particularly Chapters 10 and 11, "Design of Data Processing Systems—1 and 2."

Donaldson, Hamish. *A Guide to the Successful Management of Computer Projects.* New York: John Wiley & Sons, 1978. Note particularly Chapter 7, "Systems Design Strategy," and Chapter 8, "Specification Stage of Project Development."

Gildersleeve, Thomas R. *Successful Data Processing System Analysis.* Englewood Cliffs, New Jersey: Prentice-Hall, 1978. Note particularly Part 3, "The Functional Specifications."

Gore, Marvin and Stubbe, John. *Elements of Systems Analysis for Business Data Processing* (Second Edition). Dubuque, Iowa: Wm. C. Brown Co., 1979. Note particularly Unit Four, "The Design Phase."

Head, Robert V. *A Guide to Packaged Systems.* New York: John Wiley & Sons, 1971.

Lott, Richard W. *Basic Systems Analysis.* San Francisco: Canfield Press, 1971. Note particularly Chapter 7, "General System Design."

Lucas, Henry C. *The Analysis, Design, and Implementation of Information Systems.* New York: McGraw-Hill, 1981. Note particularly Chapters 9-12.

Martin, B.R. "Guidelines for Contracting for Computer Related Services." *Computers and Automation*, April 1970, pp. 18-25.

McLaughlin, Daniel B., Shapiro, Fred L., and Umen, Andrew J. "Designing Information Systems for Health Care Executives." *Health Care Management Review*, Spring 1980, pp. 49-57.

Riley, M.J. *Management Information Systems* (Second Edition). San Francisco: Holden-Day, Inc., 1981. Note particularly Part 3, "Designing the MIS."

9

System Implementation and Maintenance

Once a thorough systems analysis has been completed, a design approach selected, and system design specifications prepared and approved, then implementation of the hospital information system can proceed. As with all phases of system development, implementation does not just happen; it must be carefully planned in advance. Hospital administration must take the responsibility to insure that this planning occurs.

Implementing an Information System

Some erroneously equate implementation of a system with computer programming. Although programming is an important and essential part of the process, it is only one of several tasks necessary to make a system operational. The steps in implementing a hospital information system are:

- equipment acquisition
- computer programming
- training
- file conversion
- system testing
- documentation

Equipment Acquisition. In some cases, new equipment may be required for system implementation. This could range from complete installation of a general purpose computer in the hospital to the relatively simple addition of some computer terminals to an existing system. Whatever the magnitude of equipment requirements, equipment ordering and installation must be carefully planned. Sufficient lead time must be allowed to insure delivery when needed. In some cases renovations and site preparation will also be required, and good space planning must accompany all new equipment orders. A more detailed discussion of computer equipment will be found in Part II, Chapters 4 and 6.

Computer Programming. The system design specifications include requirements for computer programs that are to be written during the implementation phase of a systems project. Programming is a technical task requiring trained staff. If system requirements are documented properly, the programming task is simplified considerably.

A computer program is a set of instructions that a general purpose computer will follow in accomplishing a specified data-processing and computational task. Electronic computers are stored program devices; that is, the computer is capable of carrying out a broad array of data-processing tasks, and the specific instructions for a given job are stored internally in the memory of the machine at the time that job is executed. Programming consists of the following tasks:

1. Translating program requirements from system specifications into a logical sequence of machine operations; this is accomplished through the development of a flowchart of machine instructions for each program in the system.
2. Coding of the sequence of operations as laid out in the flowchart into a specific programming language acceptable to the computer system which the hospital uses.
3. Unit testing, or *debuggging,* of the program after it has been coded and compiled in the computer. Program testing involves the use of test data prepared by the programmer and should not be confused with system testing, which includes checking of all elements of a system, not just machine processing procedures. Test data should be realistic to insure that the program will work properly when implemented. Departmental members of the project team are invaluable sources of relevant test data for use by programmers in debugging their program.
4. Documentation of the program so that changes can be made at a later time, either by the original programmer or by a maintenance programmer.

The reader interested in more detail on the technical aspects of computer programming is referred to the Additional Readings at the end of this chapter. A discussion of programming languages (or computer software) available to hospitals is included in Chapter 5.

Training. An extremely important element of system implementation is training of hospital personnel who will operate and use the new information system. Training plans should be drawn up by the project team, and team members should take responsibility for coordinating and conducting the training sessions. These sessions should include general orientation for top management and more specific training for departmental managers and first line supervisors. Managers and supervisors, in turn, should take responsibility for training employees in their areas, and at the same time they will become more familiar with the new system. There has been considerable difficulty with many hospital information systems in the first months of operation because hospital personnel were not properly oriented and trained in advance.

File Conversion. Another task which is sometimes overlooked in implementation planning is file conversion. Many, if not most, hospital information systems will require that one or more master data files be converted from manual form to electronic storage in the computer, or that one computer system file be converted to another, before operation. For example, if a hospital is installing an order-entry system for processing and communicating orders for patient services throughout the hospital, then on the first day that the system goes into operation a master file of patient information must be created. Or if the hospital is converting its billing and accounts receivable system to the computer, the master file of open accounts must be converted to electronic storage before operating the computer system. This requires advanced planning and intensive effort during the latter stages of implementation. The magnitude of the task for large data files may require a phasing-in approach, in which a segment of the file is converted during a certain time period. For example, in the accounts receivable conversion mentioned above, one-fourth of the alphabet might be converted in week one, the second one-fourth in week two, and so on. Once again, careful planning is essential. Where conversion is from one computer system to another, the conversion should, as much as possible, be accomplished as an automatic, programmed machine conversion.

System Testing. No hospital information system should be put into operation without complete system testing. The test should be carefully planned and should cover all aspects of the new system in as realistic an environment as possible. The elements to be included in a comprehensive systems test are:

- system objectives
- output reports
- input forms and procedures

- error and correction procedures
- personnel training
- computer programs and equipment operations
- throughput times
- computer times
- cost estimates
- adequacy of system documentation

The test should be designed to determine whether specific goals and objectives can be met by the information system which has been designed and implemented. Each objective should be measured against specific test criteria. If objectives are measurable ones, as they should be (see Chapter 8), then testing of them will be possible.

The adequacy of each report and other forms of system output should be tested as well. Reports should be distributed to those who will use them and should be carefully checked to be sure that information content is accurate and formats are workable. The ability of the system to generate output data in a timely manner also should be tested.

A major element of the test is checking that data collection and input procedures are functioning properly. Is computer input generated with a minimum of errors? When errors do occur, does the system detect them and permit timely correction? Is there adequate data flow with records available for computer processing when needed? Are forms designed to be understandable and easy to use?

Error and correction procedures are important elements of any information system. Most systems will handle routine transactions without difficulty, but those few exceptions which inevitably do occur often generate confusion and frustration unless good exception procedures are built into the system design. The adequacy of these procedures must be tested thoroughly.

The system test should also be designed to check the sufficiency of personnel training. Are procedures for gathering and reporting data understood and functional? Procedures manuals should be developed before the system test begins so that they are available to hospital departments during the test period.

The test, of course, will also further check the adequacy of computer programs and machine processes involved in the system. Although a good programmer will thoroughly debug his program after it has been written, additional problems are often uncovered when a program is operated under live conditions in conjunction with all the other elements of a system.

Time measurements are also studied throughout a system test. The accuracy of computer-processing time estimates is verified, and, more important, throughput times must be recorded and analyzed. Throughput time is the total time span from collection of the first data element to preparation of the final report in a system. Since timeliness of information is such an important element of most hospital information systems, this aspect of the system test is critical.

The system test should aim at estimating as closely as possible the actual operating costs of the new system. If the costs appear to be much higher than the estimates contained in the system specifications, then hospital administrators should carefully review the entire system and decide whether or not to proceed with full implementation. The system test should mark another critical decision to proceed or not to proceed with the implementation of an information system. Implementation in the face of evidence of significant cost overruns constitutes irresponsible management.

Finally, the system test should test the completeness of system documentation, including, for example, procedures manuals, documentation of computer programs, and machine operating manuals. Documentation is the key to good system maintenance, and it should be in order before the new system goes into production.

Although every test element described above is important, the overriding purpose of a system test is to test the system as a whole. Will the various components function together in an orderly and systematic manner? To answer this question, the test should be as realistic as possible. Actual data from hospital operations should be used if at all feasible. In many cases, a parallel test may be the best way to simulate actual operation of the system. In parallel testing, the new information system operates along with the existing system, and cross-checks for accuracy are conducted on a systematic basis. Parallel testing places considerable strain on hospital operations since two systems must be operated by the hospital personnel involved. Temporary staffing often is required during this period, and it is recommended that the temporary staff be assigned to the old system so that permanent hospital employees may gain the experience of using the new system procedures. It is obvious that parallel testing requires careful advanced planning. Test plans should be approved by the department managers involved as well as the hospital administrator.

Documentation. The final aspect of system implementation is completion of all system documentation, both procedural and machine related. Documentation should be a continuous process carried out during all phases of the system project. Just before production, the project team should do a final check to insure that system documentation is adequate for effective maintenance of the new system.

System Maintenance

Hospital information systems require both scheduled and unanticipated maintenance once they are working. No matter how well a system is designed and regardless of how well it has been tested, there inevitably will be errors uncovered after the system goes into production. Systems analysts and programmers must be available to find such problems quickly and to initiate immediate corrections.

In addition, alterations in the system will be required from time to time, since hospitals are dynamic organizations subject to fairly frequent changes in operating policies and procedures. These changes flow from a variety of sources: new programs initiated by the board of trustees, changes in the composition of the community served by the hospital, expansion of facilities to meet increased demand, and ever-increasing regulation by external agencies. Information systems must be sufficiently flexible so that these changes can be accommodated, and trained technical staff must be available to initiate them.

Information systems should also be periodically evaluated. Schmitz suggests that this evaluation occur on three levels: the effect of the system on the patient, the effect of the system on the behavior of personnel in the hospital, and the economic effects of the system on the organization.[1] Improvements enabling the system to function more effectively should result from formal system evaluation.[2]

Proper staffing is required if system maintenance is to be carried out properly. Although no general rule can be stated, some systems specialists have suggested that approximately 25 percent of the total technical staff of systems analysts and programmers will need to be devoted to maintenance activities once several systems are in operation in a hospital. Failure to plan and provide for such staffing can result in many problems later. If staffing levels permit, it is also good practice to assign maintenance responsibilities to personnel not involved in the initial design and implementation of the system. The maintenance analyst or programmer should review all system and program documentation before accepting responsibility for the system, thus helping to insure that maintenance can be carried out independently of the initial design team. This can be very important in the field of computers and information systems, where qualified technical personnel are in demand and turnover can occur rapidly.

Case Study—Work Plan for System Implementation

We will now examine a case study which is designed to illustrate the principles of information system implementation. An example of a completed work plan for the implementation of a Billing and Accounts Receivable Information System will be presented. The example is fictitious and presented for illustrative purposes only. Simplifications are made in order to keep the problem size manageable. The following assumptions are made:

1. The hospital is a nonprofit community general hospital offering acute medical and surgical services.
2. The hospital already has installed a general purpose electronic computer system with on-line terminals and has developed an in-house staff capability for systems analysis and computer programming.
3. System design specifications for this system have been completed and approved.
4. The hospital is following the modular design approach, and the new billing and accounts receivable module is designed to interface with an existing system for collecting and pricing patient charges.

Implementation Work Plan
Billing and Accounts Receivable Information System

I. Equipment Acquisition

A. Three video terminals for installation in the Cashier's work area, Patient Accounting office, and administrative suite adjacent to the Controller's office.

1. Lead time for order—60 days.
2. Terminals operate on regular 110 house current, no special power requirements.
3. Hard-wiring to computer center required; allow 30 days lead time.

B. One remote printer for installation in Cashier's work area for printing of patient statements on demand.

1. Lead time for order—90 days.
2. 220 power outlet required.
3. Hard-wiring to computer center required; should be done simultaneously with video terminal in the Cashier's work area.

C. One additional random-access disk storage unit required in computer center, capacity of six million characters.

1. Lead time for order—90 days.

2. Direct installation in computer room; space available adjacent to existing disk units.

II. Computer Programming

A. Programming requirements are detailed in the system design specifications. Six new programs will be required in addition to modification of one existing program.

B. Estimated time requirements (includes individual program testing and documentation):

Program A	6 man-weeks
Program B	13 man-weeks
Program C	5 man-weeks
Program D	10 man-weeks
Program E	6 man-weeks
Program F	4 man-weeks
Modifications to Program X	2 man-weeks

TOTAL MAN-WEEKS OF PROGRAMMING–46

Three programmers to be assigned to the project; estimate four months for completion.

III. Training Requirements

A. Management orientation for hospital administrators, Controller, and members of Board of Trustees Finance Committee—two days.

B. Training of Manager of Patient Accounting Department, Chief Cashier, and other departmental supervisors—three sessions of two days each.

C. Training to be completed six weeks before system test so that department supervisors can train their own employees with assistance from project team members as necessary.

IV. File Conversion

A. Patient Accounts Master File must be converted to disk storage form before the first day of operation of the new system. Estimate 6,000 active accounts at the time of conversion.

B. Conversion plan: close down all activity ten working days prior to conversion. Temporary help to be hired to enter patient identification information and current balance figures. Details of previous account activity will be maintained on a manual basis.

C. Estimated manpower requirements for conversion: ten minutes per record to enter through computer terminals—25 man-weeks required.

FIGURE 9–1
Implementation Schedule (Conversion Date—June 30)

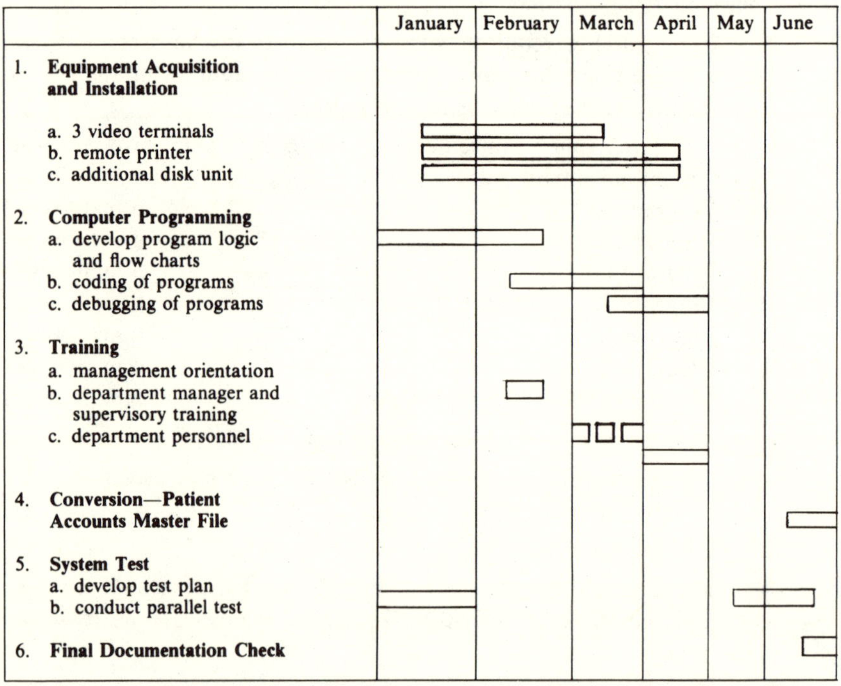

V. System Testing

A. Type of test: parallel test using a sample of 500 randomly selected accounts.

B. Duration: four weeks, with test to begin six weeks before planned conversion date.

C. Temporary manpower requirements: three additional clerical personnel to provide released time for permanent employees in Cashier's office and Patient Accounting office.

D. System test plan to be developed and coordinated by project team. Comparison of accounts from old system against computer system accounts, to be done each Saturday during test period.

VI. Documentation

A. All system documentation to be completed one week before conversion to new system.

FIGURE 9–2
Critical Path Network*

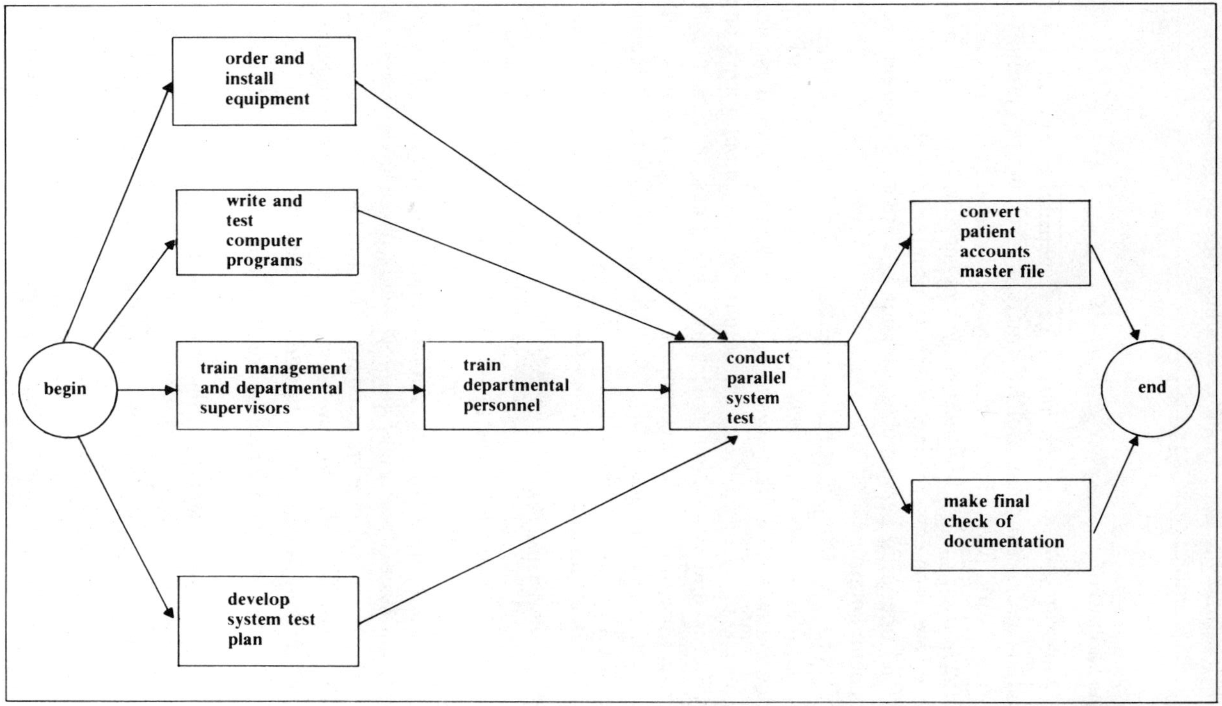

*For discussion of Critical Path Network Scheduling, see D. Michael Warner and Don C. Holloway, "Scheduling Decisions: Task Sequencing (PERT/CPM)," in *Decision Making and Control for Health Administration* (Ann Arbor, Michigan: Health Administration Press, 1978), pp. 68–78.

B. Project team leader and maintenance programmer to conduct final inspection before turning over system to the maintenance section.

SUMMARY

Hospital administration must take responsibility to insure that implementation and maintenance of information systems are carefully planned. A formal work plan should be prepared in advance of these activities. Implementation of an information system includes ordering needed data-processing equipment, writing computer programs, orientation of management and operating personnel, conversion of data files, system testing, and final documentation.

Thorough system testing is essential before implementation. In some cases, parallel testing of the new information system in comparison with an existing manual system is necessary. The system test should include a complete check of system objectives, output reports, input forms and procedures, error and correction procedures, adequacy of personnel training, computer programs and equipment operations, computer and system throughput times, adequacy of system documentation, and accuracy of initial cost estimates. If the tests show that costs are much higher than estimated or that the system is not meeting its objectives, then the hospital should not proceed with implementation.

Hospital information systems require both periodic and unscheduled maintenance after they are operational. Changing requirements in the dynamic hospital environment will also necessitate system changes from time to time. Maintenance personnel should also periodically evaluate the information system and make improvements based upon these evaluations. The information systems maintenance function in a hospital must be adequately staffed, preferably by systems analysts and programmers not involved in the original system design and implementation.

DISCUSSION QUESTIONS

9-1 Why is careful planning of the implementation phase of an information systems project so important?

9-2 What are the major steps involved in computer programming? How does programming relate to systems design?

9-3 What kind of training should be carried out before implementation of a hospital information system? Who should be trained? Who should conduct the training?

9-4 What is meant by file conversion? Why is planning for file conversion important?

9-5 What elements should be included in a system test?

9-6 What is meant by a parallel system test? How is it carried out?

9-7 What kinds of system documentation should be prepared before a system goes into operation?

9-8 What kinds of activities are included in information systems maintenance? Who should be responsible for systems maintenance?

9-9 Why is periodic evaluation of hospital information systems important?

PROBLEMS

9-1 Prepare a written work plan for the implementation of a hospital information system using in-house personnel. (You may wish to draw upon the system design specifications prepared for Problem 8-3.)

9-2 Prepare a system test plan for parallel testing of a computerized patient billing and accounts receivable system.

9-3 Assume that you are an assistant administrator of a large general hospital. The data-processing department of the hospital reports to you. Write a policy statement for your hospital detailing how information systems maintenance will be carried out.

NOTES

1. Homer H. Schmitz, "A Protocol for Evaluating Hospital Information Systems," *Hospital and Health Services Adminstration*, Winter 1977, pp. 45-56.
2. For a discussion of evaluation methodology see Russell C. Koza, ed., *Health Information Systems Evaluation* (Boulder, Colorado: Colorado Associated University Press, 1974).

ADDITIONAL READINGS

Bingham, J.E. and Davies, G.W.P. *A Handbook of Systems Analysis*. New York: John Wiley & Sons, 1972. Note particularly Chapter 21, "Planning for Implementation."

Clifton, H.D. *Systems Analysis for Business Data Processing*. Princeton, New Jersey: Auerbach Publishers, 1969. Note particularly Chapter 13, "Implementation of Data Processing Systems."

Donaldson, Hamish. *A Guide to the Successful Management of Computer Projects*. New York: John Wiley & Sons, 1978. Note particularly Chapter 12, "Implementation Stage of Project Development."

Gore, Marvin and Stubbe, John. *Elements of Systems Analysis for Business Data Processing* (Second Edition). Dubuque, Iowa: Wm. C. Brown Co., 1979. Note particularly Chapter 22, "Preparing for Implementation."

Hughes, Shirley J. "Installing a Computer-Based Patient Information System." *Journal of Nursing Administration*, May 1980, pp. 7-10.

Lucas, Henry C. *The Analysis, Design and Implementation of Information Sys-*

tems. New York: McGraw-Hill, 1981. Note particularly Chapter 14, "Testing and Installation."

Mishelevich, David J. et al. "Success Factors in the Implementation of a Comprehensive Hospital Information System." *Computers in Hospitals*, January-February, 1981, pp. 26-36.

Murdick, Robert G. and Ross, Joel E. *Introduction to Management Information Systems*. Englewood Cliffs, New Jersey: Prentice-Hall, 1977. Note particularly Chapter 9, "Implementation and Evaluation of the New MIS."

Riley, M.J. *Management Information Systems* (Second Edition). San Francisco: Holden-Day, Inc., 1981. Note particularly Part 4, "Implementing and Evaluating the MIS."

Solomon, Irving I. and Weingart, Lawrence O. *Management Uses of the Computer*. New York: Harper & Row, 1966. Note particularly Part IV, "System Installation and Operation."

10

Managing the Information-Processing Function in Hospitals

If information is to be used effectively in supporting both routine operations and management decisions in hospitals, then it is obvious that the processes by which information is collected and processed must be well managed in order to achieve these goals. This final chapter of Part III discusses the responsibilities of hospital administration in effective management of the information-processing function.

Organizing an Information Systems Department

Once a hospital has completed a master plan for information system development (see Chapter 3), it must then proceed to organize an information systems department (sometimes called a data-processing department) to take responsibility for system design, installation, and maintenance. The size and complexity of tasks to be carried out by the department will be affected by decisions on whether to develop systems in-house or to use packaged systems and software developed by commercial vendors. Regardless of the approach selected, however, the hospital must maintain a competent technical staff to guide the implementation process. The discussion in this section assumes that a hospital has chosen to develop some systems internally and has a computer system installed within the institution. Similar principles of organization apply in those situations in which hospitals use outside services, in which case only the number of technical personnel required and organizational complexity differ.

The hospital management must determine where to locate the information systems department within the organization. This decision obviously will be influenced by the knowledge, attitudes, and style of the hospital administrator, as well as by the overall organizational structure of the institution. However, careful consideration also should be given to the overall program of information system development as outlined in the master systems plan. If emphasis is to be placed exclusively on the development of business and financial applications, then consideration can be given to placing the department under the hospital controller or chief financial officer. Many hospitals have followed this organizational pattern. However, if a broader approach to information systems development is to be followed, involving the development of both financial and clinical applications with system integration to be achieved as a design criterion, then the information systems department should report directly to the hospital administrator or to one of his assistants. Klimko states the case for top management reporting:

> When the MIS function is subsidiary to financial or clinical/medical disciplines it will become a slanted, parochial organization since the MIS director has no choice but to satisfy his boss. . . . When top management realizes the cost of data-processing and the impact on the organization, placement will become more obvious.[1]

Since top management stands to gain the most from good information systems, it makes sense to place the department under the direct supervision of the chief executive officer.

A typical organization chart for a hospital information systems department is shown in Figure 10-1. The department is organized into two divisions, one concerned primarily with system development, the other with machine operations. Professional staff in the system development division are organized into three sections: systems analysis and design, computer programming, and system maintenance. The operations division includes two sections: data preparation and editing, and computer operations. If the hospital computer system operates on more than one shift, then shift supervisors are needed in the operations section.

The person selected to direct the department must be broadly skilled. He or she must have up-to-date knowledge of the technical aspects of systems analysis, computer programming, and the operation of computing and data-processing equipment and must be willing to spend the time and effort necessary to remain active in the professional field. Technical knowledge is not sufficient, however. Many hospitals have gotten into trouble by hiring a technical specialist who did not also possess the essential managerial skills required for the job. Information systems development involves major capital expenditures and substantial operating budgets. Hence, the director must be an experienced financial manager. As mentioned repeatedly throughout this book, information system development requires continuous

FIGURE 10-1
Organization of a Hospital Information Systems Department

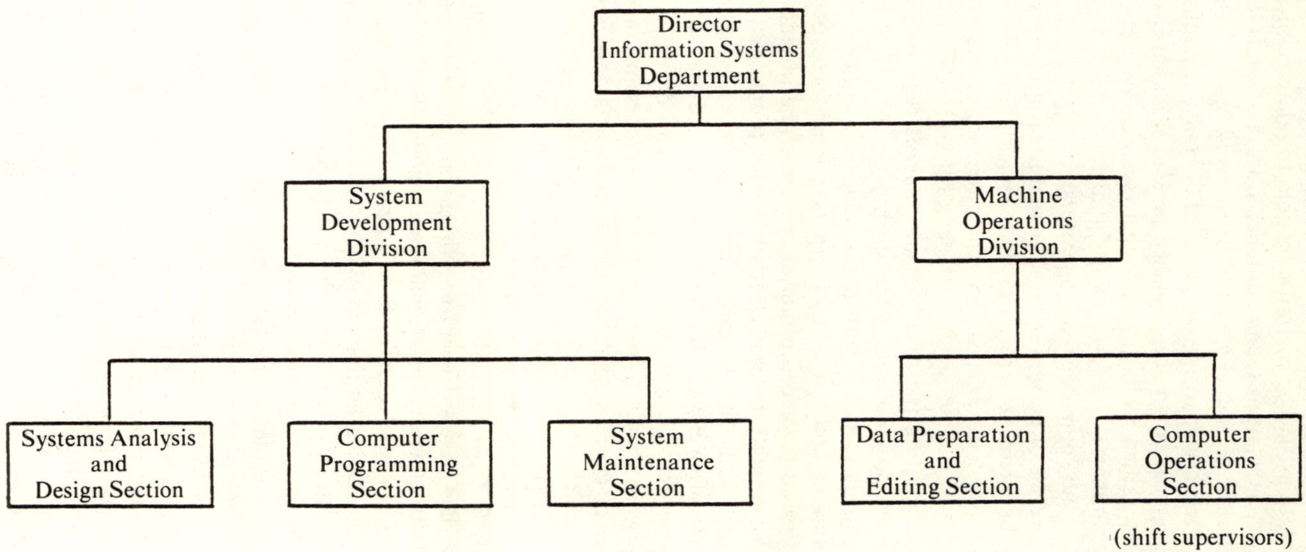

attention to human factors, and the director must also be skilled in interpersonal relations. He or she must be able to relate comfortably (and with tact) to physicians, nurses, and administrators, as well as technicians, orderlies, and clerical personnel who will be involved in one way or another with systems to be developed for the hospital. Finally, the information systems director also must be an accomplished personnel manager capable of supervising highly skilled technical personnel (systems analysts, engineers, computer programmers) and lesser skilled individuals such as data clerks, data entry clerks, and computer room operators.

Three levels of personnel must be recruited in staffing a hospital data-processing department: professional, technical, and clerical. Professional staff includes systems analysts and computer programmers, and, while it is possible to find talented persons who can fill both roles, care must be exercised in not equating the two. Systems analysis requires broad-based skills that computer programmers often do not possess. It is a highly creative process requiring someone with both technical knowledge of analytical and design techniques and also a broad organizational focus. Since most systems are complex and involve substantial man-machine interaction, the systems analyst must be able to deal effectively with people and must understand the way in which the hospital functions in carrying out its mission. Programmers often have a narrow orientation and are skilled in the technical, but somewhat routine, tasks associated with developing and maintaining the software required to carry out data-processing tasks. They are not always able to conceptualize all of the human factors and organizational constraints which are important environmental factors in the development of information systems. A small hospital will not be able to afford the costs of hiring separate staffs of systems analysts and computer programmers. Accordingly, it must carefully select those who will serve in this dual role to insure that they have sufficient knowledge and experience both in technical tasks and in broader organizational planning and development.

Technician level personnel will operate the hospital's computer and other data-processing equipment. They will work in the computer room as machine operators, often having been trained by computer manufacturers, usually at less than the baccalaureate level. The computer room supervisor must be both a skilled technician and an effective manager who can schedule the equipment and insure that it is properly maintained. Equipment maintenance is usually handled by contract with the manufacturer, who supplies periodic preventive maintenance and emergency repairs on call.

Finally, the information systems department also will include a clerical staff of data clerks, data entry clerks, and assistants to the professional and technical staff members. Some larger departments have career development programs in which talented personnel can receive further training for possible advancement to the next level of tasks in the department.

Hospitals must recruit aggressively to attract qualified systems analysts, programmers, and information systems managers—personnel in great demand by both profit and nonprofit organizations. According to one report:

> Low salaries are usually fingered most quickly as the cause of hospitals' struggle to recruit data-processing staff. But other hospital characteristics—their nonprofit orientation, the low status they assign to data-processing, the hassles caused by uncooperative physicians and the lack of career mobility hospitals provide their DP staff—may have a more debilitating effect on hospitals' recruitment efforts.[2]

To help overcome these problems, hospitals need to emphasize the life fulfillment gained from hospital work in helping others and also provide career ladder opportunities for information system professionals to assume executive management responsibilities in the organization.

An alternative to internal organization is the employment of contract management for the information systems department. A recent survey indicated that three such contract management firms were providing data-processing management services for 68 hospitals.[3]

Protecting the Privacy of Information

An important management responsibility in the modern hospital is the protection of the confidentiality of information. This generally involves two kinds of records—medical records of patients and personal information about employees. The need for privacy protection has accelerated in recent years as a result of several factors. There are continuously increasing demands for medical information about patients from such sources as prospective employers, insurance companies, third-party payers, government agencies, and, in some cases, law enforcement agencies. Countering these increasing demands for the release of information about patients and employees are even more vigorous demands from the public at large to protect the confidentiality of personal information. Public concern has been translated into legislative action at both the national and state levels. There are federal statutes which deal specifically with a citizen's right to privacy, and similar laws have also been passed at the state level. The development of modern computer technology has complicated this problem by making information more readily accessible through sophisticated electronic storage and retrieval systems. Thus, the hospital administrator and those involved in systems development are faced with the pressing need to build adequate safeguards into any information system which includes the storage of patient or employee data.[4]

There are several essential elements in a good program of information security. First, all system specifications should include procedures to be employed for the physical security of computer records of a sensitive nature. Second, carefully designed procedures are needed with regard to access to such information, particularly if the hospital is employing on-line terminals with direct access to data files. During the systems analysis phase of a project, careful study should be made to determine which employees of the hospital should have access to which data files. Once these determinations have been made, privacy protection procedures should include the following:

1. Use of carefully constructed identification codes will identify those individuals who are permitted access to certain sensitive data files.
2. Computer terminal interlock systems should prohibit terminals in certain areas of the hospital from gaining access to certain data files; for example, a terminal located in the hospital personnel office would normally not be allowed access to patient medical records files, and conversely a terminal on a nursing unit would not be able to access employee data files.
3. File interlock systems should match individual user identification numbers with sensitive data files and deny access to unauthorized inquirers.

Of paramount importance, top management in the hospital must take positive action to insure that all rules regarding information confidentiality are rigidly enforced and that penalties are imposed on those who commit infractions of these rules and procedures.

Building Controls and Audit Trails into Information Systems

Controls are necessary in all operational systems in hospitals, and they are essential in the design of hospital information systems. Controls and audit trails can help to avoid fraud and abuse and can insure that information provided by an automated system is accurate and reliable.

If possible, an internal auditor should be a member of the information system design team. Most auditors are knowledgeable about computer systems by virtue of their formal education and on-the-job training. Auditors cross departmental lines in their work and often are very knowledgeable about the total organization, its needs and problems. Hence they are very valuable members of the project team.

The objectives of an effective program of system controls should include the following:

- preventing or detecting accidental errors in a system; insuring data accuracy and completeness
- preventing or detecting fradulent manipulation of data
- preventing the misuse of sensitive or classified information
- guarding against the accidental destruction of data files and records
- providing recovery and restart procedures in the event of an operational system failure

Audit trails must be built into a system from the earliest stage of analysis and design if they are to serve their control and recovery purposes. These audit trails should include journalization of computer input, listing of all transactions including those accepted by the computer and those rejected because of input errors, and recording of changes made to system master files.

There are several items that an auditor should evaluate in assessing the adequacy of controls in an information system:

- organizational controls, including separation of system functions, particularly those involving financial transactions
- adequacy of system documentation for maintenance and troubleshooting purposes
- input and output controls, including periodic checking of reports against the original input documents which produced them
- controls programmed into the computer system itself (software controls), such as validity checking of input, data reasonableness checking, computation and checking of cross totals, and sequence checking of input data
- file safeguard and security procedures, including methods for recreating a file when necessary
- establishment of backup plans and procedures in the event of hardware failures, including agreements with outside organizations to provide backup computer time in emergency situations
- physical security and fire protection of the computer room and other hardware areas utilized in the processing of hospital information

When data are processed through on-line terminals at decentralized locations throughout the hospital, then extra efforts are needed to insure control. One such control procedure is the recording of all input transactions and maintenance of a tape file of these transactions for later checking if necessary.

As stated previously, control objectives can best be met if the internal auditor (or outside auditing consultant) is a full member of the information systems project team participating actively in the stages of analysis, design, and implementation.

EVALUATION OF SYSTEMS AND DATA-PROCESSING ACTIVITIES

Just as preinstallation planning is essential to the development of cost-effective data-processing systems in the hospital, so too management must insure that periodic post-implementation evaluation of systems is carried out. The capital investment and ongoing operational demands of sophisticated computer-based information systems place a responsibility upon the hospital to evaluate such systems continually and make improvements to them. Hospital management must take the leadership in conducting formal system evaluations.

Evaluation of data-processing activities should be conducted at two levels. Periodically, an overall management audit of the total data-processing activities of the hospital should be carried out. In addition, each major system which has been implemented should be formally evaluated to see if goals have been achieved within reasonable costs.

Chervenak calls for the conduct of periodic data-processing audits in all hospitals which have installed computer and data-processing equipment. The audit is "an independent, hard-nosed, professional examination of the effectiveness of a computer installation."[5] The audit should be supervised directly by a representative of hospital administration and should employ external consultants in order to insure objectivity. Users should be consulted extensively in the course of the review. Chervenak suggests the following 11 general areas to be examined in the course of the audit: (1) short- and long-range planning, (2) effectiveness of the hospital's organization of data-processing activities, (3) personnel policies employed, (4) effectiveness of management information generated by existing systems, (5) efficiency of machine operations, (6) professional standards employed in systems analysis and design, (7) programming standards employed, (8) efficiency of present hardware, (9) adequacy of system documentation, (10) support from equipment suppliers, and (11) cost analysis of the data-processing installation and systems installed.[6]

In addition to the overall management audit of the data-processing department, each major system should be subject to post-installation testing after sufficient time has passed and the system is functioning in a routine fashion. Systems should be evaluated in comparison with their original objectives to determine if goals are being achieved and if costs are in line with original estimates. Such reviews are essential in order for the hospital to reach decisions on whether to continue or discontinue a system, whether a system's capabilities should be expanded, or whether to make changes to improve the operating efficiency of the system. Schmitz states:

> The cost is high, so the expectations for the system are often unrealistically high, especially in the initial stages of installation. Unless a careful and thorough analysis is made which adequately treats the subject of the impact of the system at all levels of the organization and in several time frames, the user is likely to be disappointed with the system. . . .
>
> When this failure to evaluate retrospectively occurs, it makes a mockery of the evaluation and planning that was performed before the system was acquired.[7]

Although each system will have its own specific objectives against which it should be reviewed, some general questions can help provide a framework for an evaluation system. First, what impact has a given system had on direct patient care in the hospital? Second, to what extent has the system brought about beneficial changes in internal operational procedures in the institution? Third, to what extent, if any, has the system improved management information available to hospital administration? And finally, what is the economic impact of the system on the hospital?

System evaluation should be a clearly defined management responsibility of the director of information systems. A formal protocol for system evaluation should be established to guide the review process. Individual evaluations should be scheduled long enough after installation to allow the system to settle down and be operating in a routine fashion, normally a 6- to 12-month interval. Users should participate in the evaluation, and external consultants might well be employed in the case of major systems involving substantial operating costs to the hospital. If the hospital has a permanent data-processing advisory committee (as discussed in Chapter 3), this committee might be assigned the responsibility of overseeing the evaluation process. Reports of the system evaluations should be distributed to each user department and to the hospital administrator, who might also wish to share them with the hospital's governing board. Follow-up meetings should be scheduled in order to initiate action called for as a result of the findings of each study.

Management Responsibilities

The basic thesis of this book is a simple one. Information systems can be useful to hospital management provided that the process for planning, designing, installing, and operating such systems is itself well managed. Responsibilities of hospital administration have been stressed throughout this section on system analysis, design, and implementation. These are summarized in the ten points which follow.

1. Hospital management must insist on a careful planning process which precedes all major decisions related to the installation of computer equipment or the design of complex information systems. A master plan for information system development should be created and periodically updated. This plan should guide all specific implementation decisions.
2. The design of specific systems should be carried out by an interdisciplinary project team. Systems analysts and computer programmers will take the lead on technical analysis and design activities. Representatives of departments to be involved in the system should help guide the specification of system requirements and evaluate the technical design plans of the analysts. Hospital management should be involved in all major design projects to insure congruence with organizational goals and objectives.
3. Once a project team has been organized, careful systems analysis should precede any implementation decisions. Shortcuts in the systems analysis phase will inevitably lead to problems later on.
4. The preliminary design specifications for an information system should be in harmony with the master plan for information system development discussed in Step 1 above.
5. Detailed system specifications should always be required before any implementation activities take place. These specifications should be reviewed formally and approved by all user departments and by hospital administration before proceeding with the next steps in system development.
6. Throughout the analysis, design, and implementation phases of a systems project, hospital management should require careful scheduling of all activities and should receive periodic progress reports as the project proceeds.
7. During the implementation phase, thorough training of all personnel to be involved in the new system (both data-processing and user department personnel) should be carried out.

8. No system should be put into operation without first carrying out a comprehensive system test. The test should cover all phases of system operation, including machine programs and procedures, training of personnel involved in the system, ability of the system to meet original objectives, and accuracy of the initial cost estimates.
9. Provision should always be made for adequate maintenance after the system is operating. Maintenance provisions are essential to correct operational errors, to make system improvements, and to facilitate changes necessitated by changes in organizational needs.
10. As discussed in the previous section of this chapter, hospital management must insure that data-processing and computer activities are periodically audited and that all systems are formally evaluated once they are installed and operating normally.

SUMMARY

A hospital data-processing department's organizational location will be influenced by the knowledge, attitudes, and style of the administrator as well as the overall organizational context of the institution. However, the kinds of systems to be developed also should influence organizational patterns. If comprehensive clinical and financial computer applications are planned, then the director of information should report directly to the administrator or to one of his key assistants.

The director should be a person with both technical and managerial skills. In recruiting a technical staff, care should be taken to separate the very different kinds of skills required for systems analysis and computer programming. A comprehensive information systems department will include a professional staff of systems analysts and programmers, a staff of technicians for operation and maintenance of equipment, a clerical staff for data preparation and assistance to the professional and technical staff.

Protecting the confidentiality of personal information is one of the most important responsibilities of hospital administration in system development. Patient medical records, as well as personal data on employees, must be protected. A system of safeguards will include physical security of computer data files, limitation of access procedures built into the design of systems, and administrative controls with well-defined procedures and penalties for violations. Hospital management must also take the lead in insisting that the computer installation be periodically audited and that all systems are formally evaluated after they are placed in operation.

DISCUSSION QUESTIONS

10-1 What factors should determine where a hospital information systems department is located in the overall organizational structure?

10-2 What is the difference between a systems analyst and a computer programmer?

10-3 What kinds of skills should a hospital data-processing director possess?

10-4 Why is protection of confidentiality of information so important in a hospital?

10-5 Why should the data-processing department be periodically audited? What factors should be examined as part of the audit?

10-6 List some of the audit trails and controls which should be designed into an information system.

PROBLEMS

10-1 Your hospital is in the process of designing an on-line computer system for ordering patient services and storing patient information. Develop a detailed outline of a plan for security features to be included in the system to protect the confidentiality of patient information.

10-2 Six months ago your hospital installed a computerized accounts receivable and collections system which is now operating on a routine basis. Develop a plan to carry out a formal post-installation evaluation of the system. Include a list of the criteria to be used in the evaluation.

NOTES

1. William F. Klimko, "MIS Amplified" (Letter to the Editor), *Health Care Management Review*, Fall 1976, p. 6.
2. Suzanne La Violette, "More Than Low Salaries Deter Data Processing Staff from Hospitals," *Modern Healthcare*, May 1980, pp. 78-80.
3. Vince DePaolo, "Contract Management," *Modern Healthcare*, August 1980, pp. 78-80.
4. Willis H. Ware, "Old Practices in a New Age Endanger Information Privacy," *Hospitals*, October 16, 1977, pp. 133-140.
5. Larry Chervenak, "Auditing the Efficiency of Your Computer Installation," *Hospital Financial Management*, June 1970, p. 8.
6. Ibid., pp. 9-10.
7. Homer H. Schmitz, "A Protocol for Evaluating Hospital Information Systems," *Hospital and Health Services Administration*, Winter 1977, p. 45.

ADDITIONAL READINGS

Balgrosky, Jean A., Strum, Dennis W., and Bradley, Evelyn. "Information Systems: Evaluation Ensures Performance." *Hospitals*, May 1, 1982, pp. 82-84.

Chervenak, Larry. "Auditing the Efficiency of Your Computer Installation." *Hospital Financial Management*, June 1970, pp. 8-10.

Computer Security Institute. *Guidelines for Establishing a Computer Security Program*. Hudson, Massachusetts: Computer Security Institute, 1981.

Donaldson, Hamish. *A Guide to the Successful Management of Computer Projects*. New York: John Wiley & Sons, 1978. Note particularly Chapter 9, "Control Security and Privacy."

Janeura, Elise G. *Audit and Control of Computer Systems*. New York: Petrocelli-Charter, 1974.

Lindberg, Donald A.B. *The Growth of Medical Information Systems in the United States*. Lexington, Massachusetts: Lexington Books, 1979. Note particularly Chapter 5, "Evaluating the Worth of MISs."

Lucas, Henry C. *Information Systems Concepts for Management*. New York: McGraw-Hill, 1978.

Mair, William C., Wood, Donald R., and Keagle, W. Davis. *Computer Control and Audit*. Altamonte Springs, Florida: The Institute of Internal Auditors, 1976.

Milutinovich, Jugoslav and Kanter, Howard A. "Organizing the MIS Department." *Journal of Systems Management*, April 1975, pp. 36-41.

Porter, W. Thomas and Perry, William E. *EDP Controls and Auditing*. Boston: Kent Publishing Co., 1981.

IV

Information Systems in Hospitals

11

Information Systems to Support Direct Patient Care: Clinical Information Systems

In this final section of the book, attention is focused on specific information systems applications in hospitals. These applications fall into three general categories. *Clinical* (or medical) information systems (described in this chapter) involve the organized processing, storage, and retrieval of information to support patient care activities in the hospital. *Administrative* information systems (Chapter 12) are designed to assist in carrying out administrative support activities of the hospital such as payroll and patient accounting. A *fully integrated*, or *total*, hospital information system (Chapter 13) serves both of the above purposes through centralization of information storage and retrieval and data communication links throughout the hospital. *Management* information systems (Chapter 14) are designed to provide current information for management planning and control purposes.

Clinical Systems— General State of the Art

A 1976 survey by the Hospital Financial Management Association demonstrated that clinical information systems and computer applications were much less common in hospitals than administrative systems.[1] Although approximately 40 percent of the responding hospitals were involved in the use of computers to index and control medical records, no other clinical application was mentioned more than 20 percent of the time. As indicated in Figure 11-1, 17 percent of the responding hospitals have systems to sup-

FIGURE 11-1
Selected Clinical Computer Applications in Hospitals (1976)

Application	*Number of Hospitals Responding to Question*	*Computerization In-house*		*Computerization through Outside Data-Processing Service*	
		No. of Hospitals	*Percentage*	*No. of Hospitals*	*Percentage*
Medical Records Disease Index	1919	172	9	522	27
Utilization Review, PSRO	1917	141	7	194	10
Clinical Lab Reporting	1926	183	10	56	3
EKG Analysis	1917	54	3	116	6
Radiation Therapy Dosage Calculation	1896	79	4	45	2
Pulmonary Functions Reporting	1907	74	4	46	2
Inpatient Drug Profiles	1923	86	4	22	1
Multiphasic Screening	1815	32	2	23	1
Computer-aided Diagnosis	1828	23	1	27	1

Reprinted, with permission, from Hospital Financial Management Association, *The State of Information Processing in the Health Care Industry* (Chicago: The Association, 1976).

port utilization review and Professional Standards Review Organization (PSRO) activities, 13 percent have operational systems for clinical laboratory reporting, and nine percent utilize automated systems for analysis of electrocardiograms. Other applications mentioned by at least two percent of the respondents include radiation therapy dosage calculations, pulmonary function reporting, inpatient drug profiles, multiphasic screening, and computer-aided diagnosis.

A more recent (1980) survey by Dorenfest and associates indicates that financial and related administrative computer applications still overshadow clinical applications in hospitals. This is particularly true in multihospital systems, where the emphasis is on financial systems development. Larger, individually managed community hospitals are more likely to be involved in the design of patient care systems.[2] A related survey of 73 nonprofit and commercial computer shared services organizations revealed that their first priority has been offering full financial functions to hospitals, but that they also " . . . provide or plan to provide computer areas outside of finance such as . . . pharmacy, laboratory, . . . and HIS."[3]

A review of the 1980 hospital literature confirmed growing interest in the use of hospital information systems to respond to a variety of needs—management, patient care, and regulatory.[4]

A number of research-oriented and teaching hospitals have developed generalized clinical computer systems, most designed on a modular basis and some employing their own special purpose programming languages for clinical application development.[5] Not all activity has been limited to the large teaching hospital, however. With assistance from a federal grant, a 68-bed hospital in rural South Carolina developed an on-line patient information system which includes a clinical record of patient problems and treatments for access by physicians, pharmacists, and hospital staff.[6]

Giebink and Hurst conducted an extensive study of selected computer projects in health care institutions, with a special focus on information systems which support the delivery of ambulatory care.[7] Hospitals with outpatient departments were included in the study. The final report includes detailed descriptions of several medical computer projects at 19 health services organizations. Data for the study were collected through structured questionnaires and on-site interviews with project personnel. Many of the projects included in the survey involved multiple clinical applications of computers. The three most common were medical records systems, direct patient care systems, and systems of diagnostic or consultation assistance.

One of the most important findings of this study was the importance of involvement and acceptance by medical professionals, particularly physicians, to the success of a system. Equally important were the attitudes, support, and involvement of management in the system development projects examined. The more successful projects were those with active involvement of both health professionals and administrators.

Benefits were identified in the projects, both to patients and to health care providers. Patients benefited through decreased waiting times for services and through improved care which resulted from better and more accurate medical records reporting and retrieval. Benefits to providers of care included improved systems of communication of physicians' orders, more standardized protocols for diagnosis and treatment, improved medical audit procedures for quality assurance, and better planning and evaluation of health services through the availability of medical data linked to data on the social and economic backgrounds of patients treated in the ambulatory care facilities.

Several problems were noted as well. In some projects there was a lack of proper communication and interaction of medical staff and administrators in the design of systems. Some of the projects had difficulty in clarifying specific system objectives. Some of the systems had problems due to lack of proper system testing before implementation, and insufficient training and education of system users was a related problem. Uncertain funding, particularly for those projects dependent upon government grants and contracts, was also noted as a difficulty in some cases. Some projects were hampered by political problems both within the organization and outside of it. A continuing problem for some projects was users not accepting the system and being reluctant to accept change. Although software and hardware problems were minimal, some hardware problems were noted, particularly with communications equipment linked to the central computers but external to them.

In commenting on the general requirements for a medical information system, Collen notes that implementation of computer systems in other than the administrative areas of hospitals has been quite difficult.[8] He points out that planning and implementing a medical information system require extraordinary amounts of capital, personnel time and effort, and careful organization. Reliability requirements for such systems are high, and they must be designed and implemented according to careful time schedules in a modular fashion.

The need for confidentiality of patient information places special requirements on the design of clinical information systems. Employees of the hospital who will create or utilize computerized patient databanks must be carefully selected and properly trained. Adequate safeguards must be built into both hardware and software design. These should include carefully constructed coding systems for user identification, as well as terminal interlocks to insure that only authorized personnel can make inquiries into patient files. And most important of all, administrative monitoring and control is essential.[9]

In a comprehensive review of medical information systems in United States hospitals, Lindberg summarizes the major barriers to the development of clinical systems:

> Barriers . . . have been sociological and behavioral as well as technological. . . . The speed of technical change in this field has been far greater than the speed of social adaption. . . . medicine seems to suffer greatly from an administrative pattern of extreme balkanization. There are also major deficits in our understanding of basic physiological processes. Those faults have a direct influence on systems design and efficiency. Social barriers include slow adaptability by the health professions . . . and the seeking of short-term profits and earnings by both the computer and hospital industries.[10]

COMPUTER-AIDED DIAGNOSIS

Computer-aided diagnosis can best be examined within a general framework for diagnostic systems consisting of two major components: (1) systems for collecting patient data and communicating this data to the physician (including data on the patient's medical history, physical examinations, and diagnostic tests performed) and (2) systems for comparing patient-specific information with available medical knowledge to assist the physician in diagnostic decision making.[11]

Automated History Systems. Systems developed for automated medical history-taking from patients usually involve direct patient-computer communications through a computer terminal.[12] A sequence of standardized questions is presented to the patient on a video screen, and the patient responds by depressing keys on the computer terminal. Most of the questions will require only a yes or no answer. The computer program which controls the inquiry process will be designed to branch to a new question or set of questions based upon the patient's response to previous questions, in much the same way that a trained health professional would conduct a face-to-face interview with the patient. Computerized history systems generally are used as the first phase in a two-phase process. The second phase includes a personal interview by the physician, with the results of the automated history available. Hence, the physician's time is economized, and he or she can focus on specific problems for which additional information is needed. Results of standardized laboratory tests might also be available at the time of the second phase interview.

A byproduct of automated history systems is the storage of information from a large group of patients on magnetic tape or other form of computer storage. The database thus created is available for purposes of both research and patient follow-up. Research uses are particularly important, since data from a large number of patients have now been captured according to standardized protocols, thus providing the possibility of comparative studies of patient populations.

Systems have also been developed for more complete capture of patient information before consultation with a physician. The most noteworthy of these are systems for automated multiphasic screening. Such systems include computer-aided collection of both patient history and physical examination data according to standardized protocols. The computer summarizes data obtained from the screening laboratory for review by the physician in advance of a follow-up visit from the patient.

One of the best known multiphasic screening systems was developed at the Permanente Medical Group in Oakland, California. Dr. Morris Collen, principal investigator of the group which developed the system, described it as follows:

> The automated multitest laboratory provides electrocardiography, anthropometry, chest and breast x-rays, visual acuity tests, tonometry, retinal photography, audiometry, vital capacity determinations, a health questionnaire on pre-punched cards, and laboratory tests including eight blood chemistries done simultaneously with direct punched-card output. Before the patient leaves the multitest laboratory, additional indicated procedures are arranged in accordance with programmed computer 'advice' rules. When all test reports are received, the computer prints out a summary report for the physician.[13]

In recent years, questions have been raised about the effectiveness of multiphasic screening on health status of patients. In a controlled trial, major differences between screened and non-screened patients were not found. However, previously unknown abnormalities requiring retesting for confirmation were identified in 28 percent of the patients screened, leading to medical treatment in 15 percent of the cases.[14]

Computer-Aided Diagnosis. Systems designed to compare patient-specific data with available medical knowledge fall into two categories: computer systems for direct signal processing and clinical decision systems. Much of the work in signal processing has been done in two areas, interpretation of electrocardiograms and analysis of electroencephalograms. In electrocardiogram (EKG) analysis, electronic signals from EKG leads attached to the patient are recorded on tape or disk or directly transmitted to a computer for processing. The computer will first convert these analog signals (continuously fluctuating electrical impulses) to digital form (a series of numbers) for fast and accurate computation. The computer program will then compare the wave forms for a specific patient against known standards and, through a series of programmed decision rules, arrive at a differential diagnosis. The results are then printed out for the internist or consulting electrocardiographer to review.

Systems for computer analysis of EKGs have been demonstrated to be effective on a communitywide basis. Twenty hospitals with a total bed capacity of 2,387 participated in a regional system of EKG analyses by computer.[15] Data communications systems were used to link each hospital to a central computer facility, and the results were transmitted back in the same manner. The system was found to be cost-effective, but more important, in 85 percent of the cases, trained electrocardiographers agreed with the computer printout and made no change or only minor amendments to the computer output before certifying its validity. The time spent in physician interpretation of the EKG waveform was approximately half that required using manual methods.

A portable bedside EKG unit with built-in microcomputer has been used by cardiologists at Lawrence Hospital in Bronxville, New York. The unit records, analyzes, and prints the interpretation of the EKG in 80 seconds. In a test of the system, diagnosis of normal EKGs was 99 percent accurate, and the system was accurate in abnormal EKGs well over 90 percent of the time, comparing favorably with physician diagnoses.[16]

Computer processing of neural signals is similar to that of EKG analysis as far as data collection and reporting are concerned, although the analysis programs are obviously different. Several successful EEG analysis programs are described in the literature.[17]

Experimental systems also have been developed for computerized simulation of the clinical diagnostic process. These systems employ logical branching according to standardized protocols programmed into the computer. Ledley describes the possible benefits of such systems:

> the mathematical-logic formulation of differential diagnosis, makes it possible for the computer (1) to make a list of the possible differential diagnoses consistent with a patient's symptom profile, (2) to systematically group symptoms that are related with respect to one disease as distinguished from the other diseases under consideration, (3) to formulate a differential diagnosis with a minimum number of necessary tests, (4) to present a precise description of a differential diagnosis for teaching purposes, (5) to provide a systematic checklist in difficult differential diagnosis cases where possible relevant tests must not be neglected, and (6) to present classes of symptoms that may indicate certain common etiological effects from a research point of view.[18]

Computer-aided diagnosis of vascular disease has been carried out at the University of Colorado Medical Center in Denver. In a study of 160 patients, computer generated diagnostic summaries required no alteration in 86 percent of the cases, and the cost of the system compared favorably to previous methods employed.[19] Scientists at the University of New Mexico have developed a computerized database system (called DIASTU) for medical diagnostic studies of gynecological cancer. The system employs a minicomputer running with a time-sharing operating system.[20]

It should be noted that systems for clinical decision making are supportive to the physician and do not replace the judgment obtained through training and experience. The design and programming of standardized protocols is a complex task limited by currently available medical knowledge which can be universalized into standards. For these reasons, such systems are still largely in an experimental and developmental stage.

Computer-aided Treatment and Follow-up

Just as computers have been used to aid in the diagnostic process, systems have also been developed which employ computers to assist in the treatment and follow-up of patients. Three examples of computer applications of this kind are discussed: computer-generated treatment protocol and reminder systems; radiation treatment planning systems; and computerized patient follow-up systems.

Systems have been developed in which the computer serves as a recorder of routine tasks to be carried out in the rendering of medical and nursing care. Once these standardized lists have been stored in the computer, automatic reminders can be generated to assist the physician and nurse in treatment planning. Systems of this kind require that standardized treatment protocols be developed for each major diagnostic category and that these protocols be programmed into the computer.

McDonald describes one such system developed at the Indiana University School of Medicine.[21] An information system was designed to provide computer suggestions about the management of selected clinical conditions. A study was conducted to review the utilization of 390 computerized protocols by a panel of nine physicians who participated in the study. The overall study results showed that physicians responded (on average) to 51 percent of the clinical events when given computer reminders and only 22 percent of the events when not given the computer suggestions. The results were not affected by level of training of the physicians participating in the research project.

In discussing the findings, the author concludes that prospective reminders do reduce clinical errors. He points out that many physician errors relate to a person's limited ability to store and process data rather than to correctible human deficiencies. Thus, the computer can be a valuable tool in augmenting the physician's capabilities and concurrently reducing his error rate.

A study of physician attitudes toward computerized clinical consultation revealed that physicians will accept systems that enhance their patient management capabilities but will oppose applications which they perceive as infringing on their management role.[22]

Similar systems have been developed to assist the nursing care process. One such system is based upon the development of a set of uniform standards of nursing care which is programmed into computer storage. When the nurse writes a specific "care initiator" on a nursing order form, the computer responds with detailed nursing care orders and list of medications to be administered. The automated nursing care plans so developed also are available for evaluation and quality audit by nursing supervisory personnel.[23]

Computers also are being used increasingly in the field of radiation treatment planning. Computerized treatment planning permits the preparation and evaluation of individual patient treatment plans, a complex mathematical problem whose solution was not feasible on an individual patient basis before the availability of electronic computation. Given data about a patient and the location and size of a tumor, the computer can determine the exact dosage to be applied at various treatment sites while minimizing the exposure of unaffected regions of the body.

A major advancement in the field of radiation therapy has been the development of computerized transaxial tomography.[24] This expensive, but powerful, new procedure is dependent upon computer processing of reconstituted x-ray images in the computer. Automatic pattern recognition programs are utilized to describe the tumor and tumor site, and graphic picture manipulation methods are employed to show three-dimensional views of the body and the size of the tumor. The system can be used on an outpatient basis and thus eliminates the need for a number of diagnostic procedures that require hospitalization. The system also permits easy periodic reevaluation of the effects of treatment on the patient.

Computer systems have also been designed to provide periodic reminder information to both patients and health care providers on the need for follow-up review and treatment. For example, tumor registries have been developed which have two functions: they provide computer-generated notices to patients when follow-up visits are due and simultaneously generate a research database which enables researchers to study the effects of cancer treatment techniques among a described patient population. Many hospitals operate systems of this kind, and some also operate on a regional or statewide basis.

Patient Monitoring Systems

Patient monitoring systems employ the computer for continuous surveillance of a patient's vital signs and periodic display of physiological data for use by trained monitoring personnel.[25] Figure 11-2 is a graphic depiction of a typical monitoring system. The first step in the process is data acquisition from monitoring equipment attached to the patient and conversion of these data from analog to digital form for computer processing and display. Data are then stored and available for retrieval for periodic display or display on demand. Computer programs enhance the measured data through structured analysis of clinical data in accordance with programmed decision rules. Trend data are also followed to monitor changes in patient vital signs over time. Patient monitoring systems can operate at the individual patient's bedside, at a central station designed to monitor a small number of intensive care beds, or at a remote location linked back to the intensive care unit by communication equipment. Three prototype monitoring systems are described below.

A computerized monitoring system in the Intensive Care Unit of Michael Reese Hospital (Chicago) continuously monitors heart rate, blood pressure, central venous pressure, intracranial pressure, pulmonary artery pressures, temperature, and respiration. Technicians also enter laboratory results, including blood gasses, cardiac output, and pulmonary function tests. The system has proven beneficial in terms of improved patient care, improved record keeping, and improved staff utilization in the ICU.[26]

At the Pacific Medical Center in San Francisco, California, a patient monitoring system is in operation in the cardiopulmonary intensive care unit. This system utilizes an on-line computer dedicated to the monitoring function rather than a central time-shared computer. Direct measurements are made of arterial, central venous, and pulmonary artery pressures; EKG; temperature; and several pulmonary functions. The computer compiles these data and makes computations every ten minutes for display at the central monitoring station. The same data are also available for display on demand on a screen located at each patient's bedside. The system was submitted to a formal evaluation study. The study documented heavy utilization of the system by nurses and others on the monitoring stations, and personnel have come to rely upon it. The research did not demonstrate statistically significant differences in morbidity and mortality between a group of patients using the monitoring system and a control group of patients monitored by traditional methods.[27]

A system installed in three Canadian hospitals has taken a different approach, using new computer technology. The Alpha monitoring system employs microprocessors, small computers built right into the individual

FIGURE 11–2
Diagram of Patient Monitoring System

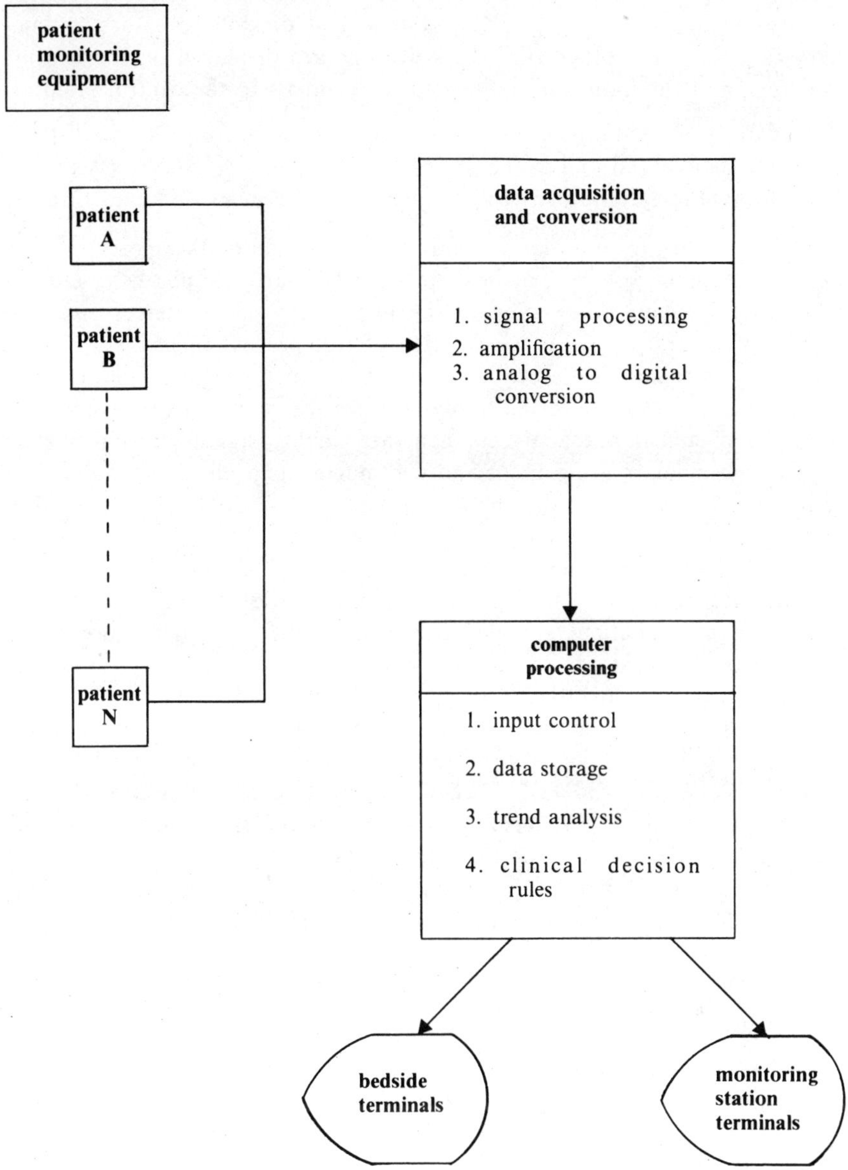

patient's bedside monitoring unit.[28] The microprocessors use changeable "plug-in" modules, electronic microcircuits which vary the monitoring program for each individual patient. The modules provide various combinations of measurements, including EKG, systolic and diastolic pressure, pulmonary functions, and other vital signs. Results are displayed on the bedside monitors, and the individual units also send signals to the central monitoring display unit.

LABORATORY AUTOMATION

Laboratory information systems constitute one of the more common clinical computer applications in hospitals. There are two phases to clinical laboratory systems: automation of the test processes themselves and processing of laboratory data. Automation of test processing involves linking laboratory instruments directly to a computer. Analog signals from the test instruments are first converted to digital form for computer processing. For example, chemical autoanalyzers generate analog signals in which slide wire potentiometers are attached to continuous strip chart recorders. The same signals which drive the chart recorders are captured and converted to digital form. The computer then carries out calculations that would be made by the lab technician in a manual system. Computer calculations include determination of peak values and computation of the concentration of the unknown patient sample. The final results are then stored in a patient laboratory data file and test results are printed.

Laboratory data processing systems can be used independently of or in conjunction with laboratory automation systems. A laboratory data processing system would include recording of test requisitions, scheduling of specimen collection and test processing, recording of the results of completed tests, preparing test reports for immediate return to the nursing units or outpatient department, periodically preparing summary reports of all tests run for a given patient, preparing statistical reports for the laboratory, and record keeping for quality control and administrative control of laboratory operations.

A complete laboratory information system would include both automation and data processing. As defined in a federal government report:

> a completely automated laboratory is . . . one which establishes positive patient-sample identification as soon as sample material is obtained from a patient and maintains this identification throughout a mechanized analytical chain and final presentation and/or recording of valid results.[29]

Whatever approach to laboratory automation a hospital may take, integration of the laboratory system with the larger hospital information system is very important. Test results must be included in central patient data files, and information on the number and types of tests completed must be transmitted to patient account files for pricing and billing.

The Automation of Medical Laboratory Sciences Review Committee of the National Institute of General Medical Sciences documents the state of the art of laboratory information science.[30] Although the report indicates that mechanized clinical laboratories have become an integral part of the practice of medicine and the delivery of health care, complete automation of the clinical laboratory has not yet been accomplished.

In discussing instrumentation requirements, this federal report states that automated instrumentation systems should:

1. be accurate, precise, and develop reproducible results;
2. perform several tests in sequence with minimum delay;
3. be capable of using small samples for pediatric patients;
4. provide for entry of emergency specimens without disrupting regular processing;
5. insure positive sample identification from input to output, a difficult problem but a very important requirement for a system of this kind.[31]

The report also points out the importance of adequate training of laboratory personnel in use of the new technology of laboratory computer systems.

In discussing the state of the art in specific laboratories, the report notes that the most advanced level of automated instrumentation is found in the clinical chemistry laboratory. Advances are also occurring rapidly in hematology, where "mechanization . . . has been quite successful in that a number of well-defined routine parameters are being measured with acceptable speed and accuracy."[32] In blood banks, most tasks are still performed manually, although data-processing systems have been applied to the logistics of blood bank operations, particularly for inventory control. Automation in the microbiology and virology laboratories has been limited to data-processing systems which process manually determined test results. Some experimental work is being carried out in the area of computer-aided organism identification.

Aikawa and Pinfield have written an excellent case study which traces the development of a laboratory computer system at the University of Colorado Medical Center in Denver, Colorado.[33] The report presents the complete chronology of events starting with the development of a punched-card data-processing system for the clinical laboratory and progressing through several stages to the installation of a self-contained, process control computer system in the laboratory. The computer system includes full automation of clinical chemistry and some automation of hematology testing. The system also provides complete record keeping for the laboratory and is linked to the central Medical Center computer for transmission of medical and administrative data for central patient files. The Colorado system is reported to be cost effective. The importance of total involvement of the laboratory staff is cited as a major factor in the system's success. All laboratory personnel were involved in an extensive training program, and one laboratory staff member received extensive training before taking on the responsibilities of chief systems designer in the laboratory.

Scalfani and Ramkissoon describe a comprehensive evaluation of a laboratory information system installed at the Hinsdale Sanitarium and Hospital in Hinsdale, Illinois. The system employs a dedicated computer system with packaged software for processing of laboratory test requisitions and results. The evaluation, conducted two and one-half years after installation, revealed that 87 percent of the specific goals stated in the original design specifications were achieved. A net annual cost reduction of $128,756 was realized, and the system development and installation costs are expected to be recovered within four years.[34]

The University of Iowa Hospitals and Clinics installed a commercial laboratory computer software package operating on a dedicated minicomputer. Considerable planning was undertaken to insure integration of this dedicated system with the central computer of this 1,090-bed teaching hospital. The system is reported to have reduced clerical work in the laboratory and improved accuracy and turnaround time of test results. The system is expected to pay for itself in the fourth year of operation.[35]

Medical Records Indexing and Retrieval

The medical record is central to all patient care activities in the hospital. It serves several important functions. First, the medical record is a guide to and continuous record of treatment while the patient is in the hospital. After discharge, it becomes an archival record available for retrieval if the patient is readmitted or requires further treatment as an outpatient. Medical records also serve as working documents for medical audit and utilization review by members of the organized medical staff. Finally, in many hospitals, particularly teaching hospitals, the depository of medical records serves as a database for research studies. If all of these functions are to be accomplished well, then good records management is essential.

The computer can be used to assist in medical records management. Systems have been developed in which computer files are maintained to keep track of the current location of medical charts in the hospital. Some systems also track the completion status of records, generating notices for the attending physician when final diagnostic and treatment information is needed.

Medical records management systems usually include a procedure for indexing of the records by patient identification number, by disease classification, and by other demographic factors so that records can be retrieved upon demand for medical audit review and research purposes. Some systems also include an on-line retrieval capability whereby abstracts of patient records are available for display on a video terminal in the emergency room, outpatient clinics, and admitting department.

The abstract will contain demographic information about the patient, a resume of recent medical history and treatment, along with critical medical information such as drug sensitivities and allergies. Systems such as these are particularly useful in large public hospitals serving as primary care centers for large patient populations, where continuity of care is a constant problem.

It should be noted that no operational computer system has yet been developed whereby electronic storage completely eliminates the need for a paper record. There are some advanced, fully integrated systems of hospital communication and data-processing which approach this capability, and these are discussed in Chapter 13. However, even in those few cases where system capability for eliminating all or part of the traditional paper record exists, the systems are not yet acceptable to the culture of the medical enterprise. Medical professionals still seem to prefer the security of the paper record to the mystique of the cathode-ray tube display.

Parkland Memorial Hospital in Dallas has implemented a system for medical records control which incorporates on-line chart completion, chart location, and clinic appointment scheduling. The system was developed as a result of concern about incomplete charts (15,000 according to a 1979 study) and the need to maintain control over chart location in this 755-bed teaching hospital with extensive outpatient activity. According to the system designers, after one and one-half years of operation, the number of incomplete charts has declined by approximately 50 percent and chart availability has improved substantially.[36]

An automated utilization review system is in operation at the Miami Heart Institute in Florida. The internally developed system provides daily reports for attending physicians and periodic summaries for the hospital's Utilization Review Committee and Professional Standards Review Organization (PSRO) office. This automated medical records system is an integral part of a comprehensive hospital information system at the Institute. Evaluation after six years of operation indicated significant clerical savings and adequate acceptance by physicians.[37]

Wirtschafter and Mesel contend, however, that most medical records systems do not lend themselves to quality of care evaluation, either prospectively or retrospectively.[38] They propose a more structured record approach which is specific to a particular medical problem or patient care goal. To accomplish this, *minimum care assurance data sets* would be appended to each medical record. These would be standardized protocols and reminder lists for treatment of particular problems and would be both patient-specific and problem-specific. The data sets would guide the appropriate treatment and care regimens for the patient and would facilitate both concurrent and retrospective review.

Pharmacy Information Systems

There is a large data-processing task to be carried out in the hospital pharmacy. Good records must be maintained in order to control carefully the ordering, stocking, and distribution of drugs and to avoid medication errors to the maximum extent possible. Accurate records are also important for billing and hospital revenue generation.

The two basic approaches to the design of computer applications in the hospital pharmacy include development of stand-alone pharmacy systems and integration of pharmacy activities with a larger hospital information system. Stand-alone pharmacy systems have been developed for control of dangerous drugs (paticularly narcotics), for drug ordering and inventory control, for control of drug distribution to patients, for storage and retrieval of drug information, for the construction of patient drug profiles, for the maintenance of the hospital's formulary, and for generation of charges for patient billing.

Pharmacy systems integrated into a larger hospital information system will typically involve the entering of medication orders on computer terminals at the nursing units of the hospital. These orders are then communicated automatically to the pharmacy, where worksheets are generated, patient profiles are updated, and labels are prepared. Such systems usually also will include automatic updating of the drug inventory and automatic generation of patient charges from the medication orders.

Virginia Mason Hospital in Seattle, Washington, conducted an extensive cost-benefit analysis of an automated pharmacy information system. A Request for Proposals (RFP) was developed and submitted to 18 computer vendors for bidding. Anticipated savings in cost of operations after five years were estimated to be approximately $437,000, with system payout projected during year three.[39]

The pharmacy information system developed at Kingsbrook Jewish Medical Center in Brooklyn, New York, employs a dedicated minicomputer installed in the pharmacy department with the aid of consultants. A user task force conducted an extensive needs analysis and developed specifications for the system. The system includes unit dose distribution, preparation of patient drug profiles, inventory control, and provision of a database for drug utilization studies and quality assurance. Use of the hospital's central computer system was rejected in favor of the dedicated minicomputer approach.[40]

Computers also are being used to monitor medications administered in hospitals. Current drug orders are checked against patient profiles to insure proper dosage, monitor contraindications, and protect against drug allergies and sensitivities.[41]

SUMMARY

Clinical information systems and computer applications are less common in hospitals than are administrative systems. Computers are used extensively in the indexing and control of medical records, but they are used less extensively in other direct patient care activities.

Involvement of physicians and hospital administrators is a key element in the success of hospital clinical computer applications. Such systems, when properly designed and implemented, have brought benefits to patients and to health professionals in terms of both patient convenience and improved health care.

Problems identified by hospitals involved in the development of clinical computer applications include difficulty in clarifying system objectives, insufficient system testing prior to implementation, inadequate training of hospital staff in utilization of new systems, and lack of proper communication among system designers, medical staff members, and administrators in the hospital.

Protection of the confidentiality of patient information is a critical requirement in the design of clinical computer applications. Safeguards must be built into the system in the design of computer hardware and software and through careful training of hospital personnel.

Systems have been developed to aid in medical diagnosis. Such systems are of two types: systems for collecting patient data and communicating these data to the physician, and systems for examining patient-specific information within the context of available medical knowledge to assist the physician in diagnosis.

Computers have also been applied to assist physicians, nurses, and other health professionals in patient treatment and follow-up. Examples of such systems include computer-generated treatment protocols, computerized nursing care systems, radiation treatment planning systems, and follow-up systems for patients with chronic illnesses such as cancer.

Patient monitoring systems employ computer technology in the continuous surveillance of vital signs and the periodic display of physiological data for observation by trained personnel. Computer programs enhance the monitored data through structural analysis and computation of trends over time.

Laboratory information systems are one of the more common clinical applications of computers in the hospital. Systems have been developed in which several of the test processes are automated, and other applications involve processing of laboratory information on test requisitions, test results, and patient charges.

Medical records are central to all patient care activities in the hospital. Systems have been developed for the indexing, management, and location control of medical records. No operational systems have yet been implemented whereby computer storage eliminates completely the need for a paper medical record. Computerized medical records systems also facilitate the work of medical audit and utilization review committees, and provide a depository for medical research purposes.

The hospital pharmacy has a large data-processing task to perform. Pharmacy computer systems have been developed for control of dangerous drugs, for drug ordering and inventory control, for control of drug distribution to patients, for storage and retrieval of drug information, for construction of patient drug profiles, for formulary construction and maintenance, and for generation of patient charges for billing purposes.

Dedicated minicomputers and microcomputers are being used increasingly in clinical applications. Some medical instruments employ built-in microcomputers for computation and storage of information. Hospitals must guard against uncontrolled proliferation of small computers through central planning and control. Dedicated systems in clinical departments should be designed in modular fashion so they can communicate with the overall hospital information system (see Chapter 13 for further discussion of system integration).

DISCUSSION QUESTIONS

11-1 Why have clinical computer applications been less common in hospitals than administrative applications?

11-2 What are some of the benefits which have accrued to hospitals as a result of installing clinical information systems?

11-3 What are some of the problems which system designers have encountered?

11-4 Why is involvement of medical professionals and hospital administrators so important to successful system implementation?

11-5 Discuss mechanisms for insuring confidentiality of patient information in automated systems.

11-6 To what extent have computers been utilized to assist in the diagnostic process? Discuss some specific applications.

11-7 Briefly discuss the application of computers to medical treatment protocols.

11-8 Describe the functioning of a typical automated monitoring system for patients in an intensive care unit.

11-9 What kinds of information systems have been developed in the hospital clinical laboratory? Briefly describe typical applications.

11-10 Have computer storage devices successfully replaced the medical records in a hospital? Why or why not? In what ways have computers assisted the medical records department?

11-11 Discuss the application of computers in the hospital pharmacy.

NOTES

1. Hospital Financial Management Association, *The State of Information Processing in the Health Care Industry* (Chicago: The Association, 1976).
2. Sheldon I. Dorenfest, "Computer Shared Services: Hospital Chains Become Important Providers," *Modern Healthcare*, November 1981, pp. 77-84.
3. Sheldon I. Dorenfest, "Computer Time Sharing: 73 Groups Provide Full Financial Functions," *Modern Healthcare*, October 1980, pp. 71-78.
4. Gary A. Mecklenburg, "Types and Uses of Hospital Information Systems Expand," *Hospitals*, April 1, 1981, pp. 112-119.
5. See, for example: Douglas C. Johnson and G. Octo Barnett, "MEDINFO: A Medical Information System," *Computer Programs in Biomedicine*, Vol. 7, 1977, pp. 191-201; Jan R. Schultz and Layton Davis, "The Technology of PROMIS," *Proceedings of the I.E.E.E.*, September 1979, pp. 1237-1244; Darrell L. Ward, David J. Mishelevich, and J. Robin Richmond, "Medical Applications in the TANDEM-16 Multiple Computer System Environment," *Journal of Medical Systems*, Vol. 3, Nos. 1-2, 1979, pp. 7-18; Homer R. Warner, "Knowledge Sectors for Logical Processing of Patient Data in the HELP System," in *Proceedings of the Second Annual Symposium of Computer Applications in Medical Care* (New York: Institute of Electrical and Electronics Engineers, November 1978), pp. 401-409.
6. Charlotte A. Johnston and Athalene B. Mole, "Patient Care Computer in 68-Bed Hospital," *Journal of American Medical Records Association*, August 1980, pp. 28-36.
7. Gerald A. Giebink and Leonard L. Hurst, *Computer Projects in Health Care* (Ann Arbor, Michigan: Health Administration Press, 1975).
8. Morris F. Collen, "General Requirements for a Medical Information System (MIS)," in *Proceedings of a Conference on Medical Information Systems* (Washington, D.C.: U.S. Department of Health, Education, and Welfare, Health Services and Mental Health Administration, January, 1970).
9. J.F. Brandejs, M.A. Kasowski, and G. Pace, "Information Systems. Part IV: Protection of Health Care Confidentiality," *Canadian Medical Association Journal*, October 4, 1975.

10. Donald A.B. Lindberg, *The Growth of Medical Information Systems in the United States* (Lexington, Massachusetts: Lexington Books, 1979), p. 105.
11. See Lee B. Lusted, "Computer Techniques in Medical Diagnosis," in *Computers in Biomedical Research*, Vol. I, R.W. Stacy and B.D. Waxman, eds. (New York: Academic Press, 1965), pp. 319-338.
12. See, for example, Warner V. Slack et al., "A Computer-Based Medical History System," *New England Journal of Medicine*, January 1966, pp. 194-198.
13. Morris F. Collen, "Periodic Health Examinations Using an Automated Multitest Laboratory," *Journal of the American Medical Association*, March 7, 1966, pp. 142-145.
14. Donna M. Olsen, Robert L. Kane, and Paul H. Proctor, "A Controlled Trial of Multiphasic Screening," *New England Journal of Medicine*, April 22, 1976, pp. 925-930.
15. *The Computer-Assisted EKG—From Laboratory to Community* (Washington, D.C.: U.S. Department of Health, Education, and Welfare, Public Health Services, Health Resources Administration, September 1973), Publication No. (HRA) 74-3104.
16. Mark Marshall, "The Bedside Computer Takes ECG, Analyzes and Prints the Interpretation in 80 Seconds," *Hospital Topics*, March-April 1980, pp. 23-24.
17. See, for example, F.H. Lopes da Silva, "Signal Analysis in Neurology," in *Biomedical Computing*, ed. W.J. Perkins (Baltimore: University Park Press, 1977), pp. 5-12.
18. Robert S. Ledley, "Aids to Medical Diagnosis," *Journal of the American Medical Association*, June 13, 1966, p. 936.
19. Daniel H. Lowenstein, et al., "Computer Diagnosis in a Vascular Diagnostic Laboratory," *Computers and Biomedical Research*, Vol. 14, 1981, pp. 592-605.
20. I.I. Rosen et al., "A Computerized Database System for Medical Diagnostic Studies," *Computer Programs in Biomedicine*, Vol. 12, 1980, pp. 249-261.
21. C.J. McDonald, "Protocol-Based Computer Reminders, The Quality of Care and the Non-Perfectability of Man," *New England Journal of Medicine*, December 9, 1976, pp. 1351-55.
22. Randy L. Teach and Edward H. Shortliffe, "An Analysis of Physician Attitudes Regarding Computer-Based Clinical Consultation Systems," *Computers and Biomedical Research*, Vol. 14, 1981, pp. 542-558.
23. June B. Somers, "A Computerized Nursing Care Systems," *Hospitals*, April 16, 1971, pp. 93-100.
24. See, for example: T. Sandor et al., "Automated Tissue Analysis from Computerized Axial Tomographic Scans," *Computers and Biomedical Research*, Vol. 14, 1981, pp. 125-130.
25. L.C. Sheppard and N.T. Kouchoukos, "Computers as Monitors," *Anesthesiology*, August 1976, pp. 250-259.
26. Elizabeth Beckmann, Ben F. Cammack, and Barbara Harris, "Observation on Computers in an Intensive Care Unit," *Heart and Lung*, November-December, 1981, pp. 1055-1057.
27. M. Hilberman et al., "An Evaluation of Computer-Based Patient Monitoring at

Pacific Medical Center," *Computers and Biomedical Research*, October 1975, pp. 447-460.
28. K.I. Christopherson, "Microprocessor Technology Adds New Dimension to Patient Monitoring Systems," *Hospital Administration in Canada*, May 1976, pp. 50-51.
29. Thomas D. Kinney and Robert S. Melville, eds., *Mechanization, Automation, and Increased Effectiveness of the Clinical Laboratory* (Washington, D.C.: U.S. Department of Health, Education, and Welfare, Publication No. (NIH) 77-145, p. 7.
30. Ibid.
31. Ibid., pp. 8-9.
32. Ibid., p. 63.
33. Jerry K. Aikawa and Edward R. Pinfield, *Computerizing a Clinical Laboratory* (Springfield, Illinois: Charles C. Thomas, Publisher, 1973).
34. John J. Scalfani and Reuben A. Ramkissoon, "The Acquisition of a Laboratory Information System," *Journal of Medical Systems*, Vol. 5, No. 4, 1981, pp. 281-303.
35. Delane A. Wycoff and James R. Wagner, "Integration of a Laboratory Computer Into a Hospital Information System," *American Journal of Clinical Pathology*, September 1978, pp. 390-399.
36. David J. Mishelevich et al., "Medical Records Control and the Computer," *Topics in Health Record Management*, December 1981, pp. 47-55.
37. Alberta Budkin et al., "An Automated PSRO-Utilization Review System," *Journal of Medical Systems*, Vol. 6, No. 2, 1982, pp. 139-147.
38. David D. Wirtschafter and Emmanuel Mesel, "A Strategy for Redesigning the Medical Record for Quality Assurance," *Medical Care*, January 1976, pp. 68-75.
39. Ted Neal, "Pharmacy Analyzes Costs, Savings of Computer Information System," *Hospitals*, February 1, 1981, pp. 70-74.
40. Bruce G. Kay et al., "How to Get the Computer Into the Pharmacy," *Hospitals*, July 16, 1980, pp. 113-117.
41. Deborah J. Brown et al., "A Hospital Medication Monitoring System," *Journal of Medical Systems*, Vol. 3, Nos. 3-4, 1979, pp. 143-151.

ADDITIONAL READINGS

Clinical Systems: General

Barnett, G. Octo et al. "MUMPS—An Evolutionary Commentary." *Computers and Biomedical Research*, Vol. 14, 1981, pp. 112-118.

Brandejs, J.F., Kasowski, Margaret Ann, and Pace, Graham. "Information Systems," Part I: The medical record; Part II: The medical record; Part III: Methodology and long-term applications; Part IV: Protection of health care confidentiality; Part V: What the users think; Part VI: What the computer can do for the primary care physician; Part VII: Problem-oriented medical record for family practice; Part VIII: Impact on the medical profession. *Canadian Medical Association Journal*, October 4, 1975.

Covvey, H. Dominic and McAlister, Neil Harding. *Computers in the Practice of Medicine*, Vol. 2, "Issues in Medical Computing." Reading, Massachusetts: Addison-Wesley Publishing Co., 1980.

Giebink, Gerald A. and Hurst, Leonard L. *Computer Projects in Health Care*. Ann Arbor, Michigan: Health Administration Press, 1975.

Johnson, Douglas C. and Barnett, G. Octo. "MEDINFO—A Medical Information System." *Computer Programs in Biomedicine*, Vol. 7, 1977, pp. 191-201.

Ledley, Robert S. *Use of Computers in Biology and Medicine*. New York: McGraw-Hill, 1965.

Lincoln, Thomas L. and Korpman, Ralph A. "Computers, Health Care, and Medical Information Science." *Science*, October 17, 1980, pp. 257-263.

Lindberg, Donald A.B. *The Growth of Medical Information Systems in the United States*. Lexington, Massachusetts: Lexington Books, 1979.

Perkins, W.J., ed. *Biomedical Computing*. Baltimore: University Park Press, 1977.

Schultz, Jan R. and Davis, Layton. "The Technology of PROMIS." *Proceedings of the I.E.E.E.*, September 1979, pp. 1237-1244.

Shires, David B. *Computer Technology in the Health Sciences*. Springfield, Illinois: Charles C. Thomas Publisher, 1974.

Stacy, R.W. and Waxman, B.D., eds. *Computers in Biomedical Research*. 2 Volumes. New York: Academic Press, 1965.

Sterling, Theodor D. and Pollack, Seymour V. *Computers and the Life Sciences*. New York: Columbia University Press, 1965.

Ward, Darrell L., Mishelevich, David J., and Richmond, J. Robin. "Medical Applications in the TANDEM-16 Multiple Computer System Environment." *Journal of Medical Systems*, Vol. 3, Nos. 1-2, 1979, pp. 7-18.

Computer-aided Diagnosis

Brazier, May A.B. "The Application of Computers to Electroencephalography," in *Computers in Biomedical Research*, Vol. I, ed. Ralph W. Stacy and Bruce D. Waxman. New York: Academic Press, 1965, pp. 295-315.

Clayton, R.D. et al. "A Radiology Reporting System Based on Most Likely Diagnoses." *Computers and Biomedical Research*, Vol. 13, 1980, pp. 258-270.

Collen, Morris F. "Periodic Health Examinations Using an Automated Multitest Laboratory." *Journal of the American Medical Association*, March 7, 1966, pp. 142-145.

Ledley, Robert S. "Computer Aids to Medical Diagnosis." *Journal of the American Medical Association*, June 13, 1966, pp. 115-125.

Lowenstein, Daniel H. et al. "Computer Diagnosis in a Vascular Diagnostic Laboratory." *Computers and Biomedical Research*, Vol. 14, 1981, pp. 592-605.

Olsen, D.M., Kane, R.L., and Proctor, P.H. "A Controlled Trial of Multiphasic Screening." *New England Journal of Medicine*, April 22, 1976, pp. 925-930.

Rosen, I.I. et al. "A Computerized Database System for Medical Diagnostic Studies." *Computer Programs in Biomedicine*, Vol. 12, 1980, pp. 249-261.

Taylor, T. R. "Clinical Decisions Analysis." *Methods of Information in Medicine*, October 1, 1976, pp. 216-224.

U.S. Department of Health, Education, and Welfare. *The Computer-Assisted EKG —From Laboratory to Community*. Publication No. (HRA) 74-3104. Washington, D.C.: Public Health Service, Health Resources Administration, September 1973.

Utyamyshev, R.I. "Development of Automatic Medical Diagnostic and Medical Information Systems." *Biomedical Engineering*, November 1974, pp. 5-7.

Wilson, Linda O. "Computerized Triage of Pediatric Patients: Automated Triage Algorithms." *Annals of Emergency Medicine*, December 1981, pp. 636-640.

Computer-aided Treatment and Follow-up

Budkin, Alberto et al. "On-Line Management of Cardiac Surgical Data." *Journal of Medical Systems*, Vol. 3, Nos. 3-4, 1979, pp. 133-142.

Marshall, C.H. "Principles of Computer Tomography." *Postgraduate Medicine*, August 1976, pp. 105-109.

McDonald, C.J. "Protocol-Based Computer Reminders, The Quality of Care and the Non-Perfectability of Man." *New England Journal of Medicine*, December 9, 1976, pp. 1351-55.

Moreland, M.S. et al. "Maire' Fringe Topography of the Human Body." *Medical Instrumentation*, March-April 1981, pp. 129-132.

Sandor, T. et al. "Automated Tissue Analysis from Computerized Axial Tomographic Scans." *Computers and Biomedical Research*, Vol. 14, 1981, pp. 125-130.

Smoller, Sylvia Wassertheil, Bell, Bertrand, and Blaufox, M. Donald. "Computer Aided Management of Hypertensive Patients." *Medical Care*, December 1975, pp. 1044-1054.

Sofaly, Kathleen J. "The Nurse and Electronic Data Processing." *Medical Instrumentation*, May-June 1981, pp. 169-170.

Somers, June B. "A Computerized Nursing Care System." *Hospitals*, April 16, 1971, pp. 93-100.

Teach, Randy L. and Shortliffe, Edward H. "An Analysis of Physician Attitudes Regarding Computer-Based Clinical Consultation Systems." *Computers and Biomedical Research*, Vol. 14, 1981, pp. 542-558.

Intensive Care Monitoring

Ackmann, James J. "A Computer System for Neurosurgical Patient Monitoring." *Computer Programs in Biomedicine*, Vol. 10, 1979, pp. 81-88.

Anderson, G.B. et al. "A Monitoring and Trending System for Intracranial Pressure." *Medical Instrumentation*, May-June 1981, pp. 191-194.

Beckman, Elizabeth, Cammack, Ben F., and Harris, Barbara. "Observations on Computers in an Intensive Care Unit." *Heart and Lung*, November-December, 1981, pp. 1055-1057.

Christopherson, K.I. "Microprocessor Technology Adds New Dimension to Patient Monitoring Systems." *Hospital Administration in Canada*, May 1976, pp. 50-51.

Hilberman, M. et al. "An Evaluation of Computer-Based Patient Monitoring at

Pacific Medical Center." *Computers and Biomedical Research*, October 1975, pp. 447-460.

Johnson, Dickey S. et al. "A Computerized Alert Program for Acutely Ill Patients." *Journal of Nursing Administration*, June 1980, pp. 26-35.

Raimer, Daniel et al. "A Metabolic Monitor: An Application of the Computer to Critical Care Instrumentation." *Journal of Medical Systems*, Vol. 5, No. 4, 1981, pp. 337-343.

Sheppard, L.C. and Kouchoukos, N.T. "Computers as Monitors." *Anesthesiology*, August 1976, pp. 250-259.

Laboratory Automation

Bloch, Daniel M. "Computer-Generated Management Tools for the Clinical Pathology Laboratory." *Journal of Medical Systems*, June 1982, pp. 305-310.

Blois, M.S. "Incorporation of Clinical Laboratory Information Systems into the Hospital Information System." In *Computers in Laboratory Medicine*, ed. D. Enlander. New York: Academic Press, 1975, pp. 35-41.

Giles, Ian G. "An Introduction to Microcomputers in Biochemistry." *International Journal of Biochemistry*, Vol. 13, 1981, pp. 673-680.

Hasenfang, Grace and Frable, William J. "Development of a Hospital Information System for Cytopathology." *Acta Cytologica*, April 1981, pp. 185-192.

Hogman, C.F. and Ramgren, O. "Computer System for Blood Transfusion Service." *Transfusion*, May-June 1970, pp. 121-132.

Keen, W.H. "Use and Efficiency of a Computer System in the Hospital Laboratory." *Pathologist*, January 1976, pp. 14-19.

Levine, Glenn B. "Advantages of Computer Systems in the Clinical Laboratory." *Hospital Progress*, June 1976, pp. 66-69.

Scalfani, John J. and Ramkissoon, R.A. "The Acquisition of a Laboratory Information System." *Journal of Medical Systems*, Vol. 5, No. 4, 1981, pp. 281-303.

U.S. Department of Health, Education, and Welfare. *Mechanization, Automation, and Increased Effectiveness of the Clinical Laboratory*. Publication No. (NIH) 77-145, ed. Thomas D. Kinney and Robert S. Melville. Washington, D.C.: Public Health Service, National Institutes of Health, 1976.

Winrich, Lonny B. and Hobbie, Russell K. "Computer Interpretation of Laboratory Test Results: An Annotated Bibliography." *Journal of Medical Systems*, Vol. 5, No. 3, 1981, pp. 219-223.

Medical Audit, Quality Assurance, Utilization Review, PSROs

Benford, Linda H., Floyd, Ronald F., and Stansel, Edward H. "UR/PSRO Long Term Care Data System." *Medical Record News*, June 1976, pp. 22-31.

Budkin, Alberto et al. "An Automated PSRO-Utilization Review System." *Journal of Medical Systems*, Vol. 6, No. 2, 1982, pp. 139-147.

Huber, G.A. et al. "Evaluating Computerized Screening as an Aid to Utilization Review." *Inquiry*, September 1974, pp. 188-195.

Schmitz, H.H. and Schoenhard, W.C. "Automated Utilization Review is Timely, Accurate, Efficient." *Hospital Progress*, July 1976, pp. 73-77, 98.

Witt, A.G. and Konicek, F. "MAL—Medical Audit Language: How One Hospital Used a Computer to Simplify Data Retrieval." *Quality Review Bulletin*, August 1976, pp. 25-28.

Medical Records Indexing and Retrieval

Ayers, W.R. et al. "Mobilizing the Emergency Room Record." *Computers in Biology and Medicine*, September 1973, pp. 153-163.

Ball, Marion J. and Shannon, Roger H. "The Medical Record Scientist as a Health Care Computer User." *Medical Record News*, June 1980, pp. 12, 108-111.

Buckley, J.D. et al. "A Computer Based Medical Record System." *Methods of Information in Medicine*, July 1973, pp. 137-142.

Collen, M.F. et al. "Problems of Computerization of Large Computer Medical Record Systems." *Medical Informatics*, April 1976, pp. 47-53.

Donahoe, A.M. "Computer System Provides Flexible Control." *Hospitals*, June 16, 1973, pp. 114-121.

Groves, William E. and Davidson, W. Ross. "A Computerized Chart Management System for Medical Records." *Computer Programs in Biomedicine*, Vol. 11, 1980, pp. 158-164.

Mishelevich, David J. et al. "Medical Records Control and the Computer." *Topics in Health Record Management*, December 1981, pp. 47-55.

Weyl, Stephen et al. "A Modular Self-Describing Clinical Databank System." *Computers and Biomedical Research*, June 1975, pp. 279-293.

Wirtschafter, David D. and Mesel, Emmanuel. "A Strategy for Redesigning the Medical Record for Quality Assurance." *Medical Care*, January 1976, pp. 68-75.

Pharmacy–Drugs

Brown, Deborah J. et al. "A Hospital Medication Monitoring System." *Journal of Medical Systems*, Vol. 3, Nos. 3-4, 1979, pp. 143-151.

Cohen, S.N. et al. "Computer Based System for Prospective Detection and Prevention of Drug-Drug Interactions." *Drug Information Journal*, January-June 1972, pp. 81-86.

Frieburn, Richard B. "Operations Analysis Applied to a Drug Distribution System." *American Journal of Hospital Pharmacy*, May 1976, pp. 452-458.

Gouveia, W.A. "Computer Applications in the Hospital Pharmacy." *Hospitals*, January 1, 1971, pp. 80-83.

Kay, Bruce G. et al. "How to Get the Computer Into the Pharmacy." *Hospitals*, July 16, 1980, pp. 113-117.

Mahoney, C.P., Lausier, J.M., and Jeffery, L.P. "Development of a Computerized Drug-Drug Interaction Retrieval System." *American Journal of Hospital Pharmacy*, December 1973, pp. 1153-1156.

Neal, Ted. "Pharmacy Analyzes Cost, Savings of Computer Information System." *Hospitals*, February 1, 1981, pp. 70-74.

Reeme, P.D. "A Basic Computerized Hospital Pharmacy System." *American Journal of Hospital Pharmacy*, March 1974, pp. 281-284.

Simon, G.I. et al. "Computerized Pharmacy Services in a Large Community Hospital." *American Journal of Hospital Pharmacy*, May 1976, pp. 459-463.

12

Information Systems to Support Administrative Operations in Hospitals

Most hospitals enter the data-processing field through the development of information systems which support administrative operations. This chapter discusses typical administrative applications in hospitals, focusing on systems which function primarily at the departmental level as an aid to routine operations. The use of computers and organized information systems for management planning and control is the subject of Chapter 14.

Administrative Systems— General State of the Art

There are several alternative approaches to the development of administrative information systems in hospitals. Some hospitals have installed medium- to large-scale general purpose computers, with administrative systems typically the first applications implemented on these systems. With the rapid advancement of minicomputer technology, some hospitals, particularly smaller ones, have installed dedicated minicomputer systems in the business office. These systems generally are sold with preprogrammed application packages for inpatient and outpatient accounting, accounts receivable, payroll accounting, general ledger accounting, and processing of accounts payable. A third approach, followed by an increasing number of hospitals, is participation in a shared computer system. Computer services can be purchased from a commercial vendor, or the hospital may choose to participate in a nonprofit shared-services organization such as those offered by state hospital associations, Blue Cross plans, local hospital councils, and corporate offices of hospital systems.

Administrative applications also are indicated in large-scale fully integrated hospital information systems. Chapter 13 discusses the state of the art of integrated hospital information systems and presents a description of a typical system.

The 1976 computer applications survey conducted by the Hospital Financial Management Association (HFMA) indicated that hospitals are much more active in developing administrative systems than they are in using computers to assist in clinical work. Figure 12-1 summarizes the more common administrative applications. Payroll accounting and reporting leads the list with 86 percent of the hospitals responding to the survey indicating that they utilize computers for payroll processing. Accounts receivable and patient billing applications follow close behind. Computers also are used extensively for producing the daily inpatient bed census and to a lesser extent for processing inpatient preadmissions and for scheduling outpatient clinic appointments.

Administrative systems also are used to support materials management in hospitals. Sixty-three percent of the survey respondents reported the use of data-processing equipment for processing of accounts payable vouchers, and more than 25 percent utilize computers for capital equipment and central stores inventory. Information systems for general accounting are also common, including general ledger record keeping, cost accounting, preparation of financial statements, and comparison of expenditures against budgeted amounts.

The HFMA survey also demonstrates the alternative routes which hospitals have followed in the development of administrative information systems. Approximately 60 percent of the hospitals using computers for administrative purposes have installed in-house computer equipment. Of these, 25 to 30 percent use minicomputers for business office applications. The remaining 40 percent utilize outside data-processing services for administrative applications.

More recent surveys by Dorenfest and associates revealed that 73 shared services organizations (nonprofit and commercial) are providing 2,219 community hospitals with a complete range of financial applications.[1] A related interview survey of 250 community hospitals (1979) indicated that 216 were computer users, with administrative applications dominant.[2]

Ball describes two levels of operational hospital information systems.[3] LEVEL I systems are capable of data collection and message switching, processing of requisitions for service, capturing of patient charges, capturing of financial data, and preparation of routine reports such as payroll vouchers, daily bed census, aged accounts receivable, and the like. LEVEL II systems have all of the above capabilities and include a computerized patient medical record, with the system programmed to handle clinical information as well as service requisitions and charges.

FIGURE 12-1
Selected Administrative Computer Applications in Hospitals (1976)

Application	*Number of Hospitals Responding to Question*	*Computerization In-house*		*Computerization through Outside Data-processing Service*	
		No. of Hospitals	*Percentage*	*No. of Hospitals*	*Percentage*
Payroll Accounting and Reporting	2072	812	39	965	47
Accounts Receivable	2070	959	46	657	32
Inpatient Billing	2080	947	46	626	30
Emergency Room Billing	2029	854	42	592	29
Outpatient Clinic Billing	2002	768	38	528	26
Inpatient Daily Census	2040	712	35	565	28
Inpatient Pre-admission	1993	133	7	87	4
Outpatient Clinic Appointment	1927	43	2	31	2
Accounts Payable Voucher and Payment	2055	771	38	519	25
Capital Equipment Inventory	1989	302	15	466	23
Central Stores Inventory	1984	288	15	195	10
General Ledger Accounting	2062	774	38	582	28
Financial Statements	2010	576	29	500	25
Budget Comparisons	2016	536	27	495	25
Cost Accounting	1970	203	10	280	14

Reprinted, with permission, from Hospital Financial Management Association, *The State of Information Processing in the Health Care Industry* (Chicago: The Association, 1976).

The literature also contains a substantial amount of criticism of hospitals and their apparent inability to develop effective information systems. Herzlinger is critical of the use of data-processing systems in nonprofit organizations, including hospitals.[4] Herzlinger characterizes the state of information systems in most nonprofit organizations as "dismal," stating that few such systems are of equal quality to those found in profit-oriented corporations: "Computer graveyards are most often found in larger hospitals and welfare departments . . . [and] the technical problems of programming and operating such a system are sometimes beyond the capability of the organization . . ."[5] The causes of this problem are several. According to Herzlinger, many administrators in hospitals are "not comfortable with numbers." They lack adequate technical skills, particularly in the use of management control techniques and in understanding financial data. Frequently, top managers are not involved in the design of information systems, particularly the important task of content specification. Hospitals and other nonprofit organizations tend to underfund information systems at their inception and then are shocked when system development costs are higher than expected. Many systems have not been adequately tested before being put into operation, with severe problems the result. Finally, information systems in many hospitals have been underused by top managers, perhaps the key to all of the above problems. As Herzlinger states, "An information system used regularly by top management for making such key decisions as budget allocation will eventually overcome any initial flaws of design and installation."[6]

Facility Utilization and Scheduling Systems

Efficient utilization of facilities is a *sine qua non* of effective hospital administration. The need to contain costs in an era of rapid inflation and diminishing resources is an important reason for every hospital to utilize facilities and resources fully. Utilization review is now mandated both by regulatory agencies and by insurance companies which provide payment for services rendered in the hospital. Administrators are also charged with the responsibility of insuring that services are available when needed, and effective scheduling of services is essential to this end.

In response to these demands for efficient facility utilization, several hospitals have developed computerized monitoring and scheduling systems. Systems have been developed to monitor inpatient occupancy rates, clinic and emergency room activity, and utilization of individual service facilities such as the operating suite. Some systems provide the capability for advanced booking and scheduling of facilities, both for patient convenience and for efficient allocation of resources, particularly personnel staffing.

Advance bed booking and preadmissions systems are particularly useful in those situations in which a substantial proportion of admissions are elective and can be scheduled in advance (for example, a specialized surgical facility). Computer programs can project average length of stay for each elective admission to the hospital once historical data (including diagnosis, surgical procedure, age, and sex of patient) have been accumulated on average length of stay. After admissions are scheduled and entered into the computer files, the system keeps track of projected occupancy levels for each day during a future scheduling period.

A system of this type was installed at the Massachusetts Eye and Ear Infirmary in Boston.[7] The system was initiated after a special task force identified several problems related to facility utilization. Bed occupancy ranged from 30 percent to 100 percent and, as might be expected, was low on weekends. Similarly, surgery utilization varied from a low of 25 percent to a high of 79 percent. Daily admissions did not approximate daily discharges, and cancellations were not being refilled at an adequate rate.

After approximately one man-year of development effort, a system was designed in which the computer keeps running projections of preadmissions two months in advance of the patient's arrival at the hospital. Several reports are produced to aid the admitting office personnel in more efficient scheduling of inpatients. A bed availability report is produced showing projected occupancy for each day of the scheduling period (up to two months in advance). A similar advanced schedule is also maintained for surgery. The system produces an admissions list for the following day to aid hospital personnel in work planning. A monthly list is also provided to each physician showing his or her patients scheduled for admission during the next two months.

As a result of installation of the computerized system, average daily census is reported to have increased by four percent, and weekend occupancy is up six percent over previous figures. Interestingly, average length of stay has decreased, presumably because of more physician participation in the new system. Of perhaps greater benefit, workload has stabilized, there is now more rapid replacement of cancelled bookings, and in general there is better planning for staffing and utilization of services within the hospital.

Acute general hospitals must maintain an accurate accounting of bed census and occupancy if they are to survive. One important purpose of census data is to facilitate monitoring of income against budgetary projections. Hospital administrators must also follow demand for specific services and make adjustments in staffing and facilities as demand patterns change.

Long Island Jewish Hillside Medical Center has developed a computerized bed census system typical of that found in many hospitals.[8] Census reports are prepared both geographically within the hospital and also by major service areas and subservice specialties. The latter reports permit detailed analysis in comparing actual occupancy against projections. Reports provide cumulative comparisons for the current month and for the year to date. They also include a calculation of what average occupancy will be required for the remainder of the year if initial projections are to be realized. The system has resulted in improved financial planning through monitoring of income against projections and has also permitted the hospital to plan and allocate resources better in response to changing demand.

A computerized system for scheduling surgery was developed at Michael Reese Hospital in Chicago. The hospital was concerned with the need for more efficient use of the operating suite, which for several years was available by "oral command of surgeon and manual write-in of clerks." Using the basic system design developed at the Massachusetts Eye and Ear Infirmary (see above), the computerized system schedules 13 operating rooms for 200 surgeons performing 10,000 procedures per year.[9]

The Michael Reese system provides advance booking for each of the operating rooms. In the process of scheduling these facilities, data are accumulated on actual utilization of the operating rooms by service, by individual physician, and by procedure performed. Variations in each of these statistics can be examined by time of day, day of week, and season. Although some initial resistance on the part of surgeons was reported, the system is now said to be well accepted. It provides more efficient utilization of facilities, combined with personalized scheduling.

Brockton Hospital in Massachusetts has developed a computerized hospital operating room log and data system designed to provide complete and accurate statistical data for auditing, supply scheduling, and planning decisions. Reports generated by the system are used by the surgical suite supervisor, the O.R. committee, the tissue committee, the anesthesiology department, the infection control committee, and the management personnel who monitor utilization. Benefits of the system include more efficient scheduling, improved quality assurance, and better facility utilization.[10]

Outpatient clinic appointment scheduling systems are becoming more common, particularly in hospitals with large clinic volumes. Computer systems have been designed to maintain continuous records of appointments made and appointment times available. In addition, computer files accumulate data on no-show rates, with variations by clinic, type of patient, time of day, and day of week available for analysis. Such data can be particularly helpful for scheduling of hospital personnel. Scheduling systems also provide automatic planning data, including lists of patients to be seen tomorrow, for use in pulling medical records for the clinics.

An automated appointment system at Duke University Medical Center processes 40,000 patient visits annually and permits health care providers in the various clinics to control their own schedules. Patients request appointments through a receptionist, who operates a video terminal on-line to the system. The system provides activity reports to hospital management which are used for productivity analysis, development of scheduling standards, and allocation of resources.[11]

Riverside Methodist Hospital in Columbus, Ohio, developed a central outpatient registration system serving 11 outpatient service areas. The system handles patient registration, outpatient billing, and management reporting. A direct link to a Blue Cross Plan computer permits immediate determination of whether a patient's outpatient services will be reimbursed by that plan. The system is reported to have improved patient satisfaction while providing a more efficient administrative system.[12]

Financial Information Systems

The development of one or more financial information systems provides the initial excursion into computers and data-processing systems for most hospitals. In the face of demands for accountability and cost containment (while still providing high quality services), hospital administrators are acutely aware of the importance of sound financial management in their institutions. Financial information is essential to assist management in guiding operational performance in the hospital. The purposes of a financial management program include (1) providing hospital administration with quantitative data for making least cost investment decisions, (2) developing operational financial subsystems which are effective and efficient, and (3) providing management information for controlling and evaluating operations.[13]

The development of a financial information system is dependent upon a good hospital accounting system which must be in place first. Berman and Weeks define accounting as "the art of collecting, summarizing, analyzing, reporting, and interpreting, in monetary terms, information about the enterprise."[14] Systems analysts must work closely with the hospital controller and his staff in modifying existing accounting procedures for computer processing. To do so, a cooperative systems approach is essential. Buldak describes the importance of a system approach in one financial area of the hospital, accounts receivable:

> A systems approach to accounts receivable management is necessary to maintain the financial integrity of hospitals. This approach begins prior to each admission and continues until the account has a zero balance. The foundation on which this approach is built is well-written policies and procedures. . . .[15]

There are two basic approaches to the development of a hospital financial information system. The hospital may choose to design individual financial applications, independent of one another, which provide categorized data to the various components of the hospital's financial management and accounting organization. Alternatively, a hospital may decide to develop a fully integrated financial information system, in which the computer brings related information together for planning, monitoring, and control.

Individual financial subsystems which have been developed include the following:

- payroll preparation and accounting (with possible linkage to a personnel data system)
- processing of accounts payable (with possible linkage to a purchase-order processing system)
- collecting charges, patient and third party billing, and accounts receivable processing
- general ledger accounting
- cost allocation system for proration of the costs of nonrevenue-generating activities and items of general overhead
- preparation of financial reports for operating supervisors, hospital administration, board of trustees, external regulators and financers
- budgeting and budget control

The University of California at Los Angeles Hospitals and Clinics developed a fully integrated financial information system in order to provide management at all levels with timely and comprehensive financial information. The system was designed on a modular basis because of the complexity of operations and the long time that would be required to develop a total information system. Ten man-years of development and programming time were involved in completing the system, which includes 65 major computer programs and produces 36 different financial reports.

The designers of this system report that the following benefits have been realized: (1) much of the drudgery associated with routine accounting operations is now eliminated; (2) managers of revenue-generating departments are more cost-conscious since they now have exact information about the cost of services which they provide; (3) hospital departments no longer find it necessary to keep their own sets of books; (4) hospital management receives a complete and timely set of financial reports; and (5) the hospital can respond readily to new requirements for information imposed by government and other external agencies.[16]

Computers also are being used for financial planning and modeling. Miami Valley Hospital, an 800-bed teaching institution in Dayton, Ohio, employs such a system. The hospital subscribes to the Hospital System Library, a financial modeling package offered by Amherst Associates, Inc. of Chicago. The system, which is accessed by time-sharing terminals located throughout the hospital, provides capabilities for forecasting, budgeting, management reporting, and cost analysis. A reported strength of the financial modeling system is its ability to simulate various assumptions in the budget and provide effects of these assumptions on the profit and loss statement for contingency planning purposes.[17]

Rush-Presbyterian-St. Luke's Medical Center in Chicago (approximately 1,200 inpatient beds and one million outpatient visits annually) uses a computer system for determining the unit cost of hospital services. Microcosting has been implemented in 30 diagnostic and therapeutic areas of the hospital as a managerial planning tool. Stated benefits of the system include: improved understanding of the components of the cost of providing services, improved pricing decisions, identification of profit and loss leaders, and measurement of the effects of various changes in services on hospital costs.[18]

Amato and Nadler describe a computer simulation model for forecasting the financial implications of capital construction projects in hospitals. Baseline data and future assumptions are provided by those using the model. The assumptions can be varied and the effects of alternative courses of action studied. The model provides annual forecasts of cash flows, patient costs, and the overall financial structure of the hospital under alternative planning assumptions.[19]

In developing financial information systems or subsystems, hospitals can choose from the same alternatives mentioned earlier: in-house system development, use of preprogrammed packages from commercial vendors, or use of outside service or sharing arrangements. Various commercial packages are available in the financial area, and hospitals considering their use should evaluate them carefully according to the principles discussed in earlier chapters of this book.

Materials and Facilities Management Systems

Computers have been used to aid hospitals in more effective management of materials and physical facilities. Examples of such systems include computerized purchasing, inventory control systems, computerized menu planning and food service management, monitoring of preventive maintenance, energy management, and project scheduling and control systems (particularly useful in construction and remodeling projects).

Requisitions for supplies and materials constitute the input to computerized purchasing systems. Requisitions are entered into the computer and matched against budgetary authorization for financial control. Overdrafts on supply accounts are flagged and sent to the appropriate supervisor for follow-up action. Once requisitions are cleared, the computer will generate purchase orders. As materials are received, receipt notices are entered into the computer and matched against an open order file. Many automated purchasing systems also include direct linkage to the hospital's accounts payable system, if system integration has been planned in advance. Some systems also provide the capability for automatic reordering of selected items.

Phoenix Baptist Hospital operates an automated inventory control system for 1,000 standard stock items, ranging from office supplies to medical and surgical supplies.[20] A packaged computer system was purchased, thus minimizing the time involved in system development. The system generates a weekly inventory analysis report which includes for each item the current cost, purchase quantity, stock on hand, reorder point (computed automatically), out-of-stock conditions, and other information. The system automatically generates purchase orders for all items whose current inventory is below the reorder point. Monthly departmental distribution reports provide data to department supervisors on current usage and costs of supplies and materials.

The hospital has been able to eliminate one purchasing clerk's position as a result of adding the computer system. The system costs 30 cents per line item, and the net dollar savings is reported to be $130 per month. Perhaps of greater importance, nonquantifiable benefits include more realistic inventory levels, reduction in the number of back orders required, and an improved purchasing cycle.

Computerized menu planning has become more common in hospitals in recent years. Minimum nutritional and dietary requirements of patients, food items available and their costs, and decision rules on factors other than nutrition and food costs are input into the computer in order to insure that balanced and aesthetically pleasing meals are served to patients. The computer responds to this information by presenting a set of least cost menus meeting the constraints imposed by the nutritional model. Good packaged programs are available to hospitals for computerized menu planning.[21]

Computerized systems have been developed for preventive maintenance scheduling and reporting. The Medical Engineering Laboratory of Strong Memorial Hospital (University of Rochester Medical Center) developed a computerized system which supports service scheduling and preventive maintenance of approximately 6,000 pieces of patient care equipment. The system was developed in-house at a cost of $6,000, with monthly computer charges averaging between $100 and $200. The system produces inspection reports, inventory control for spare parts, and billing for service to other hospital departments.[22]

Massachusetts General Hospital employs a management information system to coordinate maintenance activities in the hospital's maintenance department. Administrators use the system to allocate manpower, assess employee performance, and control utilization of resources.[23]

Energy conservation has become a critical problem for hospitals as it has for all major industries in the United States. Computer packages have been developed to assist hospitals in monitoring energy utilization. Actual utilization figures are compared against calculated requirements, and possibilities for reduced consumption are highlighted by the computer model. Khosla describes four levels of energy management and control systems in hospitals, ranging from a dedicated microcomputer that controls one device (Level 1) to centralized computer systems that provide building-wide central monitoring and control of energy consumption (Level 4).[24]

Hospitals frequently are involved in capital construction and major remodeling projects. Systems have been developed to aid in project management. One such system, Program Evaluation and Review Technique (PERT), employs computer programs to assist in project scheduling and control. Users of the system must first construct a network which shows (1) all activities required to complete the project, (2) the relationships of these activities to one another (including those which can be carried out simultaneously and those which must follow a time sequence), and (3) time estimates for completing each activity. The computer responds with a schedule which shows the critical path for project completion. As activities are completed, actual completion times are entered back into the computer system, the program is rerun, and new schedules are prepared for the remaining work. The system is an excellent tool for dynamic scheduling and control of major projects in the hospital. Good packaged programs are available.[25]

Personnel Data Systems

The employees of a hospital constitute its most important resource. Most hospitals expend 60 to 70 percent of their operating budgets on employee salaries and benefits. Thus a good personnel information system is very important to assist hospital management in manpower planning and productivity analysis. There are several important functions which a hospital personnel data system can perform, including:

- maintaining and updating the employee permanent records file
- retrieving information from this file upon demand

- providing automatic position control
- producing labor analysis reports for each cost center of the hospital
- producing reports for analyzing personnel problems, such as turnover and absenteeism
- maintaining an inventory of special skills and certifications of employees
- producing labor cost allocations with linkage to the hospital's payroll system
- providing information on employee productivity and quality control (assuming that appropriate labor standards have been developed).

The Youngstown Hospital Association (Ohio) installed an automated personnel information system serving the two units of this 832-bed system.[26] The objectives of the system are (1) to provide accurate labor information for use in union negotiations, (2) to stabilize or reduce labor costs, (3) to reduce paperwork, particularly at the departmental level, and (4) to provide quantitative data for the personnel department to use for budgetary projections, staffing analyses, development of quality control and productivity standards, and analysis of absenteeism.

Input into the system is centralized in the personnel department. Forms were simplified during systems analysis and design, and one new form now handles 85 percent of all transactions generated at the departmental level. The central personnel records computer file is updated by on-line terminals. Sixty-four elements of information are included for each employee, and all data in the file are available for display at the computer terminals.

Reports produced by the system include a monthly labor analysis by cost center, quarterly absenteeism reports, departmental productivity reports produced each pay period, and miscellaneous reports available upon demand through the on-line computer terminals. The system is said to be less expensive than its predecessor, a manual system, and it has proved to be very useful during labor negotiations.

Systems also have been developed to analyze workload data and predict hospital staffing needs.[27] At the 1,000-bed University Hospitals of Cleveland, a computer simulation study was carried out to determine the number of full-time registered nurses required for delivery of nursing services in a 20-bed medical intensive care unit. The reports produced by the system permit management to evaluate alternative staffing levels while complying with standards for safe levels of care.[28]

One particularly interesting use of personnel data has been accomplished by Mount Sinai Hospital in New York City, which developed a manpower allocation system for use during labor strikes.[29] The system draws input from the hospital's personnel and payroll database and from questionnaires completed by each nonunion employee. Computer programs match data from an available-employee file against data from a requirements file, and assignments are made to fill critical operating positions during the strike period. The program takes into account such factors as age, sex, and medical status of available employees and their personal preferences, shift preferences, and special skills. The system thus provides maximum preparedness for staffing during a critical strike period.

SUMMARY

Hospitals make extensive use of computers and data processing systems to support administrative operations such as financial management, personnel administration, monitoring and scheduling of facilities, and materials management. Administrative applications typically are the first to be designed when hospital computer systems are installed. In addition, some hospitals have installed business office minicomputers, and others utilize outside service bureaus or computer-sharing arrangements for administrative data processing. The most common administrative applications in hospitals are payroll accounting and reporting, patient billing and accounts receivable, inpatient daily census preparation, accounts payable processing, and general ledger accounting.

Hospitals have been criticized for their slowness in making effective use of information systems. Frequently, top administrators are not involved and comfortable with the development of such systems. Administrative interest and involvement is an essential element for success.

Increasing pressure for cost containment makes efficient utilization of facilities essential in the modern hospital. Several hospitals have developed computerized monitoring and scheduling systems in such areas as advance bed booking and preadmission of inpatients, preparation of bed census and occupancy reports, scheduling of service facilities such as the operating rooms, and scheduling of patients in outpatient clinics.

Most hospitals enter the data-processing field through the development of financial information systems. Some accomplish this by developing individual financial systems in functional areas, while others have designed total financial information systems, in which complete integration of data collection and financial reporting is achieved. Financial data are essential for making least cost investment decisions, for providing good services to patients, and for providing management with information for planning, controlling, and evaluating operations.

Financial systems developed in hospitals include payroll preparation and accounting, processing of accounts payable, collection of patient charges, billing, and accounts receivable, general ledger accounting, cost allocation, financial reporting, and budgeting and budget control. Computer models are also being developed to assist hospital administrators in financial planning and forecasting.

Computers are being used increasingly in the management of materials and facilities. Systems have been developed for computerized purchasing, inventory control, menu planning and food service management, scheduling and monitoring of preventive maintenance, energy management, and construction project scheduling and control.

Employees constitute the most important resource which hospitals possess. Personnel data systems can assist in manpower planning and labor analysis. Systems have been developed which maintain employee records files, provide position control, produce labor analysis reports, analyze personnel problems such as turnover and absenteeism, maintain inventories of employee skills and certifications, produce labor cost allocations, and provide information on employee productivity.

DISCUSSION QUESTIONS

12-1 Describe some of the alternative approaches to the development of administrative information systems in hospitals.

12-2 What are some of the more common administrative computer applications in hospitals?

12-3 Why are administrative computer applications more common than clinical applications in hospitals?

12-4 Discuss some of the barriers to development of effective administrative information systems in hospitals.

12-5 How can computers assist hospital administration in achieving more efficient utilization of facilities?

12-6 Why do most hospitals enter the data-processing field by developing financial systems? What alternative approaches to systems design have been employed?

12-7 Describe typical financial computer applications in hospitals.

12-8 Briefly discuss computer applications in the area of hospital materials management.

12-9 In what ways is information important to effective hospital personnel administration? Describe some of the personnel data systems which have been developed.

NOTES

1. Sheldon I. Dorenfest, "Computer Time-Sharing: 73 Groups Provide Full Financial Functions," *Modern Healthcare*, October 1980, pp. 71-78.
2. Sheldon I. Dorenfest, "Hospitals' Computer Costs Will Rise Dramatically During Next Five Years," *Modern Healthcare*, May 1980, pp. 73-76.
3. Marion J. Ball and Stanley E. Jacobs, "Information Systems: The Status of Level I," *Hospitals*, June 16, 1980, pp. 179-186.
4. Regina Herzlinger, "Why Data Systems in Non-Profit Organizations Fail," *Harvard Business Review*, January-February 1977, pp. 81-86.
5. Ibid., p. 84.
6. Ibid., p. 86.
7. C. T. Wood and A. Lamantagne, "Computer Assists Advance Bed Bookings," *Hospitals*, March 1, 1969, pp. 67-69.
8. H. Light et al., "Monitoring Occupancy Rates," *Hospitals*, November 16, 1972, pp. 53-55, 110.
9. R. Bendix, et al., "Computer Scheduling for the OR," *Modern Healthcare*, June 1976, pp. 16M-16O.
10. Stephen L. Priest et al., "Computerized O.R. Log System Has Many Uses," *Hospitals*, June 1, 1980, pp. 79-82.
11. Frank J. Herpok et al., "Automated Appointment System Excels," *Hospitals*, August 1, 1980, pp. 65-67.
12. Daniel A. Witmer and Edgar O. Mansfield, "Outpatient Registration Centralized," *Hospitals*, August 1, 1980, pp. 68-70.
13. Howard J. Berman and Lewis E. Weeks, *The Financial Management of Hospitals, Fifth Edition* (Ann Arbor, Michigan: Health Administration Press, 1982), pp. 2-9.
14. Ibid., p. 7-9.
15. R. C. Buldak, "A Systems Approach to Accounts Receivable," *Hospitals*, March 1, 1975, p. 25.
16. T. T. Thibodaux et al., "Financial Management: Computer-Based Information System," *Hospitals*, March 16, 1973, pp. 51-56.
17. Tim Jackson et al., "Financial Modeling: One Hospital's Experience," *Computers in Hospitals*, May-June 1981, pp. 18-25.
18. Bruce C. Campbell and Michael Armer, "Using Computers to Determine Unit Costs," *Hospital Financial Management*, December 1981, pp. 44-49.
19. Frank C. Amato and Michael R. Nadler, "Computer Simulation Models for Long Range Financial Planning," *Hospital Progress*, October 1975, pp. 52-56.
20. D. L. Bankes, "Computer Keeps Inventory at Optimum Stock Level," *Hospital Financial Management*, July 1973, pp. 40-41.
21. Marie Balsley, "Minicomputer Updates Food Prices Weekly," *Hospitals*, September 1, 1980, pp. 76-77.
22. Robert H. Stiefel and Patricia Welker, "A Computerized System for Equipment Control and Preventive Maintenance," *Medical Instrumentation*, January-Feburary, 1981, pp. 24-26.
23. Cengiz Tanverdi and William L. Clemons, "Management Information System Ensures Maintenance Coordination," *Hospitals*, January 1, 1979, pp. 79-81.

24. Naresh K. Khosla, "Systems for Energy Control, Management," *Hospitals*, October 16, 1980, pp. 109-118.
25. For more details on PERT see D. Michael Warner and Don C. Holloway, *Decision Making and Control for Health Administration* (Ann Arbor, Michigan: Health Administration Press, 1978), pp. 68-78.
26. C. L. Packer, "Automation in the Personnel Department," *Hospitals*, October 1, 1971, pp. 45-48.
27. See, for example, Myron E. Hatcher, "A Micro Computer Productivity Management System," *Hospital Topics*, September-October 1981, pp. 8-11.
28. N. Duraiswamy, R. Welton and A. Reisman, "Using Computer Simulation to Predict ICU Staffing Needs," *The Journal of Nursing Administration*, February 1981, pp. 39-44.
29. B. T. Ross, "Computerized System Aids Staffing in Strikes," *Hospitals*, September 16, 1975, pp. 50-52.

ADDITIONAL READINGS

Administrative Systems: General

Balgrosky, J. A., Strum, D. W., and Bradley, E. "Information Systems: Evaluation Ensures Performance." *Hospitals*, May 1, 1982, pp. 82-84.

Ball, Marion J. and Boyle, Thomas M. "Hospital Information Systems: Past, Present and Future." *Hospital Financial Management*, February 1980, pp. 12-24.

Herzlinger, Regina. "Why Data Systems in Non-Profit Organizations Fail." *Harvard Business Review*, January-February 1977, pp. 81-86.

Kelliher, Matthew E. "An Effective Information System." *Hospital Topics*, September-October 1981, pp. 12-15.

Mecklenburg, Gary A. "Types and Uses of Hospital Information Systems Expand." *Hospitals*, April 1, 1981, pp. 112-119.

Schmitz, Hower H. *Hospital Information Systems*. Germantown, Maryland: Aspen Systems Corp., 1979.

Yasaki, E. K. "Wide Variety of Computer Based Systems Available to Hospitals." *Datamation*, March 1975, pp. 115-121.

Admissions, Discharge, Transfer; Facility Utilization; Scheduling

Chase, Mark, Loszlo, Charles, and Uyena, Dean, "Modelling a Hospital Entrance System." *Dimensions in Health Service*, January 1980, pp. 16-20.

Crook, W. J. and Syrett, D. "Computerized Admissions Means Automatic Efficiency." *Dimensions in Health Service*, September 1975, pp. 26-30.

Herpols, Frank J. et al. "Automated Appointment System Excels." *Hospitals*, August 1, 1980, pp. 65-67.

McGee, V. E., Jenkins, E., and Raunsley, H. M. "Statistical Forecasting in a Hospital Clinical Laboratory." *Journal of Medical Systems*, Vol. 3, Nos. 3-4, 1979, pp. 161-174.

Nelson, Robert A. "What is the Payoff in Computerized Appointment Scheduling?" *Medical Group Management*, July-August 1981, pp. 18-21.

Priest, Stephen L. et al. "Computerized O.R. Log System Has Many Uses." *Hospitals*, June 1, 1980, pp. 79-82.

Witmer, Daniel A. and Mansfield, Edgar O. "Outpatient Registration Centralized." *Hospitals*, August 1, 1980, pp. 68-70.

Financial System

Campbell, Bruce C. and Armer, Michael. "Using Computers to Determine Unit Costs." *Hospital Financial Management*, December 1981, pp. 44-49.

Clarkin, John F. and Chizever, Sheldon D., eds. "Accounts Receivable Management." *Topics in Health Care Financing*, Spring 1982, pp. 1-71

Fetter, R. B., Thompson, J. D., and Mills, R. E. "A System for Cost and Reimbursement Control in Hospitals." *Yale Journal of Biology and Medicine*, Vol. 49, No. 2, 1976, pp. 123-136.

Fournet, B. A. and Shoemaker, P. "Hospital Chain Slices Business Office Costs With Shared Financial System." *Modern Healthcare*, Vol. 10, No. 10, 1980, pp. 88-91.

Gimmelman, Frank J. "Computerized Cash Management: The New Frontier." *Health Care Management Review*, Vol. 4, No. 2, 1979, pp. 33-39.

Jackson, Tim et al. "Financial Modeling: One Hospital's Experience." *Computers in Hospitals*, May-June 1981, pp. 18-25.

Materials Management, Physical Plant, Preventive Maintenance

Balsley, Marie. "Minicomputer Updates Food Prices Weekly." *Hospitals*, September 1, 1980, pp. 76-77.

DeJong, J. "Cost Savings in Hospital Planning Using Computer Simulation." *Hospital Topics*, Vol. 58, No. 6, 1980, pp. 18-21.

Gillette, Paul E. "Micros Have Power to Save Energy." *Modern Healthcare*, April 1982, pp. 108-110.

Mitchell, Shelby G. "Computer System Reduces Energy Costs." *Hospital Progress*, November 1979, p. 40.

Rabbie, H. M. and Korte, R. L. "A Computer System for Biomedical Equipment Maintenance Reporting." *Journal of Clinical Engineering*, Vol. 4, No. 3, 1979, pp. 237-241.

Sharp, Ray. "Hospital Uses Small Computer to Contain Big Energy Bills." *Southern Hospitals*, Vol. 48, No. 4, 1980, pp. 7-9.

Stiefel, Robert H. and Welker, Patricia. "A Computerized System for Equipment Control and Preventive Maintenance." *Medical Instrumentation*, January-February 1981, pp. 24-26.

Personnel Systems

Bendix, Jeff. "Computer Helps Unit Justify Staffing Pattern." *Modern Healthcare*, April 1982, p. 113.

Duraiswamy, N., Welton, R., and Reisman, A. "Using Computer Simulation to Predict ICU Staffing Needs." *Journal of Nursing Administration*, February 1981, pp. 39-44.

Hatcher, Myron E. "A Micro Computer Productivity Management System." *Hospital Topics*, September-October 1981, pp. 8-11.

Henney, Christina R. and Bosworth, Richard N. "A Computer-based System for the Automatic Production of Nursing Workload Data." *Nursing Times*, July 10, 1980, pp. 1212-1217.

13

Fully Integrated Hospital Information Systems

The previous two chapters have discussed individual clinical and administrative computer applications in hospitals. This chapter reviews the efforts of selected hospitals and vendors to develop fully integrated, or total, information systems. In these systems, all major information-processing functions are carried out in a coordinated fashion. The importance of such system integration has been stressed throughout this book.*

The term *hospital information system* can take on several different meanings. In an effort to reduce the confusion surrounding terminology, Veazie and Dankmyer have suggested the following definitions:

- *Hospital Information System*: an on-line communications vehicle for the entire hospital which is designed to facilitate day-to-day operations.
- *Medical Information System*: the collection and processing of medical data to produce various medical interpretations, including suggested diagnoses and possible treatments.
- *Management Information System*: the storage and processing of data to assist management in decision making, planning, and controlling hospital operations.
- *Database Management System*: a collection of interrelated data stored with as little redundancy as possible and independently of the programs which use the data; and stored in a general format available for retrieval and formatting into special reports on demand.[1]

---

*For a review of alternate approaches to achieving integration in system design see Chapter 3.

FIGURE 13–1
Fully Integrated Hospital Information System

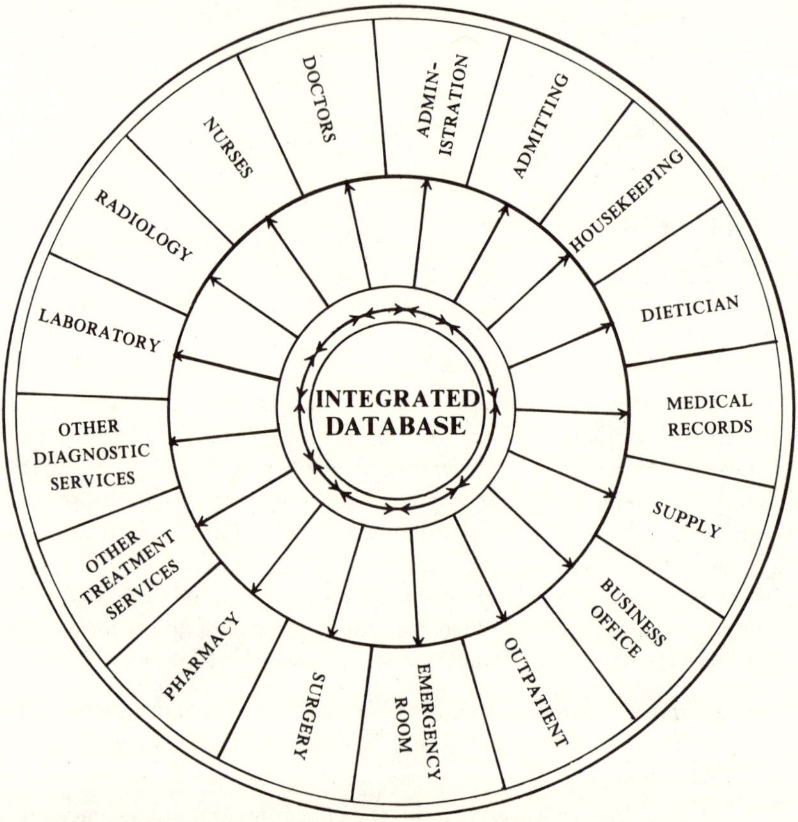

1. On-line data entry, retrieval, and display on specialized terminals
2. Program-controlled message switching for communicating information throughout the hospital
3. Integral part of the hospital's day-to-day operations
4. Fully integrated system design

Note that hospital information systems can exist without incorporating either medical or management information, but elements of both are usually present to some degree. Most hospital information systems also employ database management techniques in the construction and maintenance of data files. Thus the term *hospital information system* as it is used in this chapter includes the following components (see Figure 13-1):

- on-line data entry and on-line retrieval and display of data through specialized terminals installed at key locations throughout the hospital

- automatic (program controlled) message switching for communicating information throughout the hospital
- incorporation of the system as an integral part of day-to-day operations in the hospital
- employment of a fully integrated system design, including coordination of data files, use of common data definitions, and automatic generation and communication of data from one subsystem to another as needed; for example, a requisition for a laboratory test generates a charge to the patient's account

Historical Review of Hospital Information Systems

There has been interest in the development of total hospital information systems since the early 1960's, when computers first came into use in U.S. hospitals. Unfortunately, these early efforts often were characterized by overly optimistic claims by vendors, and several hospitals experienced false starts and resultant disappointments. Summarizing the work done during this period, Singer concluded:

> Highly developed computer-based hospital information systems are not currently in general use and will probably not be developed for general use within the next two or three years . . . The cost of developing an integrated system is high . . . Operational costs of on-line, real-time systems are high.[2]

Fortunately, the situation improved substantially as a result of work done during the 1970's. New technology has reduced the cost of on-line computing and communications systems, and several firms have developed comprehensive, fully integrated hospital information systems. Ball, writing in 1973, described 15 such systems then available on the commercial market.[3]

In a more recent review, Lindberg points out that comprehensive systems have been developed both by university medical centers and by commercial firms: "Fine systems are available commercially . . . offered by competing vendors in a substantial range of comprehensiveness. The sophistication of these [commercial] systems in the medical sphere is distinctly below that of the best of the university-based systems."[4] Because of the earlier inflated claims and severe disappointments experienced at some hospitals, many administrators remain cautious about the installation of these fully integrated systems in their institutions.

The most recent development in the quest for fully integrated hospital information systems is the development of minicomputers, which are lower in cost than some of the larger systems available to hospitals. Some designers are striving to develop systems with decentralization of processing through the use of multiple minicomputers, with integration to be achieved through the design of a communications network linking the minis for information sharing (distributed processing as described previously).

COMPREHENSIVE SYSTEMS: IN-HOUSE DEVELOPMENT

Comprehensive information systems have been developed by a number of hospitals and health science centers, most of them university-based. These systems tend to place priority on clinical data handling (as opposed to management functions) and often are designed to support clinical research projects in a university medical school.

The HELP system at Latter Day Saints Hospital in Salt Lake City, Utah, employs an automated patient medical record system with a patient care database to assist the physician in clinical decision making.[5] The system incorporates patient care information from the various service areas of the hospital into an integrated database that, when combined with standardized acute care protocols (called *alerts*), provides information to the physician for use in detecting and preventing crises in seriously ill patients.

The COSTAR system at Massachusetts General Hospital incorporates medical, administrative, and financial information obtained from a single source document into a comprehensive, centralized database.[6] The system supports ambulatory care and management decisions at the Harvard Community Health Plan in Boston. Functions of this fully integrated system include patient registration; medical records storage and retrieval; diagnostic aids, including a computer generated flowchart showing the course of a disease and variation in clinical findings over time; appointment scheduling in the clinics; and patient billing and accounts receivable. COSTAR utilizes commercially supported software that is being made available for installation on minicomputers for use in group practices.

As a final example of a university-developed system, the Problem-Oriented Medical Information System (PROMIS) at the University of Vermont incorporates a problem-oriented medical record with a central database in order to support direct patient care. On a retrospective basis, the central database provides the information necessary to carry out epidemiological studies, medical audits, financial audits, and programs of medical education in the hospital.[7]

Comprehensive Systems: Commercially Developed

Comprehensive hospital information systems have also been developed by a number of commercial firms, including manufacturers of computer hardware (for example, IBM, Burroughs, General Electric, NCR) and specialists in systems and software development (for example, Shared Hospital Systems, Medicus Medical Systems, Technicon Corporation, National Data Communication, Inc.). Two of the latter systems are described in this section to illustrate what is available on the commercial market.

The Technicon System. El Camino Hospital, a 464-bed general acute facility located in Mountain View, California, initiated a project in 1965 aimed at the design and installation of a total hospital information handling system. The project gained national recognition in 1971, when the hospital was awarded a $1.2 million contract from the Department of Health, Education, and Welfare for a comprehensive evaluation of the system being developed by the Technicon Corporation (formerly Lockheed Information Systems). The federal support ran from 1971 to 1974. In August 1974, the hospital administration made a permanent commitment to the new system by entering into a contract with Technicon for the system's continuing operation. The final report of the hospital's evaluation was published in December 1975.[8] The government also contracted with the Battelle Memorial Institute for an independent evaluation; the first Battelle report was published in 1976.[9]

The El Camino system includes entry of orders for patient services and tests through remote terminals, with program-controlled message switching and transmission of orders to the appropriate service departments. Previously entered orders and results of diagnostic tests are accessible to hospital employees in terminal displays. The system generates some of the data required for the patient's medical chart. Subsystems related to the order entry and communications system include admissions, accounts receivable, accounts payable, general ledger accounting, budgetary control, inventory control, payroll, and labor distribution.

The system has been extensively evaluated. One measure of success is obtained by examining the attitudes of hospital staff toward it. Nurses generally have accepted the automated El Camino system and most are enthusiastic about it. Physicians' attitudes have been mixed. Early technical difficulties produced much animosity among physicians, and some of this is reported to have continued even after the problems were solved. Hospital staff report that physicians have become more enthusiastic over time, and there is now majority acceptance. In August 1974, the medical staff was asked in a mail ballot whether the hospital should make a permanent commitment to the system; 56 percent voted yes (to accept), 35 percent voted no, and nine percent expressed no opinion. "Management attitudes," Giebink and Hurst state, "range periodically from pessimistic to optimistic. The major breakthrough as far as management was concerned occurred when nursing became enthusiastic."[10]

Operational problems (or system "bugs") were reported to be prevalent in the first two years of operation (1972 and 1973), but decreased considerably since then. System downtime has not been a major problem, but the hospital staff reports that periods of downtime exceeding 15 minutes cause user frustration and occasional patient inconvenience: "There are periodic recurrences of intermittent system slowdowns, which usually are symptomatic of an undetected problem. . . . Consistent system monitoring is required to detect this kind of slowdown, and only if identified early can serious response time degradation be avoided."[11]

The designers of the El Camino system offer the following general advice to hospitals considering the development of a total hospital information system:

> Hospitals considering the installation of a comprehensive medical information system with the expectation of achieving cost effectiveness should be prepared to commit the necessary level of administrative and staff support, including that of an adequate and competent management engineering organization.
>
> Institutions intending to install a medical information system should seriously consider a system that is comprehensive, integrated, fully developed and tested, and user accepted. . . .
>
> As the principal beneficiary of hospital cost savings, Government should facilitate and encourage the installation of medical information systems which are designed for direct professional use, are comprehensive in scope, and for which cost benefits have been proved.[12]

The NADACOM System. National Data Communications, Inc. (NADACOM) of Dallas, Texas, has developed a comprehensive, fully integrated hospital information system that is operating successfully in several hospitals throughout the United States. Development began in 1968, and many improvements and extensions have been added as the system has matured. The system handles virtually all routine communications related to a patient's stay in the hospital.

The admissions-discharges-transfers subsystem includes preadmission processing, updating of bed status files in real time, and preparing all census reports. Orders for patient services and treatments are entered through specially designed video terminal units (Figure 13-2). When an order is entered, the system automatically updates the patient's medical chart, prints a hard copy of the order at the appropriate service department, and produces a nursing station hard copy of the order. Simultaneously, the sys-

FIGURE 13-2
Input Terminal

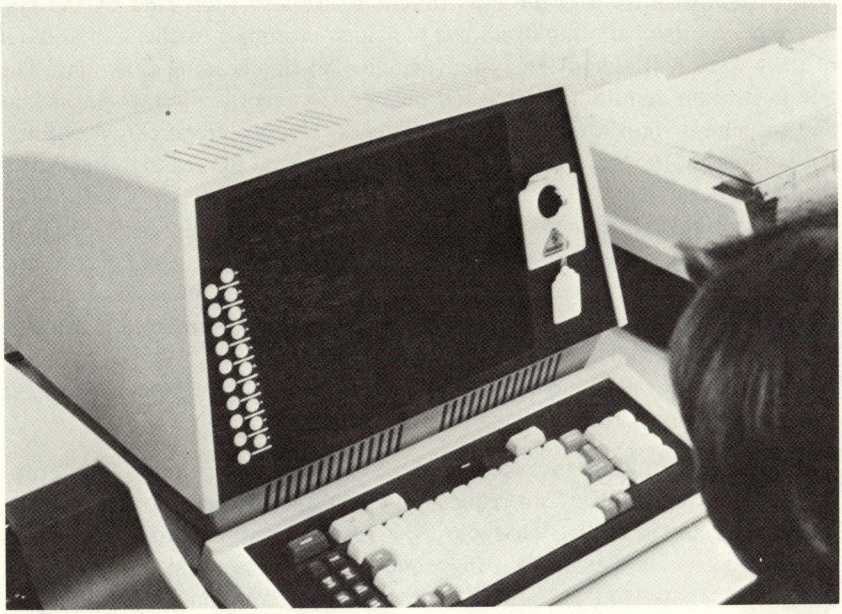

tem prepares schedules and reminder lists for tests and treatments which have been ordered, and every order entry generates real-time billing transactions and general ledger entries in the financial subsystem.

Physicians can call up records of current inpatients using any terminal, including one in the doctors' lounge. Thus a complete record of all orders and chart entries is available to the physician, who can view, write, and sign orders through the terminal if he or she so desires.

For all drug orders transmitted to the hospital pharmacy, the system calculates the proper supply of medication to be sent to the nursing unit, following rules established by the pharmacist. Orders are printed automatically on gummed labels, and the system also prepares medication lists for use by nurses on the floor. All pharmacy orders are automatically subtracted from the inventory; when supplies fall below a specified amount, they are automatically added to the reorder list in the computer files.

For departments providing diagnostic and therapeutic services, the system records orders and stop-orders, prepares worksheets for each service department, and has the capability for interfacing with automated laboratory or diagnostic equipment. For the medical records department, the system keeps track of incomplete charts; abstracts census reports from data on admissions, discharges, and transfers; and maintains special catalogs and indices, such as a current list of staff physicians.

Administrative and business functions are also supported by the system. For example, all employees use the video terminals to check in and out of their work shifts, and the system handles all timekeeping functions. The administration can add, delete, and change the records of staff physicians and suspend or reinstate admitting privileges. Housekeeping can view nursing station bed status, enter changes, and clear beds for reassignment after they have been cleaned.

The materials management functions of the system include creation of purchase orders, inventory control, requisitions processing and control, and on-line records for the central supply department to use in viewing quantities on hand and on order. A complete supply catalog is maintained in the computer files of the system.

The system also includes a complete financial management package which encompasses the following subsystems:

1. Patient billing and accounts receivable: through the on-line terminals, the cashier can request and view the current status of patient accounts, adjust charges, and retrieve entry listings; accounts receivable personnel can request statements, post payments on accounts, and perform all active account transactions through the terminals.
2. Payroll, personnel, and wage and salary: these are tied to the employee timekeeping procedures described previously.
3. General ledger accounting: the system permits real-time collection and posting of all patient transactions to the general ledger; it also can create and change general ledger entries and accounts, handle payables and inventories, perform all general accounting functions, view vendor files, request checks, maintain budgetary records, and produce a variety of financial reports for use by hospital administration and trustees.

An outpatient subsystem has been added which performs functions similar to those described above, in addition to scheduling facilities in the ambulatory service.

The NADACOM system was installed at Huntington Memorial Hospital (565 beds) in Pasadena, California, in response to a request for proposals developed by the hospital administration. The system is reported to have reduced the rate of personnel cost increases throughout the hospital and to have reduced paperwork substantially, thus freeing time of hospital personnel for patient care and the provision of administrative services.[13]

Database Management

Fully integrated hospital information systems usually rely on the development of a central database, in which one repository of information serves multiple organizational purposes. Database technology has developed rapidly in recent years, with software packages available for file updating and maintenance as well as retrieval of information via remote terminals.

Taggart describes the components of a database management system as follows:

- A *data description language*, through which the user describes the logical data structure and characteristics of the physical storage unit to be employed
- A *data dictionary-directory* that specifies the name and definition of each data element to be included in the database
- A *data manipulation language* that allows the user to add and change records in the database (some systems also include a report-writing component for simplified user specification of printed reports)
- A *query language* for use in retrieving specific records or sets of records at remote terminals
- A *database manager* that controls the entire process and provides a direct linkage to the computer's main operating system[14]

Wiederhold has prepared a comprehensive review of the application of database technology to the delivery of health care. He points out that, in many institutions which employ database management systems, a new position will be required—that of database administrator, who will be responsible for review of database reliability, adaptation to changing needs of the organization, planning for future growth, and periodic technical updating of the system.[15]

Distributed Data Processing and Networking

Minicomputers have been used for several years as independent processors in various areas of hospitals, notably in laboratory information systems. Rapid improvement in hardware and software, as well as reductions in cost, appear to make multiple small computers more attractive in meeting a hospital's total information-processing needs. The suggested advantages of a distributed processing approach include: hardware economy, reliability (one processor can fail without endangering the remainder of the network), phased development of subsystems through distributed computing, and the option of a tailored hardware configuration for each functional area of the network.[16] The key question, however, and one that overrides all of the above advantages, is: to what extent can distributed processing through multiple minicomputers be integrated into a total hospital information system?

Wasserman points out the problems of system integration with distributed processing.[17] Data as well as computers are distributed throughout the hospital. System designers must decide which data should be stored in which system, which data should be duplicated and stored in multiple systems, and which computers should have access to which data files. The overall complexity of a distributed system is greater than that of a centralized system, and software requirements are very demanding. The apparent cost advantages of minicomputer hardware might well be offset by increased communications costs and the costs of developing the software necessary for creating and maintaining the network. Good planning is essential for hospitals selecting this approach, and a commitment must be made in advance. As Wasserman states, "The significant problems associated with integrating these independent subsystems into a hospital information system are only partially alleviated by intelligent planning and equipment selection."[18]

One example of the use of multiple minicomputers in the design of a total hospital information system is the CHAMPS system installed at Canyon General Hospital in Anaheim, California.[19] The system maintains patient charts, handles orders of supplies and services for patients, schedules use of the operating rooms and other facilities, and keeps track of charges accumulated. Ten minicomputers are employed.

At the Veterans Administration Medical Center in San Francisco, a prototype medical computer network has been developed by the cardiology service. Each computer system in the network utilizes a different operating system and supports a different programming language, but the three major systems (cardiac catheterization computer system, the intensive care unit's monitoring computer, and the pacemaker surveillance clinic computer system) are capable of complete intercommunications and sharing of information through the use of a coordinated network under central control.[20]

CONCLUSION

The state of the art of fully integrated hospital information systems has improved significantly in recent years. Good generalized systems are available, and they are affordable to hospitals with 150 or more beds. One objection to such systems is that they require standardization and acceptance of generalized procedures included in the basic system design. However, a powerful argument can be made that hospitals are more similar in many of their functions than they are different, and good standardized systems can be successfully installed as long as some flexibility is included in the basic design.

One observer of the field has described the state of the art as follows:

> It is still a young field, and many of the problems . . . are simply hallmarks of an industry that is changing so quickly—in terms of user and vendor alike—that no one could really be expected to keep up with everything that is going on. However, most observers agree that the HIS has now passed from the experimental stage to being an extremely helpful tool—and may well be on its way to being indispensable.[21]

Summary

Integration of information systems is important to hospitals because of the highly interrelated nature of the functions performed in providing patient care. Fully integrated, or total, hospital information systems are designed to provide comprehensive and coordinated information to operating personnel throughout the hospital.

A fully integrated hospital information system includes the following elements: (1) on-line entry, retrieval, and display of information through specialized terminals; (2) automatic message switching for communicating information throughout the hospital; (3) a system that facilitates day-to-day operations in the hospital; and (4) a fully integrated design approach, including common data definitions, central data files, and automatic communication of data from one functional subsystem to another.

Total hospital information systems have been slow to develop. The situation has improved significantly, and a number of comprehensive, fully integrated hospital information systems are now available on the commercial market.

Recent technological improvements in the design of minicomputers have resulted in increased interest in the use of a distributed network of small computers to carry out hospital information-processing functions. Advantages of this approach include hardware economy, backup available from multiple central processors, phased development of subsystems, and tailored hardware configurations for each functional subsystem. However, the complexity of designing a distributed network of multiple minicomputers makes the question of effective system integration difficult. The apparent hardware economies of multiple minicomputers might well be offset by the increased costs of software development and the costs of sophisticated communications equipment required to make the network function effectively.

DISCUSSION QUESTIONS

13-1 Define the terms: (1) *hospital information system*, (2) *medical information system*, (3) *management information system*, and (4) *database management system*.

13-2 What are the distinguishing characteristics of a fully integrated hospital information system?

13-3 Why were there inflated claims and resultant disappointments about total hospital information systems in the 1960's?

13-4 What is meant by the term *distributed processing*?

13-5 What are the possible advantages of a distributed network of minicomputers in the design of an integrated hospital information system?

13-6 Why is system integration difficult to achieve when a distributed minicomputer network approach is employed?

PROBLEMS

13-1 Describe five comprehensive, fully integrated hospital information systems available on the commercial market. For each system include a discussion of:

a. system objectives

b. functions performed

c. hardware components

d. software design

e. cost factors

f. reported benefits and savings

g. locations of hospitals where operational installation can be found.

13-2 Develop a report to a hospital board of trustees outlining the rationale for installing a fully integrated information system. Include in your report an outline of steps to be followed in selecting and installing the system.

NOTES

1. Stephen Veazie and Todd Dankmyer, "HISs, MISs, DBMSs: Sorting Out the Letters," *Hospitals*, October 16, 1977, pp. 80-84.
2. J. Peter Singer, "Computer-Based Hospital Information Systems," *Datamation*, May 1969, pp. 38-45.
3. Marion J. Ball, "Fifteen Hospital Information Systems Available," in *How to Select a Computerized Hospital Information System*, ed. Marion Ball, Basel, Switzerland: S. Karger, 1973, pp. 10-27. For each system, the article includes information on computer terminals, central processing unit, programming languages, mode of access to data files, and location of hospitals where operational installations can be found.

4. Donald A. B. Lindberg, *The Growth of Medical Information Systems in the United States*. Lexington, Massachusetts: Lexington Books, 1979, p. 37.
5. Homer R. Warner, "Knowledge Sectors for Logical Processing of Patient Data in the HELP System," *Proceedings of the Second Annual Symposium on Computer Applications in Medical Care*, Washington, D.C., November 5-9, 1978, ed. F. H. Orthner. New York: Institute of Electrical and Electronics Engineers, November 1978, pp. 401-409.
6. G. Octo Barnett et al., "COSTAR—A Computer-Based Medical Information System for Ambulatory Care," *Proceedings of the I.E.E.E.*, September 1979, pp. 1226-1237.
7. Jan R. Schultz and Layton Davis, "The Technology of PROMIS," *Proceedings of the I.E.E.E.*, September 1979, pp. 1237-1244.
8. U.S. Department of Health, Education, and Welfare, *Demonstration and Evaluation of a Total Hospital Informations System*, by John E. Gall et al., Public Health Service, Health Resources Administration, National Center for Health Services Research, Washington, D.C.: December 1975.
9. U.S. Department of Health, Education, and Welfare, *Evaluation of the Implementation of a Medical Information System in a General Community Hospital*, by James P. Barrett et al., Final Report, Battelle Columbus Laboratories, Contract HSM 110-73-331, Health Resources Administration, National Center for Health Services Research, NTIS Publication No. 248340. Washington, D.C.: December 19, 1975.
10. Gerald A. Giebink and Leonard L. Hurst, *Computer Projects in Health Care*. Ann Arbor, Michigan: Health Administration Press, 1975, p. 190.
11. U.S. Department of Health, Education, and Welfare, *Demonstration and Evaluation of a Total Hospital Information System*, p. 47.
12. Ibid., p. 34.
13. Robert Spaziano, "A Hospital Cares," *Datamation*, June 1980, pp. 156-166.
14. William M. Taggart, *Information Systems: An Introduction to Computers in Organizations* (Boston: Allyn & Bacon, Inc., 1980), pp. 192-201.
15. Gio Wiederhold, "Database Technology in Health Care," *Journal of Medical Systems*, Vol. 5, No. 3, 1981, pp. 175-196.
16. Morton D. Schwartz, "Analysis of Hospital Computer Networks," *Journal of Clinical Engineering*, October-December 1980, pp. 311-320.
17. A. I. Wasserman, "Minicomputers May Maximize Data Processing," *Hospitals*, October 16, 1977, p. 120.
18. Ibid., p. 128.
19. Donald M. Carren, "Multiple Minis for Information Management," *Datamation*, September 1975, pp. 54-58.
20. Paul D. Keltz et al., "A Minicomputer Network for Diverse Operating Systems and Languages," *Journal of Medical Systems*, Vol. 4, No. 2, 1980, pp. 305-315.
21. Emily Friedman, "Information Systems: The Systems Need Some Solutions," *Hospitals*, May 1, 1982, p. 80.

ADDITIONAL READINGS

Ball, Marion J. "Fifteen Hospital Information Systems Available." In *How to Select a Computerized Hospital Information System*, ed. Marion Ball. Basel, Switzerland: S. Karger, 1973, pp. 10-27.

Carren, Donald M. "Multiple Minis for Information Management." *Datamation*, September 1975, pp. 54-58.

Dotson, C. William and Hinson, Irene R. "Hospital Moves From Totally Manual to Computerized Information Systems in Seven Years." *Hospitals*, October 16, 1981, pp. 131-140.

Northcutt, Douglas B. "New Hospital System Option: Distributed Data." *Hospitals*, August 16, 1980, pp. 123-126.

Potter, James G., Terrill, Thomas E., and Brown, James H. "Health Information Networks: A Coming Trend?" *Hospitals*, January 1, 1981, pp. 65-68.

Said, William F. "Distributed Data Processing and Networking Can Form a Comprehensive HIS." *Hospitals*, October 16, 1981, p. 138.

Schwartz, Morton D. "Analysis of Hospital Computer Networks." *Journal of Clinical Engineering*, October-December 1980, pp. 311-320.

Spaziano, Robert. "A Hospital Cares." *Datamation*, June 1980, pp. 156-166.

U.S. Department of Health, Education, and Welfare. *Demonstration and Evaluation of a Total Hospital Information System*, by John E. Gall et al. Public Health Service, Health Resources Administration, National Center for Health Services Research. Washington, D.C.: December 1975.

________. *Evaluation of the Implementation of a Medical Information System in a General Community Hospital*, by James P. Barrett et al. Final Report, Battelle Columbus Laboratories, Contract HSM 110-73-331. Health Resources Administration, National Center for Health Services Research, NTIS Publication No. 248340. Washington, D.C.: December 19, 1975.

Veazie, Stephen and Dankmyer, Todd. "HISs, MISs, DBMSs: Sorting Out the Letters." *Hospitals*, October 16, 1977, pp. 80-84.

Wasserman, A. I. "Minicomputers May Maximize Data Processing." *Hospitals*, October 16, 1977, pp. 119-128.

Wiederhold, Gio. "Database Technology in Health Care." *Journal of Medical Systems*, Vol. 5, No. 3, 1981, pp. 175-196.

Williamson, H. Stephen. "Designing a Total Hospital Information System." *Osteopathic Hospitals*, April 1976, pp. 14-16.

14

Information Systems for Hospital Management Planning and Control

The overviews in Chapters 11 through 13 indicate that hospitals have achieved some success in the design and installation of information systems. Moderate to good progress has been achieved in utilization of computers and automated systems for direct patient care. Some clinical systems have been extended beyond the research and development stage and are in use in hospitals and other medical facilities. Systems to support routine administrative operations are now commonplace, and fully integrated systems for the first time appear to be cost-effective for many hospitals. These integrated systems, however, are still oriented primarily toward day-to-day administrative operations rather than toward management planning and control. The development of systems for the latter purpose is still in a relatively primitive stage, a matter for further discussion in this chapter. The importance of extending available information systems technology to the next level of sophistication—management decision making—cannot be overstated. As Davis and Freeman have said, "The availability and use of information in the decision making process is not just one prerequisite for efficient and effective management in the health care field; it is *the* prerequisite."[1]

Management Information Systems: General Concepts

A management information system must be designed to support decision making in the organizational environment in which it will function.

Thus, an effective system must be more than a communication and data-processing system; it must have the capability of providing *control* to management personnel using the system. Principles of control systems were discussed extensively in Chapter 2. Management control requires both standards and quantitative measurement of actual performance measured against the standards. Hancock lists the following essential elements of a hospital control system:

- a prediction of future events, an "expectation"
- a method of measurement in the same units as the expectation
- a method of determining if exceptions exist
- a method of reporting exceptions
- the corrective actions to remove the exceptions so that expectations can be achieved[2]

The characteristics of useful management information were also discussed in Chapter 2. They are listed once again here because of their relevance to the current discussion.

Characteristics of Useful Management Information

1. Information—not data: Data must be processed intelligently in accordance with predesigned plans before they become information useful to hospital management.
2. Relevant: Data collected must be appropriate for the use to which they will be put.
3. Sensitive: Data must provide discrimination and meaningful comparison for operating managers.
4. Unbiased: Information should not be collected or analyzed in such a way as to meet the self-fulfilling prophecies of hospital management.
5. Comprehensive: All important elements or components of a system should be visible to those charged with decision-making responsibility.
6. Timely: Data must be available in advance of the time when decisions or actions are required.
7. Action-oriented: Data should be synthesized in such a way as to facilitate the decision process rather than just presenting passive facts about current operations.
8. Uniform: Data systems should provide hospital indicators that can be compared over time, both internally (against previous

performance) and externally (against the experience of other hospitals).

9. Performance-targeted: Data elements should be designed and collected in reference to predetermined goals and objectives.
10. Cost-effective: The anticipated benefits to be obtained from having the information available should exceed the costs of collecting and processing that same information.

Design of a management information system will require the development of a management database including the elements (1) units of service produced, (2) resources consumed in producing those services, (3) data for assessing the quality of services provided, and (4) indicators of the effectiveness of services provided in meeting perceived community health needs. As mentioned previously, the above categories of data should be measured against predetermined standards and expectations of performance whenever and wherever possible.[3]

Alter discusses the types of decision support systems presently installed in American industry.[4] He categorizes these computer systems in terms of what the users of the systems actually do with them, as follows:

- systems in which the users retrieve isolated data items
- systems which are used as a mechanism for ad hoc analysis of data files
- systems which provide prespecified aggregations of data in the form of standard reports
- systems which assist in estimating the consequences of proposed decisions
- systems which propose decisions to management
- systems which make decisions according to predetermined decision algorithms[5]

Systems in the first three categories hardly can be classified as management information systems, but the latter three types are designed with the needs of management in mind.

Management Information Needs in the Hospital

While there are various management information needs in the modern hospital, they can be categorized into the following five groupings:

Information to Assist in Setting Objectives and Conducting Long-

range Planning. Effective goal setting within the hospital requires information on community health needs; current problems indicators, both direct and indirect; existing service programs designed to meet these needs, both within the hospital and elsewhere in the community; and resources available to mount new programs in response to community needs.[6]

Information to Assist in Short-term Demand Forecasting and Work Planning. Forecasting requires data on historical utilization patterns, demographic data on the population being served by the hospital, projections of future changes in community demography, and comparative data from other hospitals providing similar services.[7]

Information to Assist in Resource Allocation and Cost Control. In addition to short-term demand forecasts, data on manpower, costs of meaningful service units, and capital requirements are needed in order to accomplish this objective.[8]

Information to Assist in Performance and Quality Control. Data requirements in this category include output measures, usually in the form of program statistics, quality control standards, work sampling measurements to match against standards, and data from medical audit and utilization review activities.[9]

Information to Assist in Program Evaluation. Data similar to those described in item 1 above are required; that is, programs should be evaluated in reference to original goals and long-range plans. Hence information on *changes* which have occurred in community health needs, such as problem indicators and utilization patterns, should be collected. Additionally, the management information system should facilitate cost-benefit analyses to determine if benefits achieved by the programs are worth the costs of resources consumed in providing services.

APPROACHES TO MANAGEMENT INFORMATION SYSTEM DEVELOPMENT

There are two basic approaches possible in the development of a hospital management information system. The hospital may design and install its own, personalized system, or it could choose to utilize generalized systems which are available for this purpose.

If a hospital decides to design its own system, it can do so by designing a completely separate, stand-alone management system, or it can draw on existing operational data-processing systems as sources of data, provided that these systems were designed with management information requirements in mind. Some of the current limitations in the development of management systems are discussed in the section which follows.

Several generalized management information systems are available for use by hospitals, including the following:

HAS(MONITREND)—Hospital Administrative Services System. Developed by a division of the American Hospital Association, HAS provides centralized computer processing of accounting data provided by participating hospitals. Periodic reports, which include comparative statistics and trend data on direct expenses, resource utilization, and a limited set of output measures, are returned to the hospital. Comparative statistics are provided which allow the hospital to measure itself against other institutions of similar function, size, and geographic location.[10] In 1979, HAS introduced the MONITREND program. Clients receive monthly reports containing more than 300 operational indicators for management decision making.

PAS—Professional Activity Study. PAS was developed by the Commission on Professional and Hospital Activities, Ann Arbor, Michigan. Hospitals participating in the PAS system provide case abstracts for every hospital discharge. The forms contain data on patient identification, diagnoses, surgical or obstetrical treatments rendered, investigative tests performed, nonsurgical management, and additional information specified by the hospital. These abstracts are processed on centralized computer facilities, and periodic reports are returned to the participating hospitals. The PAS system produces reports for each hospital summarizing clinical activities for a specified period. These reports can be used for indexing medical records, for providing general statistical data on hospital activity, and for utilization review and quality control.[11] In addition, PAS provides comparative data with other hospitals.

CASH—Commission on Administrative Services in Hospitals. Originally established by the Hospital Council and Blue Cross of Southern California, CASH is a nonprofit corporation which provides generalized systems for determining staffing requirements and for assessing quality in hospitals. These systems employ industrial engineering techniques in the establishment of standard time and performance measures which then are applied to a specific case mix in each participating hospital. Quality control reports produced by the system are used by hospital mangement in ongoing quality assessment.[12]

Hospital Association Systems. Several hospital associations at the state and regional levels have also developed generalized management information and reporting systems. For example, the Ohio Hospital Association has developed a service-cost index, a set of 29 indicators of quantitative measurement relating to cost, utilization, manpower effectiveness, and other factors of daily hospital operation.[13]

PBCS—Hospital Planning, Budgeting and Control System. With support from the W. K. Kellogg Foundation and the Duke Endowment, the Hospital Research and Educational Trust (HRET) initiated a project to create tools that will enable hospital managers to integrate clinical and administrative decision making and thereby extend their management capabilities. The project involves merging significant features of two existing systems, PAS and HAS (described above). Four major sets of products are included in the project: (1) a planning system drawing on the PAS database; (2) a budgeting system drawing on the HAS database and providing utilization forecasts, manpower budgets, sensitivity analysis, revenue projections, and capital budgeting; (3) an integrated database combining medical and financial data; and (4) case mix analysis of hospital operating costs.

Commercial Packages. Although most of the packaged software developed for hospitals has been for administrative and clinical computer systems which support day-to-day operations, some vendors are beginning to turn their attention to the development of software for management planning and control purposes. Most of these packages concentrate on financial control systems for hospital management.

There are advantages and disadvantages to the use of generalized management information systems in hospitals. Generalized systems minimize developmental time and costs for the hospital. They provide standardized data definitions which can be used for trend analysis and interhospital comparison. These systems are usually well documented and are relatively simple to use. On the other hand, generalized systems are not tailored to the individual hospital and its specific needs and information requirements. Often, there are reporting time lags involved since the data must be sent to a centralized computer facility for processing. Operating costs for these systems may be higher than comparable costs of a well-designed internal system, and generalized systems are less flexible and more difficult to change than systems which hospitals design themselves. Nonetheless, the need is so great for standardized performance indicators which facilitate interhospital comparisons that efforts such as those described above need to be given continued support and encouragement.

Current Limitations in the Development of Management Information Systems in Hospitals[14]

A variety of factors has limited progress toward the development of effective management information systems in hospitals. *In increasing order of importance* these are: (1) technological limitations, (2) economic factors,

(3) external factors, (4) conceptual limitations, and (5) managerial shortfall.

Technological Limitations. Management information systems development has been slowed by gaps in system design knowledge and technical skills and also by current limitations in computer technology.

Inadequate systems analysis is perhaps the most common failure.[15] User needs must be fully understood and analyzed before system design and installation. Problems often develop when "the system designer focuses on the 'how' of streamlining paper flow but not the 'why' of rethinking functions, policies, and decision processes."[16] It is the designer's responsibility to pose these questions, and the administrator's responsibility to provide the answers.

Hospital information systems have also suffered from poor technical design. Performance failures are most likely to occur when design teams focus too much on sophistication in computing technology at the expense of user-oriented reports and data retrieval capabilities.

Computer technology has developed dramatically in recent years, and systems are less likely to be constrained by equipment limitations than by lack of imagination in the design process. However, there are some hardware limitations that must be overcome, particularly the continuing high cost of data communications equipment. Hospitals have tended to follow fads in computer hardware and software, to reach for the latest advance in sophisticated computer technology when a much more modest approach would suffice.

A final technological problem is the need for better ways to protect the confidentiality of personal information, a major social issue which has emerged in recent years. The Privacy Protection Study Commission has called for complete control of patient records by hospitals and the establishment of legally enforceable requirements for confidentiality.[17] Computerized hospital information systems compound this problem, and major efforts are needed to shape improved security features for hospital information systems.[18]

Economic Factors. A major problem in the development of hospital management information systems has been undercapitalization of the developmental effort. Initial underfunding of a project leads inevitably to later dissatisfaction when time and cost estimates are not met and repeated requests for incremental funding are submitted by system designers. Careful and realistic cost analysis before initiation of a project can help to overcome this problem. Failure to evaluate alternative design strategies on a cost-benefit basis has also resulted in the implementation of information systems which are not cost effective. System designers must present accurate cost estimates to hospital management before implementation of new systems. The administrator should analyze these estimates carefully and then commit the necessary funds once a decision to proceed has been made.

External Factors. Demands on hospitals to report to external agencies are growing exponentially. As the hospital industry becomes increasingly regulated, these demands can be expected to continue.[19] Information is required to satisfy the reporting requirements of myriad local, state, and federal governmental agencies, as well as the various third-party financing organizations with which the hospital interacts. Unfortunately, there is little coordination among these agencies, so the hospital must provide individually tailored reports to each. The cost of external reporting is a significant item in the hospital's budget, not to mention the opportunity costs incurred when hospitals must divert attention from meeting internal data needs to satisfying those of the external regulators and financiers.[20]

Phillips states that external reporting demands have had the following impact on hospitals:

- continued requirement for enlarging the databases
- uncoordinated requests for data from multiple users at federal, regional, state, and local levels
- increased demands for data derived from the integration of data sources and bases
- expanded expectations regarding data processing capabilities
- increased pressures for hospitals to achieve uniformity
- increased concern over the costs of data processing[21]

Conceptual Limitations. Management information systems in hospitals also suffer from conceptual limitations in their design. One such problem is the tendency to gather data for the sake of gathering data. This is often accompanied by a rush to computerize before the fundamental design questions have been addressed. Speaking from the perspective of a practicing administrator, Connors states:

> The information systems in our hospitals are, by and large, obsolete, fragmented, and poorly conceived . . . [and] the field does not seem interested or willing to spend money and resources in tackling the fundamental questions of what information is required, for what purpose, by whom, and with what frequency and accuracy.
>
> Could not information scientists back off from the rush to computerize, develop third generation hardware and software, to creation of elaborate subsystems with questionable use, and join with managers of our hospitals in a fundamental reassessment of information requirements.[22]

Hospital information systems are too often designed to collect and aggregate data rather than to serve as decision support systems. These will not spring automatically from existing data-processing systems in hospitals. Rather, decision support systems must be planned in advance according to a model or format specified by the managers who will use the systems. Scott suggests the use of a standardized format for organizing information for decision making in hospitals. The format includes a statement of the goal to be accomplished as a result of the decision and a minimal measure of goal attainment, resource requirements and resources currently available, costs and benefits, alternatives that are possible, and timetable and procedures for implementing the decision.[23]

There are also conceptual problems with the way in which data are employed in hospital decision making. These include overly simplistic use of information, inability to combine clinical and administrative data, and lack of reference standards against which to measure performance. Information systems designed to produce periodic operating statistics for hospitals often simply aggregate pieces of data rather than breaking them down into meaningful categories. The best examples of this continue to be per diem costs and length-of-stay statistics. These measures merely tell us how long it takes hospitals to perform imprecise activities. Unless measures of hospital performance are derived which specify the effects of precise clinical activities on resource consumption, attempts at utilization review, quality assessment, and the explanation of hospital costs will remain misdirected. Thompson and his colleagues at Yale have developed a method which identifies resource consumption as a function of diagnosis, clinical procedures, and demographic factors. This level of precision permits the identification of case costs. The general analytic strategy of combining clinical and administrative data results in the quantification of hospital outputs in standardized service units called diagnosis related groups (DRGs).[24]

Perhaps the major conceptual problem in the design of hospital management information systems is the shortage of standards against which to measure performance. Managerial control requires that productivity and quality control standards be developed for all phases of hospital operations. Although there are several efforts under way at the national level directed at the development of uniform standards for hospital reporting, as yet these systems are not sufficiently performance-oriented to provide good measures of hospital efficiency and effectiveness. Until such standards are developed and agreed upon by those in leadership positions within the hospital industry, comparability and compatibility of hospital information systems will not be achieved. The need for standardized data definitions and sharing of information for interhospital comparisons is essential for community health planning. Increasingly, standards are being established by regulatory agencies, and this trend can be expected to accelerate.

A final limitation in the design of management information systems for hospitals is the failure of many hospitals to integrate data adequately from systems developed haphazardly on an application-by-application basis. Management planning and control require administrative and clinical information drawn from all parts of the organization. When communication among systems does not exist, the integrated information required for management decisions cannot be produced.

Managerial Shortfall. Many, if not most, of the conceptual and technical problems discussed above result from an organizational gap that exists between the technical knowledge of system designers and the perspectives of chief executive officers on key decision needs and related systems requirements. In short, there continues to be inadequate involvement and apparent lack of sophistication of top hospital management in system planning and design. Anthony and Herzlinger state:

> Support means more than acquiescence. Although top management's time is precious, it must be willing to allocate a significant amount to the system development effort. It must understand the objectives and general concepts of the proposed system well enough to see the benefits accruing to each individual, and must explain to the principal subordinates how it will help them and the organization as a whole.[25]

Other key hospital personnel must also be involved in system planning decisions, particularly physicians. Since physicians directly control the flow of revenue in most hospitals, their involvement and support is essential.

A major cause of system failures in hospitals is inadequate top management control of the system development process. There are numerous cases in which management has failed to hire a competent technical staff; has allowed poor and unprofessional practices to be followed in systems analysis, design, and implementation; has failed to set priorities for system development based upon organizational objectives; has failed to monitor projects adequately to insure that they are completed on time and within budget limitations; has failed to provide for maintenance of information systems after they have become operational; and has failed to evaluate operational systems periodically.

Characteristics of Effective Management

This is a strong indictment of managerial activities in the hospital field. Managerial shortfall relates not to lack of motivation on the part of hospital chief executive officers, but rather to a knowledge gap and shortage of technical skills in managerial control and systems technology.

Consider some of the characteristics of effective management required for information systems to succeed in supporting management planning and control in hospitals.

First and foremost, hospital administrators must have adequate knowledge of control processes and procedures if they are to provide effective leadership in their organizations:

> Many of these managers have little acquaintance with the technical aspects of management, such as accounting, finance, or data processing. It is not unusual to find administrators of mammoth health facilities who are unable to read their own financial statements.
>
> This lack of training not only means that the managers are unable to take an active position in shaping the management control systems in their organizations, but also that they are insecure in doing so and, at times, so intimidated by the technical staff who work for them that the managers abdicate their leadership position in designing, installing and operating these systems.[26]

According to Harvey's study, managers in organizations with successfully implemented information systems were sophisticated, future-oriented, sensitive to environmental change, favorable to innovation, and oriented toward decision making.[27] Given adequate knowledge and sufficient motivation, we return once again to the most important variable of all, involvement by top management in system planning and design. Rockart states that the single most important factor in successful implementation of an information system is "for the abstraction to be that of the decision makers who must use the information."[28]

Health Services Research and Information Systems

Hospital information systems now function at the operational feedback level described by Katz and Kahn,[29] representing nothing more than the quantification of what individual operating units of the hospital are presently doing. Lacking environmental sensitivity, these systems typically become ends unto themselves. However:

> This is still the basic institutional form of information upon which many organizations rely. They will supplement it in various ways: i.e., through the insight, observations, and wisdom of men in leadership positions; through the use of consultants; or even through an occasional special investigation or research project. Though these supplementary means of intelligence gathering may prove of great value in critical situations, they do not provide an organization with a reliable means for getting adequate information about its prospects for survival and effectiveness in a changing world.[30]

Hospitals need to bring their information systems to a more sophisticated level so that they will provide a systemic view of the organization to decision makers, focusing on long-term trends and forecasts, environmental changes, the effectiveness and quality of services rendered, and similar measures that transcend the functioning of any one element of the organization.

Before this can happen, however, certain fundamental problems must be solved. Paramount among these is the need to develop better and different kinds of performance and utilization measures which are standardized among hospitals for comparative purposes.

Case Mix Analysis

Fetter, Thompson, and Mills have designed an information system which merges patient data with administrative data.[31] Their system illustrates very well the importance of generating standardized, decision-oriented information which at one level explains individual hospital performance and, when aggregated across hospitals, provides precise comparative measurements for fiscal and utilization review by state and regional bodies. Their system includes the following components and capabilities:

- a uniform accounting and reporting system providing standard data to the regulatory agency on costs and budgets
- a set of processes for capturing patient abstracts and charges as inputs to a central statistical system
- a system to generate uniform financial reports and budget analyses
- a classification and reporting system to provide individual and comparative measures of hospital performance and utilization
- a system to provide information to hospitals and regulatory agencies to aid in the evaluation of quality of care
- an information and reporting system to support a basic rate setting and reimbursement capability equitable to consumers, providers, and third-party payers.

Effective information systems will have all these capabilities. It is important to emphasize that the critical ingredients of the information system outlined by Fetter et al. are the actual measurement of case mix and its consequences for case costs, and implications for quality review.

From the work on case mix analysis has sprung the development of DRGs, diagnosis related groups. These are patient classification units which group patients according to diagnosis, severity of illness, and common demographic characteristics.

> Diagnosis related groups are constructed so as to be 'statistically coherent' and 'medically meaningful.' Statistically coherent means that patients in a DRG tend to consume similar amounts of hospital resources. Medically meaningful means that patients in a DRG tend to have similar clinical conditions or treatment regimens. This allows DRGs to be used by both hospital financial management and the medical staff, providing a common language between these two groups.[32]

Much attention has been devoted to the development of a standard set of DRGs for cost control and reimbursement purposes. Kropf and Greenberg contend that case mix techniques are essential " . . . to control hospital capital expenditures in a rational, clinically sound manner. . . . This strategy for controlling hospital costs is powerful, proven, inexpensive and has high political feasibility. . . ."[33]

Current researchers of health service utilization must consider carefully the relative utility of the quantification of further *description* (e.g., formulating utilization rates and cost rates with more precise population data in the denominator) versus the explanatory power gained from newly formulated *analytic units* such as case mix and case cost. Both approaches result in standardized quantification and the development of elegant and expensive information systems, but the latter explains service use while the former simply counts it.

Summary

Although substantial progress has been made in the use of computerized information systems for clinical and administrative purposes in hospitals, the development of systems to support management decision making is still in an early stage.

Management information systems must provide more than just communication and data-processing capabilities; they must assist the administrator in controlling productivity and assessing quality of services rendered. Useful management information must be relevant, sensitive, unbiased, comprehensive, timely, action-oriented, uniform, performance targeted, and cost-effective. A management database should include information on: (1) units of service produced, (2) resources consumed in producing those services, (3) the quality of services rendered, and (4) indicators of effectiveness in meeting perceived community health needs.

Management information needs in the modern hospital fall into the following five categories:

- information to assist in setting objectives and conducting long-range planning.
- information to assist in short-term demand forecasting and work planning
- information to assist in resource allocation and cost control
- information to assist in performance and quality control
- information to assist in program evaluation

Hospitals may choose to develop their own internal management information systems, or they may elect to participate in generalized, pre-packaged systems. Generalized systems can be installed with a minimum of developmental time and cost, and they offer the advantage of uniform data definitions that permit interhospital comparisons. Internally developed systems can be tailored more closely to a hospital's individual requirements and often provide information on a more timely basis.

Development of effective management information systems in hospitals has been hampered by technological limitations, economic factors, external factors, conceptual limitations, and managerial shortfall. The latter is the most critical of these limitations. Hospital managers must have adequate knowledge of control processes and procedures if they are to provide effective leadership in their organizations. Effective administrators will be knowledgeable, sophisticated, future-oriented, sensitive to environmental change, favorable to innovation, and decision-oriented.

Hospital information systems presently operate at the operational feedback level, providing quantification of what individual operating units are doing. They lack environmental sensitivity and need to be brought to a more sophisticated level, one on which they can focus on long-term trends and forecasts, environmental changes, and the effectiveness and quality of services rendered.

DISCUSSION QUESTIONS

14-1 Define the term *management information system*.

14-2 List the essential elements of a hospital management control system.

14-3 What are some of the characteristics of useful management information? How difficult is it to build these characteristics into the design of a hospital management information system?

14-4 What categories of information should be included in a management database?

14-5 To what extent can hospitals rely on generalized systems (e.g., HAS, PAS, CASH) to meet their management information needs? What are some of the advantages and disadvantages of using generalized systems?

14-6 How important is the development of standard data definitions for use in hospital management information systems? Why is interhospital comparison important?

14-7 What factors have limited the development of management information systems in hospitals?

14-8 What is case mix analysis? Why is it important to hospital cost control and management planning?

PROBLEMS

14-1 Assume you are the chief executive officer of a 400-bed community general hospital. Prepare a memo to a special task force of the management committee which you have appointed to develop a management information system for the hospital. The memo is to serve as a charge to the task force in carrying out this work.

14-2 Conduct an audit of the management information capabilities of a hospital in your locale. Determine the extent to which good management information is available for:

a. goal setting and long-range planning
b. short-term demand forecasting and work planning
c. resource allocation and cost control
d. performance and quality control
e. program evaluation.

NOTES

1. Samuel Davis and John R. Freeman, "Hospital Managers Need Management Information Systems," *Health Care Management Review*, Fall 1976, p. 66.
2. Walton M. Hancock, "Dynamics of Hospital Operational Control Systems," *Hospital and Health Services Administration*, Summer 1976, p. 24. See also John P. Young, "A Conceptual Framework for Hospital Administrative Decision Systems," *Health Services Research*, Summer 1968, pp. 79-95.
3. Paul B. Hofman, "Establishing Standards of Institutional Performance," *Hospital Progress*, February 1976, pp. 50-53.
4. Steven L. Alter, "How Effective Managers Use Information Systems," *Harvard Business Review*, November-December 1976, pp. 97-104.
5. Ibid., p. 98.
6. See Christopher P. O'Conner, "A Data Set for Hospital Planning," *Health Care Management Review*, Fall 1979, pp. 81-84, and Sister Mary Leila, Thomas R. O'Donavan, and Larry P. Schwartz, "Planning—A Full-Time Responsibility," *Hospital Progress*, September 1976, pp. 94-98, 124.
7. Michael B. Harrington, "Forecasting Areawide Demand For Health Care Services: A Critical Review of Major Techniques and Their Application," *Inquiry*, September 1977, pp. 254-268.
8. See, for example, D. Michael Warner and Juan Prawda, "A Mathematical Programming Model for Scheduling Nursing Personnel in a Hospital," *Man-*

agement Science, December 1972, pp. 411-422, and John D. Thompson, Robert B. Fetter, and Charles D. Mross, "Case Mix and Resource Use," *Inquiry*, December 1975, pp. 300-312.

9. See, for example, Larry E. Shear, "Ability to Measure Performance Should Be an Integral Part of Management Information Systems," *Hospitals*, October 16, 1981, pp. 123-129, and Charles J. Austin and Harry S. Carter, "Hospital Information Systems & Quality Assurance," *Hospital & Health Services Administration*, Fall 1981, pp. 42-62.
10. D. Michael Warner and Don C. Holloway, *Decision Making and Control for Health Administration* (Ann Arbor, Michigan: Health Administration Press, 1978), pp. 363-365.
11. John R. Griffith, *Quantitative Techniques for Hospital Planning and Control* (Lexington, Massachusetts: Lexington Books, 1972), pp. 337-365.
12. Ibid., pp. 304-321.
13. Walter A. Mischley and Norman Spuehler, "Complex Data in a Simple Graphic Formula," *Hospital*, December 1, 1974, pp. 46-49.
14. The sections which follow also appeared in a paper: Charles J. Austin and Barry R. Greene, "Hospital Information Systems: A Current Perspective," *Inquiry*, June 1978, pp. 104-108. Reprinted by permission.
15. John V. Soden, "Understanding MIS Failures," *Data Management*, July 1975, pp. 29-33, 46.
16. Ibid., p. 30.
17. *Personal Privacy in an Information Society: The Report of the Privacy Protection Study Commission* (Washington, D.C.: U.S. Government Printing Office, 1977). Stock No. 052-003-00395-3.
18. Willis H. Ware, "Old Practices in a New Age Endanger Information Privacy," *Hospitals*, October 16, 1977, pp. 133-140.
19. Donald F. Phillips, "Regulation and Data Systems: Questions of Demands Versus Needs," *Hospitals*, October 16, 1977, pp. 85-90, 202, and Robert N. Anthony and Regina E. Herzlinger, "Requirements of Outside Agencies," in *Management Control in Nonprofit Organizations* (Homewood, Illinois: Richard D. Irwin, 1975), pp. 325-327.
20. Regina Herzlinger, "Management Noninformation Systems in Health Care Organizations," *Health Care Management Review*, Spring 1976, p. 73.
21. Phillips, "Regulation and Data Systems," p. 90.
22. Edward J. Connors, "Hospital System Aspects," in *Operations Research in Health Care: A Critical Analysis*, eds. Larry J. Shuman, R. Dixon Speas, and John R. Young (Baltimore, Maryland: Johns Hopkins University Press, 1975), pp. 29-30.
23. Terrence J. Scott, "Formatted Decision Processes and the Use of Advocacy," *World Hospitals*, Vol. 13, No. 3, 1977, pp. 151-152.
24. Thompson, Fetter, and Mross, "Case Mix and Resource Use," pp. 300-312.
25. Anthony and Herzlinger, *Management Control in Nonprofit Organizations*, pp. 317-318.

26. Herzlinger, "Management Noninformation Systems in Health Care Organizations," p. 74.
27. A. Harvey, "Factors Making For Implementation Success and Failure," *Management Science*, February 1970, pp. B312-B321.
28. J.F. Rockart, "On the Implementation of Information Systems," in *The Management of Health Care*, eds. William J. Abernathy, Alan Sheldon, and Coimbatore K. Prahalad (Cambridge, Massachusetts: Ballinger Publishing Company, 1974).
29. D. Katz and R.L. Kahn, *The Social Psychology of Organizations* (New York: John Wiley & Sons, 1966), pp. 248-249.
30. Ibid., p. 249.
31. R.B. Fetter, J.D. Thompson, and R.E. Mills, "A System for Cost and Reimbursement Control in Hospitals," *Yale Journal of Biology and Medicine*, Vol. 49, May 1976, pp. 123-136.
32. J. Joel May, ed., "Diagnosis Related Groups," *Topics in Health Care Financing*, Summer 1982, Chapter 2, "Data Systems for Case Mix" by Leo K. Lichtig, p. 14.
33. Roger Kropf and James Greenberg, "A Case-Mix Approach to the Control of Hospital Capital Expenditures," *Health Care Management Review*, Spring 1982, p. 22.

ADDITIONAL READINGS

Anthony, Robert N. and Herzlinger, Regina. *Management Control in Nonprofit Organizations*. Homewood, Illinois: Richard D. Irwin, 1975.

Barker, W. Daniel. "Management Reports Can Help Control Costs." *Hospitals*, October 16, 1977, pp. 165-170.

Churchill, H. and Dirksen, C. "Wanted: A Uniform Reporting Systems." *Dimensions in Health Services*, February 1981, pp. 9-12.

Fedorowicz, Jane and Veazie, Stephen. "Automated DRG Systems: Unanswered Questions." *Hospital Progress*, January 1981, pp. 54-55, 71.

Griffith, John R. *Quantitative Techniques for Hospital Planning and Control*. Lexington, Massachusetts: Lexington Books, 1972.

Griffith, John R.; Hancock, Walton M.; and Munson, Fred C. *Cost Control in Hospitals*. Ann Arbor, Michigan: Health Administration Press, 1976.

Hancock, Walton M. "Dynamics of Hospital Operational Control Systems." *Hospital and Health Services Administration*, Summer 1976, pp. 23-42.

Harrington, Michael B. "Forecasting Areawide Demand for Health Care Services: A Critical Review of Major Techniques and Their Application." *Inquiry*, September 1977, pp. 254-268.

Hayes, M. and Moritz, M. "Patient Classification Systems—A Nurse Management Tool." *Dimensions in Health Services*, August 1981, pp. 22-24.

Herzlinger, Regina. "Management Noninformation Systems in Health Care Organizations." *Health Care Management Review*, Spring 1976, pp. 71-76.

Hofman, Paul B. "Establishing Standards of Institutional Performance." *Hospital Progress*, February 1976, pp. 50-53.

Kropf, Roger and Greenberg, James. "A Case-Mix Approach to the Control of Hospital Capital Expenditures." *Health Care Management Review*, Spring 1982, pp. 17-24.

Murdick, Robert G. and Ross, Joel E. *Introduction to Management Information Systems*. Englewood Cliffs, New Jersey: Prentice-Hall, 1977.

O'Connor, Christopher P. "A Data Set for Hospital Planning." *Health Care Management Review*, Fall 1979, pp. 81-84.

Scott, Terrence J. "Formatted Decision Processes and the Use of Advocacy." *World Hospitals*, Vol. 13, No. 3, 1977, pp. 151-152.

Shear, Larry E. "Ability to Measure Performance Should be Integral Part of Management Information Systems." *Hospitals*, October 16, 1981, pp. 123-129.

Shuman, Larry J., Speas, H. Dixon, and Young, John P. *Operations Research in Health Care: A Critical Analysis*. Baltimore, Maryland: Johns Hopkins University Press, 1975.

Soden, John V. "Understanding MIS Failures." *Data Management*, July 1975, pp. 29-33, 46.

Thompson, John D., Averill, Richard F., and Fetter, Robert B. "Planning, Budgeting, and Controlling—One Look at the Future: Case-Mix Cost Accounting." *Health Services Research*, Summer 1979, pp. 111-125.

Warner, D. Michael and Holloway, Don C. *Decision Making and Control for Health Administration*. Ann Arbor, Michigan: Health Administration Press, 1978.

Yoder, J.L. and Connor, R.A. "Diagnosis Related Groups and Management." *Topics in Health Care Financing*, Summer 1982, pp. 29-42.

15

Future Trends in Hospital Information Systems

This book has attempted to provide an honest appraisal of the state of the art in hospital information systems, to review accomplishments, and to describe problems which confront administrators and system designers. This final chapter looks ahead to a brief examination of the future. Any such predictions are admittedly subjective, but the trends which are discussed flow logically from the experiences of the past, insuring at least partial validity of the prognostication.

TECHNOLOGICAL CHANGE

Continued improvements can be expected in the technology which supports hospital information systems in the years ahead. Hardware will continue to improve in both capability and reliability, and unit costs will continue to decrease. Continuing advances can be expected in microprocessors, data communications terminals, and mass memory devices.

One example of the impact of these technological advances is the anticipated benefits from the application of computer-aided techniques to non-invasive diagnostic and treatment methods. Such systems offer the dual benefits of improved patient care and reduced costs through the elimination of costly (and often dangerous) surgical procedures. In a recent article on this subject, Kuntz describes new techniques of digital fluoroscopy and interventional radiology in the nonsurgical diagnosis and treatment of atherosclerosis (hardening of the arteries), a major cause of heart attacks and strokes. Digital fluoroscopy employing microprocessors ". . . will permit the detection of lesions blocking arteries and veins to the same degree presently obtained with arteriography, but without the risk."[1]

New drug infusion devices also are being developed to free patients from intervenous medication administration, eliminating the need for hospitalization as a result. These programmed drug infusion devices, about the size of a pack of cigarettes, can be worn externally to control the flow of drugs, whether continuous or at preset intervals.[2]

Lindberg describes the effects of developing technology on future medical information systems and indicates that profound changes can be expected as the result of developments in microprocessors, mass storage, communications, and the use of artificial intelligence techniques.[3] Microprocessors will support advanced clinical information-processing systems close to the patient without the need for large centralized systems. New mass storage devices (such as laser-etched disk storage systems) will remove virtually all limitations on the size of data files and offer real promise for the storage and retrieval of medical images. Advances in communications technology make medical networking more practical, thus providing health care institutions with computer terminal access to patient medical records stored in regional or national data files.

In the area of software, artificial intelligence methods of programming and system development provide the ". . . capability to enlist the enthusiasm and participation of the biomedical community because it focuses on the essence of processes (the knowledge structure) rather than the superficial appearances of the processes such as tend to be addressed in ordinary programming techniques."[4] These user-oriented, functional software systems will play a major role in the development of more sophisticated hospital information systems in the future.

Weston predicts that, by the year 2000, home computers will have a major impact on health care delivery. The home computer, linked to regional and national health data systems, will provide basic health information for the family and could be used to submit input readings on such factors as blood pressure, cardiovascular recordings, and disease symptoms for transmission to regional databanks and ultimate use for diagnostic purposes.[5]

Some observers believe that hospitals are now moving from a position of inferiority to one of superiority in information systems development. A recent study by the IBM hospital computer users organization (ECHO: Electronic Computing Health Oriented) predicts rapid developments in hospital computing during the 1980's and emergence of the hospital industry as a leader in the field of information technology.[6]

Organizational Effects

Technology also will affect the future organization of the hospital. Figure 15-1 depicts one possible organizational plan. An Administrative

FIGURE 15-1
Hospital Organization of the Future

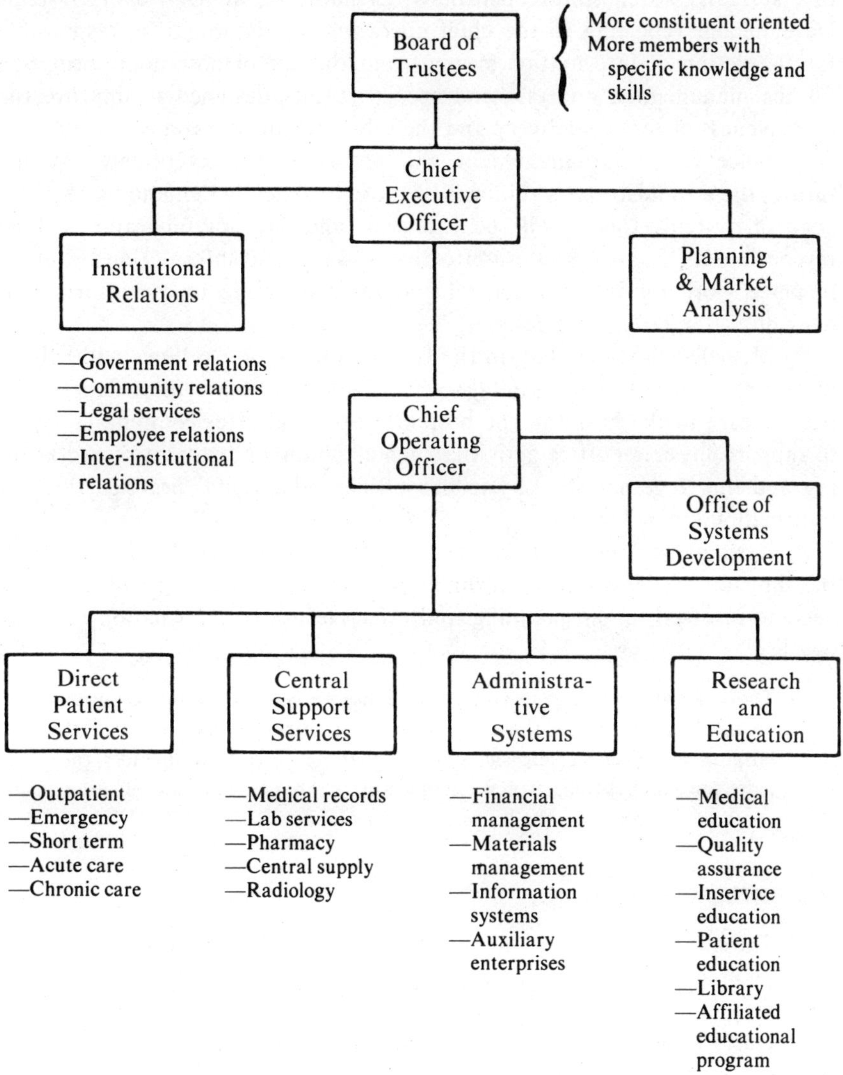

Systems Division of the hospital is charged with the design and development of hospital systems, including the effective incorporation of information systems into hospital operations. In addition, an Office of Systems Development reporting to the chief operating officer would be responsible for the design of information systems and the use of hospital information for the management analyses and special studies designed to improve the effectiveness of service delivery and the efficiency of operations.[7]

Since hospital management will be more systems oriented in the future, the administrator's role will be more technically demanding. Knowledge of systems theory will be essential, and the administrator will be responsible for insuring that an effective management information system is in place, both for internal control and for responding to the information demands of external agencies.

Mishelevich states that, in the future, information systems will help to attract physicians to join hospital staffs. In addition to providing support for patient care in the hospital, the hospital also could offer computer services to support physician office activities such as billing and patient record keeping and link together the physician's office and hospital practice through information technology.[8]

Kernaghan points out that hospital trustees will not be exempt from the impact of information technology and that board members must become involved in the planning and effective use of information technology:

> Those boards that do get involved have discovered that there is good reason to do so. Primary among these is the trustee's responsibility to ensure that the hospital has decision support systems that will enable it to meet the challenges of competition, of new methods of reimbursement, and of other influences that impinge on the hospital's survival. . . .[9]

Regional and National Databanks

The need for regional and national databanks of patient records seems to be an emerging theme among commentators on the future of health care delivery.

Gustafson and Thesen contend that traditional management information systems in the health care field are inadequate and do not furnish policymakers with the kinds of information needed for decision making. Such systems should be expanded to include *qualitative* data and capability for special studies, as needed.[10] Leary and associates state that hospitals need comparative data, generated on a regional basis, in order to keep up with the regulatory agencies:

> They need access to the kind of regional data and sophisticated analytic tools used by rate setting agencies, Blue Cross plans, health systems agencies, professional standards review organizations, commercial insurers and the federal government.[11]

Austin and Carter have developed a conceptual model for a national hospital information system. Through integration of clinical and administrative information and standardization of measurement, the proposed National Hospital Information Resource Center would produce periodic reports to each participating hospital, including: utilization of services; direct costs, computed on a case mix basis; indirect costs, computed by cost center and by case mix; time trend analyses; comparisons with other hospitals of comparable size and patient mix; productivity reports; patient satisfaction reports; and quality assessment information. In addition, the Center would produce general statistical reports by geographic region, size, and category of member hospitals.[12] Development of such systems are likely within the next 10 to 20 years.

SOCIOECONOMIC ISSUES

As the technology continues to improve, needs will increase for national policies to insure orderly incorporation of the technology within our social and economic institutions.

William Norris, Chief Executive Officer of Control Data Corporation, is concerned that we are losing the competitive edge in computer technology to other countries where government support of research and development is more commonplace. He sees the need for a United States industrial policy developed through a voluntary commission comprised of senior representatives from government, business, labor, and other sectors of society.[13]

Wessel and Kirkley point out that other countries are further along than the United States in developing national policy on computer and communications technology. They call for the development of a national information committee that would ". . . create a database, a coherent body of information about the computer/communications age we are now entering and how it is affecting our lives economically, politically and ethically."[14] Policies developed by the committee would assist in evaluating the effects of technology on social institutions and also help in forming a posture on international trade.

Without a doubt, computers increasingly will affect the lives of all of us in the future. Social scientists, technologists, and administrators must work together in order to achieve the potential of the new technology and to incorporate it effectively into organizational life as we move into this electronic age.

CONCLUSION

Hospital information systems can be expected to improve in the years ahead. Administrators and other key hospital personnel (nursing supervisors, medical directors, middle managers) will become more and more sophisticated in using information intelligently for program planning, evaluation, and management control. This sophistication will be the result of improved education and training, longer experience with the use of computer systems, and increased external pressure to have good information available.

Many problems in the planning, design, and implementation of systems will remain. Even as systems are improved, information and analysis will never replace the judgment, experience, and intuition of experienced administrators. In many situations decisions will continue to be based primarily on political considerations. However, the net result of improved information availability will be decisions which are better informed. Everyone involved in policy decisions, including the advocates of special interests, will be required to confront issues which are better defined as the result of improved information. Patients will be the ultimate beneficiaries of the improved services which will result from more informed policies.

NOTES

1. Ester F. Knutz, "Equipment Will Cut Costs and Close Some Hospitals," *Modern Healthcare*, September 1981, pp. 84-86.
2. Ibid., p. 86.
3. Donald A.B. Lindberg, *The Growth of Medical Information Systems in the United States* (Lexington, Massachusetts: Lexington Books, 1979). Note particularly Chapter 7, "Effects of Changes in Technology on Future MISs."
4. Ibid., p. 147.
5. Alan J. Weston, "Health Care Delivery and Health Data Processing in the United States," *Allied Health and Behavioral Sciences*, Vol. 2, No. 2, 1980, pp. 223-228.
6. Suzanne La Violette, "Shaking Their Inferiority Complexes, Hospitals Prepare for New Advances," *Modern Healthcare*, June 1980, p. 24.
7. Charles J. Austin, "The Hospital of the Future: How Will It be Structured?" *Health Services Manager*, October 1979, pp. 1-4.
8. David Mishelevich, "Use of Information Systems Gives Physicians Incentive to Join Hospitals," *Modern Healthcare*, July 1981, pp. 54-56.
9. Salvinija G. Kernaghan, "With Information Systems, More May Be Less If Needs Aren't Planned," *Trustee*, November 1982, p. 17.
10. David H. Gustafson and Arne Thesen, "Are Traditional Information Systems Adequate for Policy Makers?" *Health Care Management Review*, Winter 1981, pp. 51-63.
11. Robert J. Leary, Robert A. Chernow, and Henry J. Friedman, "Hospitals Need

Comparative Data to Keep Ahead of New Regulations," *Modern Healthcare*, July 1981, p. 96.

12. Charles J. Austin and Harrison S. Carter, "National Hospital Information Resource Center: A Model," *Inquiry*, Winter 1981, pp. 291-299.
13. William Norris, "Keeping America First," *Datamation*, September 1982, pp. 280-287.
14. Milton R. Wessel and John L. Kirkley, "For a National Information Committee," *Datamation*, September 1982, p. 248.

ADDITIONAL READINGS

Austin, Charles J. "Hospital Information Systems and the Development of a National Health Information System." *Journal of Medical Systems*, Vol. 6, No. 1, 1982, pp. 3-11.

Austin, Charles J. "The Hospital of the Future: How Will It Be Structured?" *Health Services Manager*, October 1979, pp. 1-4.

Gustafson, David H. and Thesen, Arne. "Are Traditional Information Systems Adequate for Policy Makers?" *Health Care Management Review*, Winter 1981, pp. 51-63.

Lindberg, Donald A.B. *The Growth of Medical Information Systems in the United States*. Lexington, Massachusetts: Lexington Books, 1979.

Pugliese, Donald F. "Hospital Medical Information Systems in 1981: Where Are We?" *MUG Quarterly*, Vol. 11, No. 4, 1981, pp. 16-18.

Salerno, Lynn M. "Catching Up With the Computer Revolution." *Harvard Business Review*, November-December 1981, pp. 8-24.

Appendix A Glossary of Technical Terms

Address. The identifier for a storage location in the computer or for an input-output unit.

Administrative information systems. Information systems which are designed to assist in the performance of administrative support activities in the hospital such as payroll accounting, accounts receivable, accounts payable and daily inpatient bed census.

ALGOL. ALGOrithmetic Language. A scientific computer programming language introduced in 1958. This language was developed by an international committee of representatives from a large number of professional organizations and in some respects resembles FORTRAN (see *FORTRAN*). ALGOL is a universal language which can be used on various types of computer systems manufactured by several different companies.

Algorithm. A step-by-step procedure for performing a task. Computer algorithms consist of logical and mathematical operations.

Analog signal. The representation of data by physical variation of some continuous variable such as temperature, pressure, rotation, voltage, speed, or electrical resistance.

Applications program. A program that performs tasks for the computer user.

Arithmetic and logic unit (ALU). The CPU circuitry which performs mathematical and logical operations. An ALU typically includes devices for adding, complementing, accumulating, shifting, and logical operations.

Array. An organized grouping of computer storage locations of the same data type. Arrays are arranged according to dimensions. Any element of an array is identified by one or more subscripts, where each subscript refers to a dimension of the array.

Assembly language. A programming language in which each statement represents one command or an established group of commands in machine language. Assembly language has advantages over machine language for programming because commands are given in mnemonic form instead of as number codes and because labels of storage locations or the starting points of parts of the program are given as names rather than as numbers. Assembly languages convert the commands, operands, and labels of a program into machine language binary code in the proper sequential order.

Assignment operator. A symbol for a command to the computer to store a value; usually := or =.

Audit trail. Provisions for a step-by-step trace of the path of a transaction through a system.

Bar code labels. Precoded marks on a printed form or plastic card which can be automatically read by specially designed computer input devices. Bar codes are extensively used in the retail food industry for product identification and pricing in a form called the Universal Product Code (UPC).

BASIC. Basic All-purpose Symbolic Instruction Code. A data processing language developed at Dartmouth University as a tool for familiarizing students with fundamental programming concepts. It is considered to be one of the easiest languages to learn and is well suited as a time-sharing language in which the user communicates directly with his data files. BASIC is a universal language which can be used on various types of computer systems manufactured by several different companies.

Batch processing systems. Systems in which data are grouped together for a specified time period and stored in machine readable form for later processing. This type of system has application where there is a high input volume, but no essential need for fast response time. Common areas of hospital application are payroll, billing, accounts payable, accounts receivable and general ledger accounting.

Baud rate. The number of bits transmitted per second. For example, if the baud rate for a communication link is given at 1,200 baud, this means that data are being transmitted over the link at the rate of 1,200 bits per second.

Binary data. Data stored or transmitted on the basis of the binary number system.

Binary number system. A base-two number system in which the only digits are 0 and 1. See *Figure 4-4* for a listing of the first 16 binary numbers (0-15) given as four-digit patterns. Place values for binary numbers are powers of two.

Bit. A contraction of binary digit and the unit of data in the notation of the binary number system.

Block. A physical record unit for data storage or transmission. Data are grouped into blocks which can be stored or transmitted more efficiently than logical records.

Blocking factor. The maximum number of logical records or characters which can be contained in a given block on disk or tape.

Boolean operation. A logical operation defined by a system of logic using binary representation. The system was formulated by nineteenth-century mathematician George Boole.

Bubble memory. A memory device based on magnetic bubbles, which are tiny cylinders of magnetic material caused by sufficiently large magnetic fields applied to a surface with an appropriate garnet film.

Bucket. A large unit of physical data storage.

Bus. A set of parallel signal connection lines which link the central processing unit with primary memory and with input–output facilities. The parallel lines of a bus permit simultaneous transmission of the bits of a single byte. Three categories of buses (control, data, and address) are used to connect the CPU to main memory and peripherals and to provide separate paths for transmission.

Byte. A binary pattern which can consist of seven or eight bits signifying a unit of data. The bits representing the data may be accompanied by an additional bit, such as a parity bit, used in error detection. In the realm of the computer user, bytes are usually equivalent to printed characters. Some bytes are used as control messages for transmission processes.

Cathode-ray tube (CRT). An electronic vacuum tube with a screen on which characters and graphic patterns may be displayed by control of a beam of electrons.

Central processing unit (CPU) (also called *central processor*). The controlling and processing center of the computer which processes data, performs the actual calculations, and supervises and coordinates the various functional units of the system.

Clinical (or medical) information systems. Information systems which involve the organized processing, storage, and retrieval of information to support patient care activities, such as indexing medical records, clinical laboratory reporting, analyzing electrocardiograms, and computer-aided diagnosis.

Clock. A time-keeping device, or an oscillator which provides the fundamental pulse frequency in order to synchronize events in the CPU.

Closed system. A completely self-contained system which is not influenced by external events (see also *system, cybernetic system, open system*).

COBOL. COmmon Business Oriented Language. An English-like data processing language which is widely used for business data processing applications. Most instructions are coded using English names instead of restricted names or symbols. This makes the language easier for the programmer to write and the user to read. COBOL is a universal language which can be used on various types of computer systems manufactured by several different companies.

Code. A computer program written according to a special structure or the use of symbols according to a special convention. See also *bar code*, *object code*, and *source code*.

Communication link. The physical means of connecting one computer to another or of connecting a peripheral device to a computer for the purpose of transmitting and receiving information. Also called a data transmission link. See also *dedicated link*.

Compiler. A computer program which translates instructions and subroutines written in a high-level language (see also *ALGOL, COBOL, FORTRAN, PL/I*) and prepares a program written in machine language ready for direct use on a specific computer system.

Computer output microfilm (COM). The direct conversion of computer output into imaging on microfilm or microfiche to provide a permanent record.

Computer programming. The process of coding a set of instructions or steps in a given data processing language which directs the computer and coordinates the operation of all hardware components.

Core memory. The special main storage unit of the computer which is an integral component of the central processing unit.

Critical Path Network (also called *CPM* or *Critical Path Method*). A tool used to define the interrelationships on a time scale for all events and activities which must be accomplished in order to complete a predetermined objective. Used as a scheduling and management control tool for major projects, the network is established by the interdependency of the events and activities and a critical path is determined to show the duration of the overall project. CPM has the ability to vary the time along the critical path to determine its effect on cost. (See also *PERT chart.*)

Cybernetic system. A self-regulating system which contains the following automatic control components: sensor, a monitor, standards and a control unit. This system uses part of its energy to feed back information to compare performance with a standard and make corrections or adjustments. (See also *system, closed system, open system.*)

Data. Facts secured from empirical observations or research. Data in and of themselves often have little value, and take on meaning only after sorting, tabulation, and processing into a more usable format.

Data type. A classification of data used in computer programming to characterize data subject to certain operations or data which can be stored in a certain fashion. For example, numeric data can be subject to arithmetic operations, such as addition and subtraction, while alphanumeric data can be subject to string analysis operations. Numeric data have traditionally been subclassified as integer or floating point. Languages such as Pascal and ADA permit user-defined data types.

Debugging. The process by which computer programs are tested and programming errors are identified and corrected.

Decision table. A tabulation or array of possible alternative actions, displayed in such a way that the conditions for each course of action are clear. The use of decision tables has been formalized as an aid in the systems analysis and program design processes.

Dedicated link. A communication link which is limited to a particular use, such as high-speed computer transmissions.

Deterministic system. A system in which the component parts function according to completely predictable or definable relationships. Most mechanical systems are examples of this type of system. (See also *system.*)

Digital signal. The representation of data as a numerical series of discrete units. Digital signals in a computer system are represented in a binary (0 or 1) coding system by the "on" or "off" condition of an electronic switch.

Direct-access computer storage (also called *random-access storage*). Data files which are stored without dependence on the location of previously obtained data. This provides direct access to any data item in a file without the need for sequential searching.

Disk directory. A disk file used to list all the program files or data files stored currently on a disk.

Disk drive. A peripheral data storage device utilizing a magnetically coated disk. The disk drive consists of a mechanism to provide rotation of the disk (spindle), a read-write head to establish and detect magnetic patterns on the surface of each disk surface being accessed, and a mechanism to position the head appropriately for access. A metal disk approximately 18 inches in diameter is common in large systems and most mainframe system disk drives are designed for disk packs consisting of stacks of such disks. This medium has the advantage of faster retrieval of data than tape drives have because of its direct (random) access capability. Microcomputers commonly use disk drives accepting single 5.25-inch or 8-inch floppy (plastic) disks. This type of disk drive also provides storage of initial load programs and diagnostic routines for large systems. See *Winchester disk technology*, *floppy disk.*

Distributed processing. A data processing system in which the workload is spread out through a network of minicomputers located in different organizational units (e.g., minicomputers in the admitting office, business office, laboratory, and outpatient department). System integration is more difficult to achieve when using distributed processing.

Documentation. Internal documentation consists of the recording of descriptive information about a computer program in the form of comments embedded in the program. This procedure assures that information vital for maintenance of the software will be available when needed. External documentation consists of programmer's manuals and guides which thoroughly describe the software and the conditions for its use.

Dump. Hexadecimal equivalents of the contents of memory, printed out to assist in the debugging process.

Facilities management. A contract arrangement providing for the management of a hospital computer system and the supply of specialized software by an outside firm.

Field. A subdivision of a record in a file system or a subdivision of a computer instruction in assembly or machine language.

Floppy disk. A thin, circular piece of coated plastic which resembles a flexible phonograph record and is used as one type of direct or random access computer memory.

Flowchart. The steps to be programmed and the sequence in which they are to be performed, displayed in the form of a graph consisting of symbolic shapes, legends, and connecting flowlines. There are two main categories of flowchart: program and system. See *Figure 5-4*.

FORTRAN. FORmula TRANslator. A programming language developed by the IBM Corporation and originally intended for use on scientific problems. This language is widely used for quantitative and statistical applications. FORTRAN is a universal language which can be used on various types of computer systems manufactured by several different companies.

Hardware. The physical components of a computer system, i.e., the electronic, magnetic, and mechanical units which comprise the central processor, memory and storage units, input–output devices, interface units, and communication links.

Hexadecimal number system. A base-16 number system. Each hexadecimal digit represents a four-bit pattern since 16 is a power of two. Hexadecimal numbers thus can efficiently and exactly represent the binary values stored or transmitted in digital computer systems and can provide compact displays of the contents of computer memory.

Hierarchy chart. A chart organized in hierarchical, top-down fashion and used to display the relationships of program modules as an aid in structured programming and documentation.

High-level languages. Computer programming languages which are independent of the limitations of a specific computer. These languages must be translated by the computer into machine language. See *Chapter 5* for descriptions of languages.

History file. An inactive file (or previously used version of a file), normally retained in off-line storage, to facilitate reconstruction of transactions or data. Periodically copied history files are commonly referred to as backup or archive files.

Hollerith code. A system of encoding alphanumeric information onto cards or of representing optically read mark patterns.

Impact printer. A kind of printer that involves physical contact with the paper, normally with an inked ribbon placed between the paper and the part of the printer that forms the characters.

Indexed file. A file containing records stored in sequence according to an index field. Access to records is gained by searching the index fields or by consulting a directory based on the indexing method.

Information. A meaningful aggregation of data or knowledge which can be evaluated for a specific use or set of uses.

Integrated circuit. An entire electronic circuit mounted on a single silicon chip and containing components such as transistors, resistors, diodes, and capacitors.

Integrated systems. A set of information systems which can share common data files and can communicate among themselves.

Intelligent terminals. Terminals that have the capabilities of microcomputers to process data independently of the main system, and thus are capable of storing valid data ranges and instructions adequate to perform some checking of data entered at the terminal.

Interactive system. Also referred to as an on-line system or a real-time system. Interactive systems have the capability of providing near-instantaneous responses to inquiries from a terminal because of the immediate access to all necessary data. In such systems, the users of information are in direct communication with their data files.

Interpreter. An interactive high-level language which analyzes source code on a statement-by-statement basis and makes extensive use of pre-established subroutines in translating source code. Examples are APL, BASIC, LISP, and MUMPS. Interpreters are particularly suited to interactive environments, such as CRT terminals and microcomputers. Interpreters offer editing features, immediate syntax-error messages, and interactive debugging, but they are less efficient than compilers in certain aspects of code translation.

Key. One or more fields of a record used in identification or location of the record.

Life cycle. The life cycle of software is the sequence of specification, design, implementation, and maintenance of computer programs. For models of computer hardware, the life cycle is the sequence in market status of development, announcement, availability, and obsolescence. The level of vendor support for hardware is high at the beginning of the life cycle, while availability of repair and spare parts degrades at the conclusion.

Light pen. An electronic, pen-like device by which the user of a video computer terminal points to data displayed on a cathode-ray tube and retrieves that information for processing purposes.

Linked list. A list where each item in the list has a pointer to the next item or to one end of the list.

Log file. A file recording all transactions occurring in a computer system. Log files are used for auditing purposes and to reconstruct data.

Machine language program. A data processing program or instruction code which can be used directly by the computer without having to be translated. This type of program is also referred to as an object program.

Mainframe. The portion of a computer system that contains the CPU and main memory, as contrasted with peripheral devices, such as input–output facilities and auxiliary memory storage. This term is used to characterize relatively large computer systems which normally have very large main memories, many on-line terminals, and extensive auxiliary memory storage.

Management information system. A set of formalized procedures designed to provide current information for management planning and control. The system may or may not be computerized. Two generalized management information systems available to hospitals are Hospital Administrative Services (HAS) and Professional Activity Study (PAS).

Manual system. An information system which operates without any type of machine processing of data.

Master file. A file of relatively permanent information, which is usually updated periodically.

Maxicomputer. A large mainframe computer system. See *mainframe; Figure 6-1.*

Menu. A list of options, displayed on a CRT screen, to allow the user to select the function to be performed or another, more specific menu.

Microcomputer. A small computer system, usually designed for a single user and capable of being set up on a desktop. See Figures 1-5; 6-1.

Microprocessors. Small computers which employ changeable "plug-in" modules. These electronic microcircuits are used for such purposes as individual patient monitoring units for critically ill patients in intensive care units. In a general sense, a microprocessor is the CPU chip, or semiconductor, component of a microcomputer.

Minicomputer. An intermediate-sized data-processing unit that contains an internal memory and can accept other peripherals such as disk storage, line printers, and magnetic tape units. See *Figure 6-1.*

Modem (modulator/demodulator unit). A data communications device that modulates and demodulates data between two or more input–output devices and a data transmission link. To modulate, the modem converts direct current signals to transmission tones. To demodulate, the modem converts transmission tones to direct current signals.

Modular design. Design of information systems as individual units or modules, following a predetermined plan which enables the modules to share information and communicate among themselves.

Module. A segment of a computer program. Modern structured programming encourages modular techniques in which individual tasks and subtasks are programmed as separate modules. Proper use of modules can contribute to software reliability and facilitate software maintenance. See *modular design.*

Multiplexing. The process of combining two or more signals into a single signal, transmitting it, and then sorting out the original signals.

MUMPS. Massachusetts General Hospital Utility Multi-Programming System. A computer programming language for application to medical computing problems which was developed by the Laboratory of Computer Science at the Massachusetts General Hospital in 1966. It is a near-English, user-oriented language with excellent capability for use in a remote access, multiuser, time-sharing environment.

Nassi-Shneiderman (N-S) charts. Charts designed to represent program logic more adequately from the standpoint of structured programming. See *Figure 5-4.*

Network. An interconnected collection of autonomous computers.

Node. A point of convergence in a diagram or PERT chart. In a distributed processing system or computer network, the interconnected elements, such as computers, terminals, peripheral controllers or multiplexers, and data communication processors. Nodes in a computer network or distributed system have addresses.

Nominal. An approximate value, such as a nominal voltage level, defined by an acceptable range of values.

Nonimpact printer. Printers using xerographic, chemical, thermal, or laser technology. Advantages of various types of nonimpact printers include high speed, favorable repair records, or reduction of noise.

Normal form. A convention for files used in database management systems. Normal forms restrict file structure to provide straightforward, unambiguous storage of data in files so that reliable access methods can be implemented.

Object code. A version of a program translated into machine code which can be relocated where needed at execution time. Object code versions of programs are cataloged and stored on disk to avoid unnecessary recompilation of repeatedly used programs.

Off-line. Peripheral equipment in a system not under the direct control of the central processing unit or data stored in a form which has been removed from direct control of the CPU. Examples of the latter are reels of magnetic tape stored and not currently mounted on the tape drive. Punched cards and paper tape also provide off-line storage of data.

Open system. A system which exchanges energy, information, or material with its environment. Thus, an open system has the capability of adjusting to the environment over time. The system is both influenced by and in turn influences the environment in which it functions. (See also *closed system, cybernetic system,* and *system.)*

Operand. Values to be processed by the computer according to the program instruction.

Operating system. A set of integrated subroutines and programs which control the operation of a computer and manage its resources.

Optical scanner. A device which uses the scanning of light patterns to generate analog or digital signals in order to report marking patterns on a document such as a card, sheet, or label. As computer peripherals, optical scanners are equipped to transmit codes to a processor for interpretation.

Order processing. All processing in a hospital computer system invoked by a physician's or nurse's order and the subsequent responses associated with it. See *Figure 6-3.*

Packaged systems. Generalized computer systems, marketed by a number of commercial firms, which are designed to fulfill the information needs of any hospital. Examples include generalized admitting and census control systems, billing and accounts receivable systems, and medical records systems.

Parallel testing. The process by which a new and an old data processing system are checked with the same input data for the same time period in order to verify that the new system satisfactorily meets the design criteria. In some cases the new system will be computerized and the system being replaced is a manual one.

Peripheral. A device attached to a computer, such as a printer, CRT display, keyboard, disk drive, or tape drive, which transfers information to and from the computer.

PERT chart. PERT is the acronym for Program Evaluation and Review Technique. It is a method which coordinates and synchronizes project scheduling, thereby minimizing delays, conflicts, and interruptions. By scheduling and budgeting resources, a predetermined job can be completed in the shortest possible time. The PERT chart is the actual network constructed on paper showing events, activities, and completion times. (See also *Critical Path Network.*)

PL/I. Programming Language. A general purpose computer programming language which incorporates some of the features of other high-level languages and provides the programmer with an application-oriented language for programming of both scientific and business needs. PL/I is a universal language which can be used on various types of computer systems manufactured by several different companies.

Plug-compatible machine (PCM). A device capable of being interchanged with an equivalent device manufactured by a different vendor. It should be possible to install and operate a PCM in place of an equivalent device without modifications.

Pointer. A field in a record containing the address (in the form of a variable name, number, or label) of data or of another record.

Program. A set of instructions to the computer. Programs are written in the instruction set of the machine (machine language), in an assembly language, or in a high-level language, and are stored in the computer as a sequence of binary numbers.

Protocol. A convention used for communication between devices about initiating or concluding a transmission, to synchronize transmissions, or to reconcile different speeds of sending and receiving. Protocols can consist of timed changes in voltage levels on certain signal lines (hardware protocols) or of the exchange of special control characters (software protocols). For example, a printer uses a protocol to communicate that it is ready for more data or that it can receive no more data.

Pseudocode. A programming aid consisting of a procedure for writing out the structure of a program in simplified English. Pseudocode specifies the detailed steps required in solving a problem and lists the required files, records, and fields to be referenced in the program.

Random-access memory (RAM). Storage which permits access to the bit pattern stored at a particular address. It is affected by loss of power and is therefore called volatile memory.

Read-only memory (ROM). Permanent instructions that cannot be altered by ordinary programming. It is not affected by loss of power and is therefore called nonvolatile memory.

Real-time. Performance of information processing within the time constraints of interaction with physical processes or immediate human use. The results of a given transaction must be delivered in time to control a physical device or to provide a response for a user waiting at a terminal.

Record. A collection of one or more fields of data on a related topic. Files are made up of records.

Redundancy. Hardware or software redundancy in a computer system refers to the replication of equipment, programs, or data sets necessary to assure continual availability of system services for users. In hospital systems, redundancy may be manifested by multiple CPUs and mirrored, closely coupled file systems. Multiple microcomputers or minicomputers in distributed processing systems, as well as distributed subsets of data in such systems, provide redundancy in case of failure of a part of the system. History, archive, and backup files provide a measure of redundancy for processing of transactions in a computer system and for software acquired or developed.

Register. A temporary storage location accommodating a byte or word of data to facilitate arithmetical or logical operations or the transfer of data. Registers can be implemented through specialized hardware features of the computer or by software reservation of space in memory for the purpose.

Sequential-access memory. A storage technique in which the stored items of information become available only one-after-the-other in sequence. Sequential-access memory has the advantage of compact storage and the disadvantage of considerable variation in time necessary to reach a particular record.

Shared systems. Information processing services used by two or more hospitals which do not have sufficient volume and/or financial backing individually to justify designing and maintaining an in-house computer system. These hospitals join together in a sharing arrangement for designing and maintaining a computer system to fit their needs.

Software. The programs which control the operation of a computer, including applications programs, operating systems, programming languages and translators. Software includes documentation of hardware and software in printed forms such as manuals and books.

Source code. The form in which programs are entered for processing by a high-level language.

Spindle. A way of referring to a disk drive. The number of spindles is often given as a rough measure of random-access auxiliary storage capacity.

SPOOLing. Acronym for simultaneous peripheral operations on-line. A technique by which output to slow devices is placed into queues on mass storage devices until transmission is possible. This allows more efficient use of the system, since programs requiring use of low-speed devices, such as a printer, can complete processing without delaying other programs.

Stub testing. A programming strategy of implementing and testing portions of a program, beginning with the main or control module of the program.

Synchronization. Control of the interaction of devices which are initiating or maintaining communication or which function at different relative speeds.

System. A network of parts or elements joined together to accomplish a specific purpose or objective. Every system must include (1) input, (2) a conversion process, and (3) output. (See also *cybernetic system, closed system, open system.*)

Systems analysis. The process of *collecting, organizing,* and *evaluating* facts about information system requirements and about the environment in which the system will operate.

Table file. A file containing tables of data consulted repeatedly by software in the system.

Tape drive. A tape recorder specifically designed to work in a computer system for recording, storage, and retrieval of data. Data stored on magnetic tape are accessible in sequential (not direct) fashion.

Throughput time. The total time span from collection of the first data element to the preparation of the final report in a given system.

Time-shared computer system. See *interactive system.*

Transaction file. A file of transactions accumulated as a batch ready for processing against a master file.

Transmission. The transfer of data from one location to another, which can utilize paths over wire or by microwave. Transmission modes used in computer communication links include asynchronous, synchronous, and binary synchronous. In asynchronous transmissions, bytes (characters) are sent and received individually and each byte is preceded by a start bit and followed by a stop bit. Synchronous transmissions involve sending data at a predetermined rate as defined by a clock. The synchronous mode of transmission offers the advantage of not needing start and stop bits for individual characters. Binary synchronous transmissions utilize special character codes which precede and follow messages and assure reliability together with a higher possible rate of sending and receiving data. The binary synchronous transmission mode is characteristic of certain large mainframe computer systems.

Truth table. A listing of all possible truth values for statements, logical expressions, or states of a function.

Variable. A symbol used in a computer program to assure consistent reference to a storage location in the computer in which various values may be stored during the execution of a program. The use of variables is a convenience for programmers using high-level languages, since they do not have to be concerned with the actual locations used by the computer to store values.

Video display terminals (VDT). Computer input–output terminals which combine a keyboard and a cathode-ray tube (CRT). Video display terminals provide direct on-line access to computer files.

Videodisc technology. A nonmagnetic data storage technology utilizing prepared discs. Videodiscs offer high data storage densities. Optical or laser videodisc systems scan the reflective surface of the disk to detect tiny pits used to encode data. Capacitive videodisc equipment electronically detects minute variations in capacitance as the disc is being played.

Virtual memory. A storage technique that permits the operating system to address more memory than is available in main memory. Disk storage is used to provide the additional memory and thus serves as an extension of main memory.

Voice recognition systems. Digital systems which can store templates of utterances and later use this information to determine whether a particular person is speaking or to identify a word or phrase. Such technology can be used for data entry or for security purposes. Advantages of voice recognition systems are that keyboard skills are not needed for data entry and that the hands can remain free for other tasks while commands are being given to the computer.

Winchester disk technology. A hard-disk technology featuring a fixed, sealed disk and head assembly. The control of air contamination helps to increase reliability and permits high recording density.

Word. A set of characters with a length the same as the storage capacity of a register or parallel transmission bus in a computer. A word is thus a convenient unit for storage of an instruction or number.

Word-processing. Software functions which manipulate data in text form. Word-processing systems are designed to edit and store documents such as letters, memoranda, tables of processed data, mailing lists, and messages. Word-processing systems can include test output formatting, file merging, file management, pagination, electronic mail, and other capabilities. Such systems normally can deliver output ready for printing or typesetting.

Appendix B
Key to Flowcharting Symbols

General

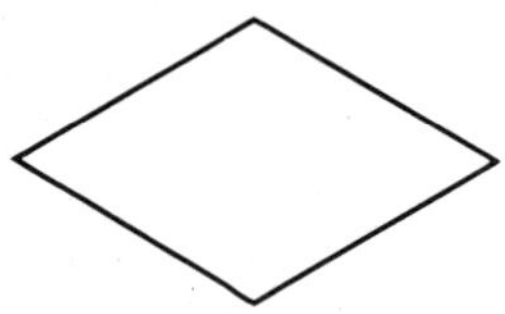

Decision

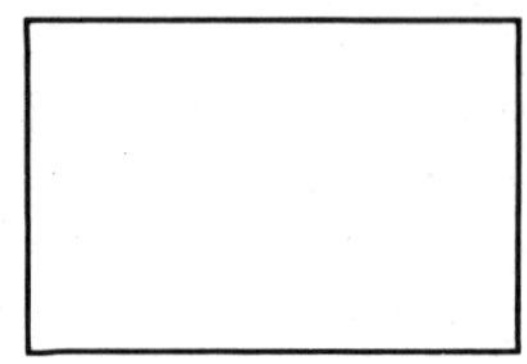

Process

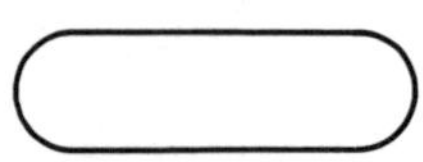

Begin, End

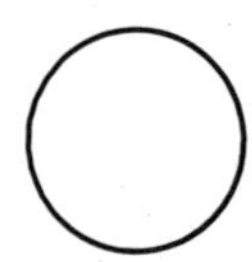

Connector

Programming

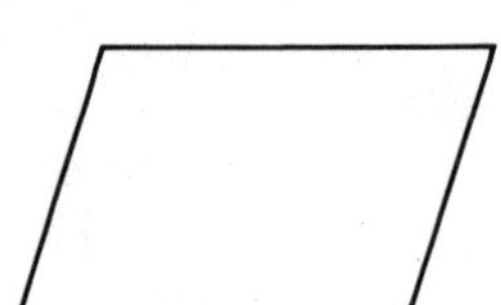

Input or Output

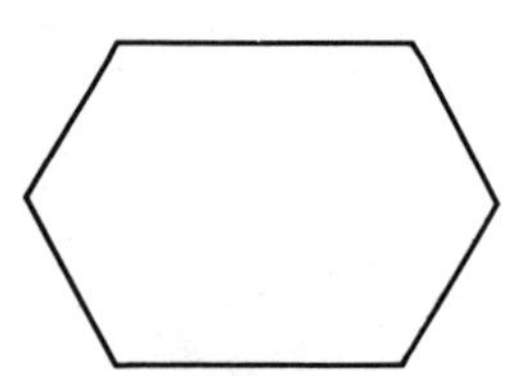

Routine or
Initialization

System

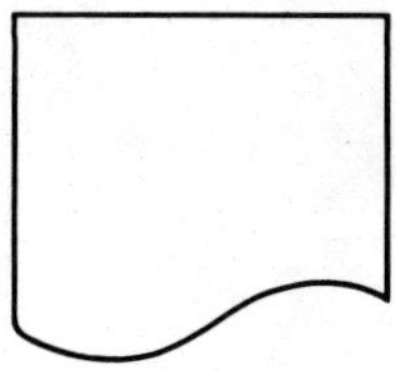

Input or
Output Document

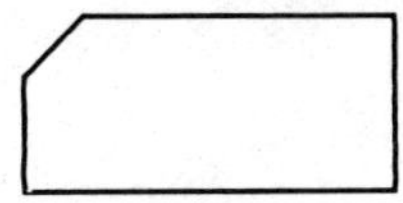

Punched Card

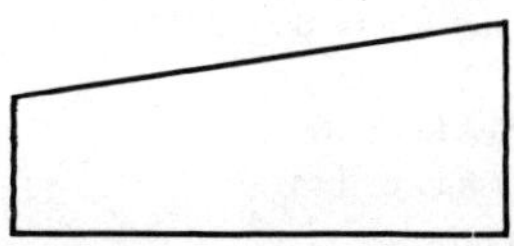

Computer Terminal
for Manual Access

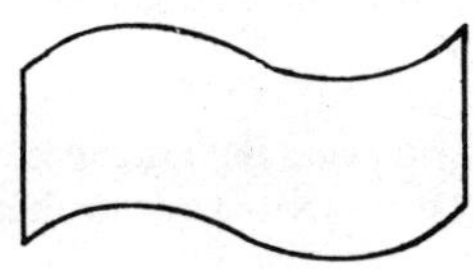

Punched Tape

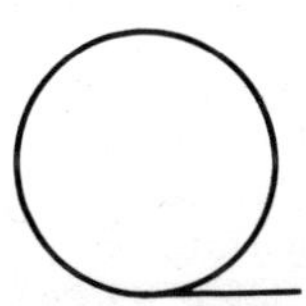

Magnetic Tape
File

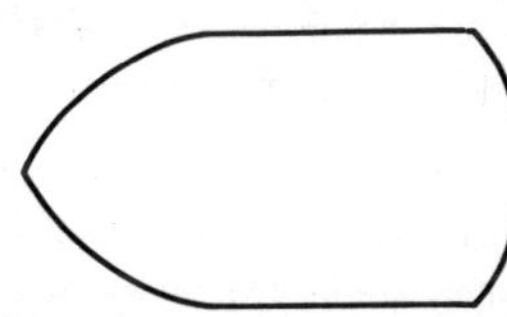

CRT Display

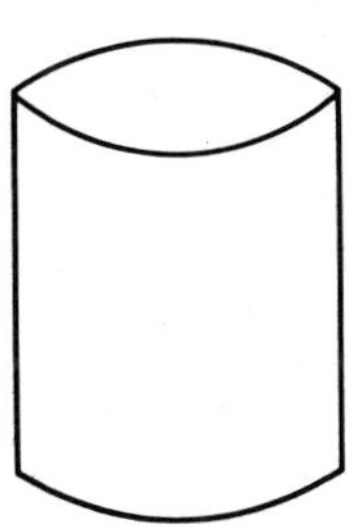

Magnetic Disk File

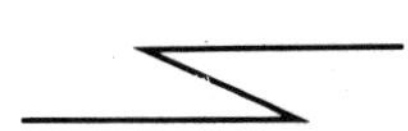

Communication
Link

Index

About the Author

CHARLES J. AUSTIN is President of East exas State University in Commerce, Texas. He also holds a faculty appointment as Professor of General Business and Computer Science. He previously served as Vice President for Academic Affairs at Georgia Southern College in Statesboro and Dean of Graduate Studies and Professor of Health Care Administration at Trinity University in San Antonio, Texas.

Before joining the Trinity University administration in 1974, Dr. Austin served in Washington, D.C. as Study Director for the Commission on Education for Health Administration and was a professor in the Graduate Program in Hospital Administration at Xavier University in Cincinnati. Dr. Austin also had various assignments in the U.S. Department of Health, Education, and Welfare, including Chief of the Information Systems Division, National Library of Medicine, with responsibility for the development and operation of MEDLARS. He has also served as Director of Computer Services and Assistant Professor of Preventive Medicine and Comprehensive Health Care at the University of Colorado Medical Center and as a systems analyst and computer programmer at Procter and Gamble.

Dr. Austin is a Fellow of the American Public Health Association, former Chairman of the Accrediting Commission on Education for Health Services Administration, and a member of numerous professional societies. He is the author of *The Politics of National Health Insurance* and numerous articles published in professional and scholarly journals and is currently Chairman of the Editorial Board of *The Journal of Health Administration Education.*

Dr. Austin has a B.S. from Xavier University in Cincinnati, an M.S. in Health Administration from the University of Colorado, and a Ph.D. in Interdisciplinary Studies (Social Sciences) from the University of Cincinnati.